Psychopharmacology and Women

Sex, Gender, and Hormones

Psychopharmacology and Women

Sex, Gender, and Hormones

Edited by
Margaret F. Jensvold, M.D.
Uriel Halbreich, M.D.
Jean A. Hamilton, M.D.

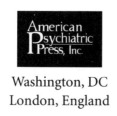

American Psychiatric Press, Inc.

Washington, DC
London, England

Note: The authors have worked to ensure that all information in this book concerning drug dosages, schedules, and routes of administration is accurate as of the time of publication and consistent with standards set by the U.S. Food and Drug Administration and the general medical community. As medical research and practice advance, however, therapeutic standards may change. For this reason and because human and mechanical errors sometimes occur, we recommend that readers follow the advice of a physician who is directly involved in their care or the care of a member of their family.

Copyright © 1996 American Psychiatric Press, Inc.
ALL RIGHTS RESERVED
Manufactured in the United States of America on acid-free paper
99 98 97 96   4 3 2 1

American Psychiatric Press, Inc.
1400 K Street, N.W., Washington, DC   20005

Library of Congress Cataloging-in-Publication Data
Psychopharmacology and women: sex, gender, and hormones / edited by Margaret F. Jensvold, Uriel Halbreich, Jean A. Hamilton.
    p.   cm.
    Includes bibliographical references and index.
    ISBN 0-88048-545-0
    1. Psychopharmacology—Sex differences. 2. Women—Physiology.
I. Jensvold, Margaret F., 1956- . II. Halbreich, Uriel, 1943- . III. Hamilton, Jean A.
    [DNLM: 1. Psychopharmacology. 2. Women's Health. 3. Psychotropic Drugs—pharmacology. 4. Women—psychology.   QV 77
P972105 1996]
  RM315.P752   1996
  615.78′082—dc20
  DNLM/DLC   95-39524
  for Library of Congress   CIP

British Library Cataloguing-in-Publication Data
A CIP record is available from the British Library.

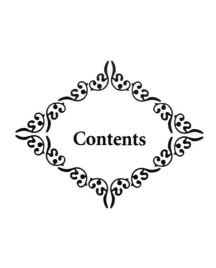

Contents

Section I
Cross-Cutting Fields

Contributors

Martha A. Brumfield, Ph.D.
Associate Director of Regulatory Affairs, Pfizer, Inc., New York, New York

Theresa L. Crenshaw, M.D.
Physician; sexual and relationship therapist; San Diego, California

James M. Ellison, M.D., M.P.H.
Associate Clinical Professor of Psychiatry, Harvard Medical School, Boston, Massachusetts; Consulting Psychiatrist, The Cambridge Hospital, Cambridge, Massachusetts; and Chief, Mental Health Department, Robert H. Ebert Burlington Health Center, Harvard Pilgrim Health Care, Burlington, Massachusetts

Merida Grant
Clinical psychology graduate student, Duke University, Durham, North Carolina

Shelly F. Greenfield, M.D., M.P.H.
Instructor in Psychiatry, Harvard Medical School, Boston, Massachusetts; and Medical Director of Ambulatory Services, Alcohol and Drug Abuse Treatment Program, McLean Hospital, Belmont, Massachusetts

Uriel Halbreich, M.D.
Professor of Psychiatry, Research Professor of Gynecology and Obstetrics, and Director of Biobehavioral Research, State University of New York, Buffalo, New York

Jean A. Hamilton, M.D.
Director, Institute for Women's Health, and Betty Cohen Professor of Women's Health, Medical College of Pennsylvania and Hahnemann University, Philadelphia, Pennsylvania; Professor of Psychology, Social and Health Sciences, and Women's Studies, Duke University, Durham, North Carolina

Wilma Harrison, M.D.
Senior Associate Medical Director, Pfizer, Inc., New York, New York; Associate Professor of Clinical Psychiatry, College of Physicians and Surgeons of Columbia University, New York, New York

David S. Janowsky, M.D.
Professor of Psychiatry, School of Medicine, University of North Carolina, Chapel Hill, North Carolina

Margaret F. Jensvold, M.D.
Director of the Institute for Research on Women's Health, Washington, D.C.; and psychiatrist in practice, Bethesda, Maryland, and Washington, D.C.

Keh-Ming Lin, M.D., M.P.H.
Director and Associate Professor of Psychiatry, Center on the Psychobiology of Ethnicity, Research and Education Institute, Inc., and the Department of Psychiatry, Harbor–UCLA Medical Center, Torrance, California

Maria Dorota Majewska, Ph.D.
Special Expert, Medications Development Division, National Institute on Drug Abuse, National Institutes of Health, Bethesda, Maryland

Martha K. McClintock, Ph.D.
Professor and Chair, Committee on Biopsychology, Department of Psychology, University of Chicago, Chicago, Illinois

James M. Perel, Ph.D.
Professor of Pharmacology and Psychiatry and Director, Clinical Pharmacology Program, Western Psychiatric Institute and Clinic, University of Pittsburgh Medical Center, Pittsburgh, Pennsylvania

Donald W. Pfaff, Ph.D.
Professor of Neurobiology and Behavior, The Rockefeller University, New York, New York

Victoria C. Plaut
Undergraduate student, Harvard College, Harvard University, Cambridge, Massachusetts; Women's Health Research Fellow, Institute for Research on Women's Health, Washington, D.C.

Jeffrey Rausch, M.D.
Professor and Vice Chairman, Department of Psychiatry and Health Behavior, Medical College of Georgia, Augusta, Georgia

Nathan Rojansky, M.D.
Senior Lecturer, Hebrew University Medical School, Department of Obstetrics and Gynecology, Jerusalem, Israel

Sally K. Severino, M.D.
Associate Professor of Clinical Psychiatry, The New York Hospital, Cornell Medical Center, Westchester Division, White Plains, New York

Barbara B. Sherwin, Ph.D.
Professor of Psychology and of Obstetrics and Gynecology, McGill University, Montreal, Quebec

Michael Smith, M.D.
Professor of Psychiatry, Center on the Psychobiology of Ethnicity, Research and Education Institute, Inc., and the Department of Psychiatry, Harbor–UCLA Medical Center, Torrance, California

Kathleen N. Stern, Ph.D.
Former graduate student in Biopsychology, Department of Psychology, University of Chicago, Chicago, Illinois; currently employed in the pharmaceutical industry

Sally Szymanski, D.O.
Clinical Research Fellow, Department of Radiology, Division of Nuclear Medicine, Johns Hopkins Medical Institutions, Johns Hopkins University, Baltimore, Maryland

Steven J. Wamback, B.Sc.
Biologist, technical writer, and Editorial Project Manager for this and other books, Biobehavioral Research Program, Department of Psychiatry, School of Medicine, State University of New York, Buffalo, New York

Katherine L. Wisner, M.D.
Director, Women's Services, Mood Disorder Program, Department of Psychiatry, and Associate Professor of Psychiatry and Reproductive Medicine, Case Western Reserve University, Cleveland, Ohio

Kimberly A. Yonkers, M.D.
Assistant Professor of Psychiatry and of Obstetrics and Gynecology, University of Texas Southwestern Medical School, Dallas, Texas

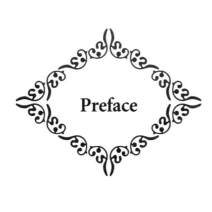

Preface

It has been well documented that sex and gender differences in the use, metabolism, and effects of drugs are understudied (U.S. General Accounting Office 1990, 1992). Nevertheless, a substantial body exists of research and clinical literature about a wide variety of such differences. This book gathers together the current knowledge base regarding sex and gender differences in psychotropic drugs and pharmacotherapy. Emphasis is placed on those aspects of sex and gender differences that are of particular relevance to women, because 1) drug research has traditionally assumed a prototypical male subject, excluding women from much drug research or failing to examine sex differences, and 2) many sex and gender differences in drug use, metabolism, and effects are directly relevant to the clinical care of women. This book will assist clinicians, researchers, policymakers, and health care consumers to incorporate knowledge of sex differences in psychotropic drugs and pharmacotherapy into current and future clinical care and research.

In the first section of the book, sex differences in the pharmacokinetics of psychotropic medications, including basic mechanisms, are reviewed by Hamilton and Yonkers. Sex differences in brain morphology and pharmacodynamics are described by Majewska. Janowsky, Halbreich, and Rausch discuss effects of ovarian and other hormones on the brain. Pfaff and Severino present molecular studies of sex differences in the brain, together with an analysis of implications for understanding of behavior, including motivation, libido, and other reproductive-related behaviors. Pharmacogenetics of sex and ethnicity differences in psychotropic medications are elucidated by Smith and Lin.

The second section of the book takes a life-cycle perspective and develops the concept of reproductive psychopharmacology. Menstrual cycling and pregnancy may influence the need for or reactions to psychotropic medications in some women. Exogenous sex steroid hormones may either alleviate or cause psychological symptoms and may interact with psychotropic medications. As the leading end of the "baby-boom generation" moves into menopause, the menopause experience is gaining greater attention in the popular media, both as a focus of research and as a cause of concern to female health consumers. Chapters by Jensvold, Wisner and Perel, and Sherwin discuss topics relevant to prescribing psychotropic medications for reproductive-age and peri- and postmenopausal women.

Drug sex differences may arise either from differences specific to the sexes (e.g., menstrual cycle effects) or from differences in the prevalence or expression of factors that can occur in either sex. Consequently, discussion of sex differences in drugs requires attention to sex differences in the prevalence and course of psychiatric conditions. In the third section of the book, sex differences of various pathophysiological entities and implications for their pharmacological treatment are discussed. Sex differences in the incidence, presentation, and course of anxiety disorders, schizophrenia, and alcoholism and other substance abuse, and pharmacological treatment of these conditions, are discussed by Yonkers and Ellison, Szymanski, and Greenfield. Meta-analytic techniques promise to yield significant new information about sex differences from the body of research already published as well as from future studies. In a model meta-analysis of imipramine studies, Hamilton, Grant, and Jensvold document a sex difference favoring males. Sexual side effects of psychotropic medications—which have been understudied in general, and particularly so in women, but which are of increasing interest to many patients—are discussed by Jensvold and colleagues.

The fourth section of the book describes improvements in research methodologies, indicating directions for advances in research and clinical care. The phases of drug development, including the U.S. Food and Drug Administration's revised guidelines for inclusion of women in drug testing, are detailed by Harrison and Brumfield. Stern and McClintock present a significantly improved method of determining the timing of ovulation and, thus, of menstrual cycle phases. A model research design for studies of menstrual cycle– and gender-related effects on drugs is outlined by Jensvold, Hamilton, and Halbreich.

The editors wish to acknowledge the invaluable and excellent assistance provided by Editorial Project Managers Rebecca Richters, at American Psychiatric Press, Inc., and Steven J. Wamback, at State University of New York, Buffalo, in preparation and editing of multiple drafts of the manuscript.

|

Section I
Cross-Cutting Fields

Gender-Sensitive Psychopharmacology: An Overview

Margaret F. Jensvold, M.D., Uriel Halbreich, M.D., and Jean A. Hamilton, M.D.

"Gender-sensitive pharmacology" incorporates knowledge of sex- and gender-related variables into clinical decision making, research, and medical education in pharmacotherapy. Here we gather in one place much of the information that is available on sex-related factors in psychopharmacology, point out where gaps in knowledge remain, and especially demonstrate the need for gender-sensitive psychopharmacology. It is our hope that this book will be of assistance to clinicians, researchers, health consumers, and policymakers.

In point of precise language, there is little in this book that is related to gender. The term *sex differences* subsumes four terms that are often used interchangeably but that should be distinguished: sex, gender, sexuality, and reproductive function. *Sex* refers to the biological categories male and female. The vast majority of people are born either male or female (although intersex variants do rarely occur). Assignment to sex categories may be determined by chromosomal, endocrinological, gonadal, nuclear chromatin, or phenotypic evidence. For any particular individual, these biological methods of determining sex are usually, but not always, in agreement and usually agree with the psychological and social determination of sex of the individual. Most of the pharmacological research to date that examines sex- or gender-related variables examines sex differences by comparing and contrasting findings in men versus women. Gender is a more complex, socially and culturally constructed variable (Deaux 1993). Gender-related factors have been identified as potentially important in pharmacology, but for the most part, they remain a topic for future research. Sex differences must be documented before conclusions can be drawn about gender differences.

Sexuality refers to sexual functioning, including sexual thoughts, feelings, and behaviors. *Reproductive function* refers to behavioral, hormonal, and other changes associated with reproductive system–related functioning (e.g., the hypothalamic-pituitary-gonadal axis, pregnancy, menopause). The term *sexual side effects* of medication has often been used to refer to two different and distinct yet overlapping sets of medication side effects: those involving *sexual function* (e.g., delayed orgasm, changes in libido) and those involving *reproductive system function* (e.g., affecting the menstrual cycle).

Until recently, women were excluded as research subjects from much pharmacological research, including the early phases of drug testing and a number of prominent large studies, as well as many smaller studies. Also, commonly, when women have been included in drug research, data have not been analyzed with regard to sex and have not been reported in a manner that allows such analyses to be performed. Factors unique to women have often been used as justification for excluding women from drug research.

Reports, during the last decade, on the need to include women in drug research (Halbreich and Carson 1989; Hamilton 1986; Hamilton and Parry 1983; Kinney et al. 1981) were, for the most part, ignored by the field until the U.S. General Accounting Office (GAO) released its report documenting that the National Institutes of Health had not implemented its own guidelines requiring that women be included in medical research (U.S. GAO 1990). The release of that GAO report on June 18, 1990, was a watershed event. A plethora of media publicity (Cotton 1990; Debrovner 1993; Jensvold et al. 1991) and changes in regulations (U.S. Food and Drug Administration [FDA] 1993) have followed. The history of pharmacological regulation shows that regulatory changes have tended to be crisis driven (Johnson and Fee 1993). For example, drug development regulations became more paternalistic and protective of fetuses after the diethylstilbestrol and thalidomide debacles several decades ago. Recent changes in FDA guidelines (U.S. FDA 1993) were made after widespread media coverage of the adverse effects on women's health care resulting from insufficient inclusion of women in research and drug development trials.

Currently, a gender-related blind spot persists in much of the litera-ture available to clinicians and researchers. The American Psychiatric Association's "Practice Guidelines for Major Depressive Disorders in Adults" makes only one mention of sex, and that is to minimize the role of sex differences in treatment of depression (American Psychiatric As-sociation 1993). A prominent conference symposium on psychotropic drugs in patient subpopulations discussed effects of age and race but made only passing reference to sex (Potter 1993). A review of citations to sex, gender, and menstrual cycle in the indexes of nine books listed under psychotropic drugs in the computerized card catalog at the Na-tional Institutes of Health library published between 1985 and 1993 re-vealed the following: one book listed 8 citations to sex; a second listed 10 citations to menstrual cycle; a third book listed 1 citation to sex, 1 to gender, and 2 to menstrual cycle; and the remaining six books made no references to sex, gender, or menstrual cycle.

A major change is, however, currently in progress. The FDA's re-cently revised guidelines recommend 1) that drug development data be analyzed with regard to sex differences and 2) that factors unique to women (effects of the menstrual cycle, and drug interactions with hor-monal contraceptives and hormone replacement therapy) be studied. As a result of policy changes, much pertinent information will doubt-less be forthcoming. Although the FDA's revised guidelines constitute recommendations rather than regulations, it is our hope that pharma-ceutical companies and university-based researchers will follow the FDA's lead.

Even with limited knowledge, increasing our understanding of sex- and gender-related factors in psychopharmacology is demonstrably important for treatment of patients. It may be particularly important for treatment of women, since women take more psychotropic medications than men, and because factors unique to women influence medication effects. About two-thirds of antidepressants and antidepressant-tranquilizers dispensed in the United States are prescribed to women (Baum et al. 1988). Women take more medications than men and more multiple medications than men (Baum et al. 1988; Domecq et al. 1980); and evidence suggests that even when corrections are made for the number of medications taken, women tend to have more side effects and more adverse effects than do men (Bottiger et al. 1979; Domecq et al. 1980). The reasons for the increased adverse effects of medications in women are not known, but most likely these effects are due, in part, to the fact that features unique to or different in women, as compared with men (e.g., Jensvold et al. 1992), have often not been taken into account in drug research or prescribing.

The greater emphasis on sex-related factors in pharmacology is part of a larger trend toward individualizing medication dosing. Age (U.S. FDA 1989) and race/ethnicity (Lin et al. 1993) as well as sex (Merkatz et al. 1993a, 1993b; U.S. FDA 1993) are receiving increasing attention as critical variables in pharmacological research and practice.

Psychotropic medications tend to have a wide range of possible effective dosages. In general, psychotropic medications must be optimized on an individualized basis to a greater extent than many other classes of medications. Cookbook-type recommendations of fixed medication dosages for all patients—very common several decades ago but less so now—are, for the most part, likely to be further replaced by recommendations for specific subgroups of the population.

The recommendation that patients be pushed rather aggressively up to the "highest tolerated dosage" came about in the 1970s when research documented that the most common reason for nonresponse to psychotropic medication was that dosages used were too low. Patients were encouraged to take higher dosages of medication and to tolerate considerable side effects. The push for patients to take the highest tolerated dosages almost certainly contributed to greater response but also contributed to heavy loads of side effects.

A trend within psychopharmacology is to temper the recommendation of automatically pushing the patient's medication to the "highest tolerated dosage," aiming instead for a dosage that minimizes side effects while maintaining therapeutic effects. The advent of newer effective medications with fewer side effects (e.g., selective serotonin reuptake inhibitors, newer antipsychotic and anticonvulsant medications), in combination with public education campaigns (e.g., the National Institute of Mental Health's Depression/Awareness, Recognition, and Treatment [D/ART] program, the American Psychiatric Association's Panic Awareness Program) and popular informative books (e.g., Duke and Hochman 1992; Kramer 1993), has resulted in greater numbers of persons seeking treatment with psychotropic medications and the hope, on behalf of many potential patients, that side effects will not be too bothersome.

Without certain technological advances, progress in reproductive endocrinology and neuropsychopharmacology would not have been possible. The development of radioimmunoassays in the early 1970s led to a vastly increased understanding of sex steroid hormones, including their rhythmic, pulsatile nature and intricate feedback mechanisms. Refinements in neuroimaging techniques in the 1980s opened the way for studies of pharmacological action in the human brain. Genetic techniques permit investigation of hormone-receptor interactions, which generally involve genetic complexes, as well as studies of genetic differences in inherited or expressed isozyme patterns, which in turn influence drug metabolism. The ability to detect pregnancy soon after conception makes it possible to include women in earlier phases of drug testing with increased safety and decreased risk (Halbreich and Carson 1989). More accurate methods of detecting the timing of ovulation (Stern and McClintock, Chapter 18, this volume) contribute to more accurate determination of menstrual cycle phases, necessary for menstrual cycle research.

Issues not addressed here include nonbiological, psychosocial, and behavioral factors pertinent to the psychopharmacology of women. Readers are referred elsewhere for discussions of these topics (Hamilton et al. 1995; Jensvold and Hamilton, in press; Mogul 1985). An extreme example of such factors includes the tendency within some family structures (and in some workplaces) for the woman to become the "identified patient," sometimes with the unrealistic wish that if that woman would "just take medication," the entire system would be cured.

There have been case reports suggesting that psychotropic medications may sometimes be used for the purpose of exploiting and victimizing women, such as by sexually inappropriate therapists (e.g., those who drug and rape women patients) (Noel and Watterson 1992). Psychiatry has often been susceptible to appropriation as an agent of social control (Group for the Advancement of Psychiatry 1993; Jensvold 1993b; Stover and Nightingale 1985). This issue may be of particular concern to women, since psychiatric patients are more frequently women, and women still often have less power than men in the social structures within which they function.

On the other hand, appropriate use of psychotropic medications is often empowering. Psychotropic medications may alleviate the limitations imposed by depression, panic, and other psychiatric conditions, helping to free the energies of the consumer of the medication for more productive use. Psychiatrist Peter Kramer (1993), in an interview, commented, "The mother's-little-helper pills of the 50s and 60s [antianxiety drugs like Miltown, Librium, and Valium] were used to make women comfortable in settings that should have been uncomfortable. The antidepressants like Prozac, in a sense, are feminist drugs, liberating and empowering" (Stone 1993, p. 62). Comas-Diaz and Jacobsen (1995) write, "the empowering approach to psychopharmacology views education as an emancipatory method aimed at helping women of color [and others] manage their situations in a self-affirming manner" (p. 86). The education of consumers as well as professionals may be advanced through concurrent treatment by a nonphysician therapist and a physician-psychopharmacologist; Comas-Diaz and Jacobsen describe the "therapeutic relationship designated as a 'therapeutic triangle' and a critical agent of change" (1995, p. 85).

Currently, substantial advances involving psychopharmacology are being made in basic research and clinical practice. New drugs with improved side-effect profiles are being introduced into the market. New indications for existing medications are being discovered. Hormonal agents are, at least temporarily, receiving more attention now than in the recent past, when there were even greater barriers to the development of hormonal technologies (Mastroianni et al. 1990). Advances in pharmacogenetics, molecular and receptor technology, and neuroimaging techniques are furthering our understanding of the means by which psychotropic drugs achieve their effects. Incorporation of analyses of sex- and gender-related factors into research and practice will contribute to a more gender-sensitive psychopharmacology and to improved care of the women and men who use psychopharmacological agents.

Sex Differences in Pharmacokinetics of Psychotropic Medications

Part I: Physiological Basis for Effects

Jean A. Hamilton, M.D.,
and Kimberly A. Yonkers, M.D.

The two broad subdivisions in pharmacology research are pharmacokinetics (which pertains to delivering the drug to and removing the drug from the site of action) and pharmacodynamics (the drug's mechanism of action, e.g., receptor functioning). This chapter and Chapter 3 comprise a two-part review of what is and is not known about sex-related differences in pharmacokinetics. In this chapter—Part I—we reexamine the physiological basis for sex-related differences in pharmacokinetics. We summarize studies specifically linking pharmacokinetic changes to 1) use of exogenous hormones such as oral contraceptives (OCs) or postmenopausal hormone replacement therapy (HRT) and exposure to endogenous hormonal changes such as those associated with 2) menstrual cycle phase or 3) menopausal status. Confounding effects of aging and coadministration of other (nonhormonal) drugs (possibly having sex- or gender-linked patterns of use or effects) are also briefly summarized. In Part II—Chapter 3—we address sex and related differences for each class of psychotropics.

Physiological Basis of Sex-Related Differences

Sex differences in pharmacology for animals and humans have been previously reviewed (Dawkins and Potter 1991; Giudicelli and Tillement 1977; Goble 1975; Hamilton 1991; Hamilton and Conrad 1987; Hamilton and Parry 1983; Kato 1974; K. O'Malley et al. 1971; K. Wilson 1984; Yonkers et al. 1992a). Nonetheless, we provide an updated, comprehensive review focused on the physiological basis of sex differences in pharmacokinetics. An understanding of the physiological substrate is important for two reasons: 1) to corroborate and provide a stronger rationale for examination of sex differences, and 2) to help clinicians organize their knowledge about sex and related differences, should these exist. The latter rationale will provide a basis for anticipating when sex and related effects are likely to occur, both for new drugs and for pathophysiologically defined conditions. Further, we assess both the preponderance and the weight of the evidence, considering, for example, the proportion of studies showing findings that are significant or in the same direction as well as the strength of various methodologies.[1]

The general topic of pharmacokinetics is a broad one. It encompasses absorption and bioavailability, distribution, metabolism, and elimination. A more general review of pharmacokinetic mechanisms is beyond the scope of this chapter, but a summary of major concepts and

---

[1] While we considered a quantitative analysis of these data, we have been advised to reserve meta-analysis for cases in which there are more than 10 studies.

principles follows.[2] In clinical psychiatric practice we are most concerned with drugs given orally. For oral administration, key factors include gastric emptying, small-intestine transit time and motility, secretion of gastric acid and enzymes, and "first pass" liver metabolism, which will affect bioavailability. *Bioavailability* refers to the percentage of unchanged drug that reaches systemic circulation. In some cases, this is affected by the rate of absorption. Perhaps the most critical factor determining a drug's serum concentration, however, is the *first-pass effect*—the amount of drug metabolized during absorption and extracted by the liver before reaching the systemic circulation. Drugs fall into two categories: high hepatic extraction or low hepatic extraction. In low hepatic extraction, clearance (CL) is more highly dependent on intrinsic hepatic metabolism.

---

[2] All types of pharmacokinetic effects depend in part on passage of the drug across (lipid) cell membranes. Important physicochemical characteristics of a drug that affect membrane passage are its molecular size and shape, its degree of ionization, the relative lipid solubility of its ionized and nonionized forms, and the medium of suspension. Important host/environment characteristics include circulation at the site of delivery; area of the absorbing surface (which varies by the route of administration); local pH and gastric acid secretion (i.e., for a weak acid or base, the nonionized form is more lipid soluble, and gastric pH will be an important factor; in contrast, completely ionized, lipid-insoluble drugs are absorbed slowly); gastric oxidation; rate of gastric emptying; gastrointestinal (GI) blood flow (especially to the main site of absorption for orally administered drugs—the small intestine); weight; volume of distribution (Vd); body composition (including lean body mass [LBM], which is directly proportional to total body water [TBW] and inversely proportional to percentage body fat [BF], with the latter implying storage of lipophilic drugs in fat as a reservoir; TBW is about 70% of body weight in lean and 50% in obese individuals); extracellular water (ECW), which is mainly plasma; intracellular and other tissue concentration; protein binding (which implies lower active, free drug); cardiac output (which depends on body surface area [BSA]); circulation to the site of action (e.g., brain blood flow, especially for psychotropics); nonsynthetic (phase 1) biotransformation reactions (oxidation, reduction, or hydrolysis); synthetic (phase 2) biotransformation reactions (conjugation, involving coupling the drug or its metabolite with an endogenous substrate); activity of various hepatic microsomal drug-metabolizing systems involved in biotransformation (which can be induced by smoking, chronic alcohol consumption, and use of other nonhormonal drugs); circulation at the sites of metabolism and elimination (including hepatic and renal blood flow); glomerular filtration rate (GFR); creatinine and other clearance (CL); renal tubular secretion and reabsorption (especially with highly lipid-soluble drugs); and excretion by other routes.

Important factors affecting drug distribution include body size, composition, and fluid volume; blood flow and tissue concentration; and protein binding. Drugs and other foreign substances are metabolized by enzyme systems in the liver, kidney, gastrointestinal (GI) tract, and lung. The most important site of metabolism is the liver. Hepatic metabolism depends on the activity of microsomal biotransformation reactions, and these are often catalyzed by P450 cytochrome oxygenases. (P450 cytochrome activity is important, as we shall see in Part II, because most psychotropics are metabolized in this way.) Lipid-soluble (usually nonionized or nonpolar) compounds are converted into water-soluble (ionized or polar) compounds that are more readily excreted in urine (Bressler 1982). Most elimination occurs by way of the kidney or feces. Drug-metabolizing capacity and CL are indexed by measures such as the elimination half-life ($t^1/_2$) and its volume of distribution (Vd).

Mechanisms Showing Sex Differences

Physiological studies in humans have long revealed sex differences in multiple mechanisms affecting drug absorption and bioavailability, distribution, metabolism, and elimination (Hamilton 1991; K. Wilson 1984; Yonkers et al. 1992a). As illustrated in Table 2–1, sex differences in physiological mechanisms underlying pharmacokinetic effects in young adult to middle-aged humans have been documented for at least the following: gastric emptying rate (also indexed by residual volume), basal gastric acid secretion, gastric oxidation, weight, body composition (lean body mass [LBM], total body water [TBW], extracellular water [ECW], and percentage body fat [BF]), brain blood flow, hepatic biotransformation, and creatinine CL (CL_{cr}). In addition, data are suggestive—albeit inconclusive—for small-intestinal or GI transit time, tissue concentration, and protein binding.

Physiological Basis for Effects of Sex

Absorption and Bioavailability

Gastric emptying.   The small intestine has greater absorptive capacity (due to greater surface area) than the stomach but is dependent on the

Table 2–1.   Sex-related effects on physiological variables: pharmacokinetic mechanisms

Absorption and bioavailability

Variable	Findings in women vs. men	Percentage effect	Predicted impact on CL and/or BL in women vs. men	Reference
Gastric emptying time (S = solids; L = liquids)	Slower	29–55 (S) 25–78 (L)	↓ BL	1
Small-intestinal transit time	(Faster?)	?	↓ BL	2
Gastric acid secretion	Lower	27–40	↑ BL (bases)	3
Gastric enzymes (ADH)	Lower (first-pass metabolism)	77	↑ BL	4

Distribution

Variable	Findings in women vs. men	Percentage effect	Predicted impact on CL and/or BL in women vs. men	Reference
Weight	Lower	16	↑ BL	5
Total blood volume	Lower	6 kg/ body weight	↑ BL	6
Absolute percentage body fat	Higher	11	(↓ BL initially) ↑ BL later (lipophilic agent)	7
Brain blood flow	Higher	15	↑ Activity	8
Protein binding	(Lower?)	?	(↑ free fraction?); possible effects if narrow TI and small Vd	9

Metabolism and elimination

Variable	Findings in women vs. men	Percentage effect	Predicted impact on CL and/or BL in women vs. men	Reference
Hepatic metabolism: side-chain oxidation	Lower	58	↓ CL (↑ BL)	10

(continued)

Table 2–1.   Sex-related effects on physiological variables: pharmacokinetic mechanisms *(continued)*

Metabolism and elimination *(continued)*

Variable	Findings in women vs. men	Percentage effect	Predicted impact on CL and/or BL in women vs. men	Reference
Hydroxylation	Lower	—	↓ CL (↑ BL)	10
Glucuronide conjugation	Lower	34	↓ CL (↑ BL)	10
Renal elimination: creatinine clearance	Lower	15	↓ CL (↑ BL)	11

Note. ADH = alcohol dehydrogenase; BL = blood level; CL = clearance; TI = therapeutic index; Vd = volume of distribution.   References:

1. Datz et al. (1987a) and Hutson et al. (1989) are the basis for percentage effect estimate.[4]
2. Rao et al. (1987) requires replication.
3. Booth et al. (1957), Grossman et al. (1963), and Yamagata et al. (1975) provide the basis for percentage effect.
4. Frezza et al. (1990).
5. Mayersohn (1982).
6. Lusseveld et al. (1993).
7. Mayersohn (1982).
8. R. C. Gur et al. (1982) and Shaw et al. (1979).
9. Jochemsen et al. (1982) and K. Wilson (1984).
10. Walle et al. (1989) requires replication, but other data support percentage effect estimate (K. Wilson 1984).
11. Cockcroft and Gault (1976) and Ouslander (1981).

delivery of compounds (i.e., gastric emptying). Slower *gastric* emptying results in higher residual volume, slower absorption, delayed peak levels (especially for bases, due to gastric acidity), and lower peak blood concentrations (Sellers 1985). In contrast, slower motility in the *small intestine* results in a greater degree of overall absorption. Gastric emptying has been studied for solids, liquids, and semisolids; data for solids may be most relevant for medications taken in pill form. Sex differences in gastric emptying have been the focus of at least 10 studies (Booth et al. 1957; Datz et al. 1987a; Horowitz et al. 1984; Hutson et al. 1989; Notivol et al. 1984; Petring and Flachs 1990; Rao et al. 1987; Shay et al. 1987; Wedmann et al. 1991; Wright et al. 1983). In premenopausal females compared with males, the decrease in gastric half-emptying ranged from 29% to 55% slower for *solids* and from 25% to 78% slower for *liquids*. The better designed studies of gastric emptying are those of Datz et al. (1987a) and Hutson et al. (1989). A methodological refinement is shown in studies by Notivol et al. (1984) and Wright et al. (1983), who considered body surface area (BSA).[3] The bulk and weight of the evidence point to slower gastric emptying in premenopausal females compared with males (for further details and assessment, see Table 2–1),[4] suggesting lower peak blood levels in females compared with males.

Small-intestinal transit time and indices of motility.   Rao et al. (1987) found that *mouth-to-cecum* transit time was 7% faster in females compared with males, although the difference was not significant. If a significant sex difference were confirmed in subsequent studies, faster transit time in the small intestine would tend to decrease absorption and, hence, bioavailability, in females compared with males.

There does not appear to be a difference between premenopausal

---

[3] The length of the intestines may be correlated with BSA, which also suggests that absorption may be lower in females.

[4] In premenopausal females compared with males, the decrease in gastric half-emptying ranged from 29% to 55% slower for *solids* and from 25% to 78% slower for *liquids*. Datz et al. (1987a) found a decrease of 55% and 78% in women for solids and liquids, respectively. For solids and liquids, slightly lower percentages of gastric emptying were found by Hutson et al. (1989) (29% and 66%, respectively) and by Notivol et al. (1984) (43% and about 25%, respectively). In a study pooling obese and nonobese subjects, another group reported a decreased rate for solids but not liquids (Wright et al. 1983), finding that differences persisted even when BSA was considered. A mixed meal and a liquid fatty meal were also emptied more slowly in women than in men (Rao et al. 1987; Wedmann et al. 1991). In contrast, four studies have found no sex-related effect on gastric emptying (Horowitz et al. [1984] for solids or liquids; Petring and Flachs [1990] for semisolids or liquids; Shay et al. [1987] for solids alone; and Booth et al. [1957] for liquids alone). However, Horowitz et al.'s (1984) study included postmenopausal women (aged 21–62 years), which may have obscured differences for solids (Hutson et al. 1989). Two of the studies specified that subjects were not using any medications (e.g., OCs); however, Shay et al. (1987) and Booth et al. (1957) were silent on this point. Neither Horowitz et al. (1984) nor Shay et al. (1987) presented data or summary statistics for nonpatient control subjects by sex.

females and males in indices of antral motility (Hutson et al. 1989). Variations in GI blood flow would affect degree of medication absorption, but this has not been investigated.

Secretion of gastric acid and gastric enzymes.   Higher gastric acidity is associated with higher absorption of weak acids, whereas lower gastric acidity (i.e., a relatively alkaline gastric environment) results in higher gastric absorption of weak bases. Basal gastric acid secretion is 33%–40% lower on average in healthy premenopausally aged females compared with males aged 20–49 years (Grossman et al. 1963). Other studies include those of Booth et al. (1957), who studied young males and females, with the latter tested in the follicular cycle phase; and Yamagata et al. (1975), who studied subjects in age groups spanning six decades. Thus, the three studies of gastric acid are consistent. Although pharmacokinetic effects have not been demonstrated directly, these data suggest increased absorption of bases (e.g., tricyclic antidepressants [TCAs], benzodiazepines, phenothiazines) and decreased gastric absorption of acids (e.g., phenytoin, barbiturates such as phenobarbital) in females.

The gastric mucosa contains alcohol dehydrogenase (ADH), which oxidizes alcohol, decreasing the amount of ingested alcohol that will enter systemic circulation. Gastric ADH activities were 70%–80% higher in healthy males than in females, corresponding to a 77% lower first-pass metabolism in females and 41% greater blood alcohol concentrations. Thus, delayed CL of alcohol (greater bioavailability) in healthy females compared with males results in part from decreased first-pass metabolism (Frezza et al. 1990).

Distribution

Body size, composition, and fluids.   Assuming an average 70-kg male and 59-kg female, adult women weigh on average about 16% less than men. Lower weight (correlated with height) results in lower BSA.[5,6]

---

[5] The DuBois height-weight equation is used to calculate BSA in square meters (m^2): (weight in kg) × (height in cm) × 0.007184 (Berkow 1982). BSA is used to calculate cardiac output in L/minute/m^2: 2.5–3.6 L/minute/m^2.

[6] Overall, older studies report that women have *proportionately* higher cardiac outputs, largely because of lower oxygen-carrying capacity of their blood and lower

For blood, the total volume is about 6% lower per kg body weight in females compared with males.[7] Females, having lower total blood volume, may show somewhat higher serum concentrations of water-soluble drugs compared with males. The ratio of ECW to TBW is lower in males than in females (Lusseveld et al. 1993).

For 25- to 35-year-old adults, the *absolute* percentage BF is on average about 11% higher in females (22% for males and 33% for females, respectively [Mayersohn 1982, p. 43]).[8] Higher percentage BF results in both lower TBW and lower LBM. Initially, drugs ingested by women will have a lower serum concentration due to a larger Vd. Over time, however, lipophilic drugs will be stored in adipose tissue and $t^{1/2}$ may become prolonged. This would lead to higher serum levels in females compared with males (Yonkers et al. 1992a).

Blood flow and differential concentration.   Seeman (1989) observed that sex differences in cerebral blood flow may affect drug redistribution to the brain, with women showing a 15% higher flow than men (R. C. Gur et al. 1982; Shaw et al. 1979), particularly during the second and third decades. This mechanism may be especially important for psychotropics, which are thought to act by altering brain function. Further, some psychotropics are concentrated in brain tissue compared with plasma (Sallee and Pollock 1990), although data are not summarized by sex. For example, the brain:adipose:plasma steady-state tissue concentration of the TCA imipramine is 12:3:1.

Protein binding.   There have been few detailed studies of possible sex-related differences in drug plasma protein binding (Hashimoto et al. 1991; Jochemsen et al. 1982; K. Wilson 1984), with a variable pattern

---

peripheral oxygen extraction (Astrand et al. 1964) and partly due to greater heart rate and stroke volume with exercise (Becklake et al. 1965). While such studies continue to be cited (O'Toole 1993), the implications for pharmacokinetics are probably negligible, except perhaps during prolonged exercise or pregnancy, when increased cardiac output might affect hepatic blood flow.

[7] But the plasma volume is similar, at 39 mL per kg body weight in males, compared with 40 in females (J. D. Wilson et al. 1991).

[8] Of course, this means that (*relative)* percentage body fat is 1.5 times higher (33% versus 22%) in females compared with males.

of results for different proteins.[9] While it is inappropriate to generalize, in some cases women of certain ages may show lower binding (C. B. Kristensen 1983). Since the amount of drug that is free is the amount available for biological activity, the amount of protein binding is an important parameter to assess. Even a small displacement of certain highly bound drugs can result in a proportionately large increase in free, active drug (e.g., if a drug were 99% bound and 1% free, then a 1% decrease in binding would double the active drug). Not only might this affect therapeutic efficacy, but greater free drug can increase toxicity. This is clinically meaningful if the drug has a narrow therapeutic index (TI: ratio of the drug required to produce a toxic effect compared with that for a therapeutic effect) along with a small Vd. Thus, changes in proteins are unlikely to be important for imipramine, but for antidepressants with a narrower TI, such as nortriptyline, this may be important.

Metabolism and Elimination

Hepatic metabolism.   The activity of various hepatic microsomal drug-metabolizing systems involved in biotransformation of drugs differs according to sex. According to K. Wilson (1984), nonsynthetic, oxidative biotransformation reactions are typically more sensitive to sex effects (e.g., hydrolysis) than are synthetic reactions such as conjugation (e.g., via glucuronic acid). The P450 cytochrome oxygenases catalyze different reactions.

The picture is further complicated in that some drugs have several avenues of biotransformation—called "partial pathways"—involved in their metabolism. Propranolol is an example of such a drug. *Side chain* oxidation of propranolol is approximately 58% less active in women than in men, and glucuronidation, typically less sensitive to sex, is 34% lower in females compared with males (Walle et al. 1989). In contrast, *ring* oxidation of propranolol is unaffected by sex. Thus, partial metabolic pathways can show differential effects of sex.

---

[9] Here we will focus on albumin, but there are also changes in lipoproteins (e.g., apolipoprotein B) and α_1-acid glycoprotein (Sallee and Pollock 1990; Hashimoto et al. 1991), among others. In a sample including premenopausal and postmenopausal females and comparably aged males, more than 40 plasma proteins were studied in relation to sex and menopausal status (Hashimoto et al. 1991), with a variable pattern of results.

Renal elimination.   Males have greater CL_{cr} than females, even when correcting for BSA. As one example, the formula for estimating true CL_{cr} in relation to age multiplies the result by 85% for females, meaning that the results are 15% lower on average for females (Cockcroft and Gault 1976; Ouslander 1981). The sex difference in CL_{cr} implies an effect on glomerular filtration rate (GFR), which could affect renal excretion of drugs. If so, there may be a tendency for females to show less CL and higher blood levels of drugs that are eliminated via the kidney.

Summary

Unfortunately, although consistencies exist in some of these data, there are gaps in knowledge, and many findings have not been replicated or extended with more intensive research. Nonetheless, the sizes of many replicated effects are of sufficient magnitude in and of themselves (e.g., on the order of a 20% effect or greater) to suggest that they may have meaningful effects on pharmacokinetics. Even if an isolated effect were not of sufficient magnitude to affect pharmacokinetics, several such effects, pushing CL or bioavailability *in the same direction*, might together have a substantial effect. Table 2–1 shows that most effects of sex are, in fact, in the same direction—that is, they have a predictable impact of increasing blood levels and decreasing CL. This is especially true for drugs metabolized by the liver, although drugs that are excreted primarily through the kidney may represent an exception. However, few empirical data are available to guide us in estimating how such factors may vary, combine, or show interactive effects within individuals.[10] We consider it likely that small-intestinal absorption is more often important than rate of gastric emptying and also that the degree of hepatic metabolism will weigh heavily in determining net effects, but these are empirical questions, particularly as they may relate to sex. Since there are numerous sex differences in the physiological substrates for pharmacokinetic effects, it would not be surprising if sex differences were observed in pharmacokinetic indices such as bioavailability, CL, $t_{1/2}$, and Vd, and

---

[10] Further, in theory, effects of sex might be washed out by variable or opposing effects of hormonal (OC or HRT) or nonhormonal drugs, hormonal status (menstrual cycle phase or menopause), age, or other confounding effects.

ultimately in steady-state plasma concentrations of some psychotropics.

As we shall see in Part II, when sex differences have been observed, women have tended to show greater bioavailability and slower apparent CL. Thus, several reviewers (Hamilton 1991; K. Wilson 1984; Yonkers et al. 1992a) have hypothesized that females will tend to show higher plasma concentrations compared with males (because of greater bioavailability, slower CL, or both). Even if plasma differences exist and are statistically significant, little is known about possible drug-concentration differences by sex in the central nervous system (CNS). The need to demonstrate whether effects are clinically meaningful remains. Even if sex differences were shown to exist in controlled studies, findings might be either masked or magnified in less well-controlled studies if there were substantial, confounding effects of OCs, HRT, and menstrual and menopausal status.

Effects of Synthetic Hormones

Hormonally related treatments and conditions, including synthetic hormones such as OCs, can affect pharmacokinetics (Hamilton and Parry 1983; Teichmann 1990). OC-induced changes in pharmacokinetics are important epidemiologically: nearly 25% of women of childbearing age (15–44 years) in the United States use OCs (Mishell 1989). Of U.S. women ages 50–65 years, 32% are using postmenopausal HRT (Harris et al. 1990).

OCs typically contain synthetic estrogen, progestin, or both. HRT has often been limited to natural (conjugated) estrogen (e.g., Premarin). However, combination preparations are increasingly used for HRT, including a "continuous combined" regimen wherein synthetic or natural estrogen and a progestin (e.g., medroxyprogesterone, norethindrone, micronized natural progesterone) are taken daily (Lobo 1993). Thus, certain HRT regimens may mimic OC effects.

Physiological Basis for Effects of Exogenous Hormones

Absorption and Bioavailability

Gastric emptying.   Several authors have suggested that OCs may alter absorption, although most such effects have been inferred rather than assessed directly (Ellinwood et al. 1984). Evidence suggests that OCs lessen the sex difference observed in gastric emptying of liquids (Wedmann et al. 1991) premenopausally (in comparison with follicular measures). In contrast, Hutson et al. (1989) found that HRT largely preserves the premenopausal sex difference in gastric emptying. Findings for OC and HRT effects are summarized in Table 2–2.

Secretion of gastric acid.   Conjugated estrogens (as in HRT) have been observed to mitigate the usual increase in gastric acid output at midcycle by about 18% (Sakaguchi et al. 1991). Estrogen level accounted for 40% of the variance in gastric acid output in young women. Cruz et al. (1951) found that exogenous estrogen or progesterone usually decreases gastric acid secretion.

Distribution

Body composition and fluids.   OCs are associated with increased fluid retention (Preedy and Aitken 1956) and edema, at least at the older, higher dosages. They may also affect aldosterone secretory rate (M. J. Gray et al. 1968). OCs have recently (presumably with modern, reduced dosages) been reported to suppress the usual menstrual effect on ECW (Lusseveld et al. 1993). Witten and Bradbury (1951) studied pharmacological doses (5 mg) of estrone (as in some HRT preparations) in women (aged 15–52 years) on indices of hemodilution, with acute injections resulting in 15%–21% increases in blood volume.

HRT may also affect body composition, at least in high-dose preparations. Jensen et al. (1986) studied three dosages of combined HRT in postmenopausal women, finding that HRT (4 mg estradiol and 1 mg norethisterone) was associated with a 13% increase in 24-hour urinary creatinine excretion. Because body weight was unchanged, this effect was thought to be due to increased muscle mass and decreased fat mass.

Blood flow and liver volume.   OCs can increase liver (blood) volume by 17%, which may affect kinetics for drugs with high rates of hepatic extraction, leading to increased CL (Homeida et al. 1978).[11] The ef-

---

[11] Six months of treatment with 30 μg ethinyl estradiol and 500 μg dl-norgestrel was associated with a 21% decrease in antipyrine CL. OC use reduced drug-metabolizing capacity by 33%, and OC discontinuation resulted in normalization of drug-metabolizing capacity.

Table 2–2.   Effects of oral contraceptives (OCs) and hormone replacement therapy (HRT)

Absorption and bioavailability				
Variable	Findings in women vs. men	Percentage effect	Predicted impact on CL and/or BL in women	Reference
Gastric emptying time (S = solids; L = liquids)	Slower with OC (but lessens sex difference)	18 (L)	Less ↓ BL than with sex alone	1, 2
	Slower with HRT	30 (S), 60 (L)	↓ BL	
Gastric acid secretion	Lower acid with 1.25 or 2.5 conjugated estrogen; or progesterone	18	Effect ↑ BL (bases) similar to that of sex alone	3
Distribution				
Variable	Findings in women vs. men	Percentage effect	Predicted impact on CL and/or BL in women	Reference
Protein binding	e.g., lower plasma albumin	3–12	↑ free BL	4
Liver (blood) volume	Higher	(17?)	(↓ BL in drugs with high extraction)	5
Metabolism and elimination				
Variable	Findings in women vs. men	Percentage effect	Predicted impact on CL and/or BL in women	Reference
Hepatic metabolism: hydroxylation	Lower (especially when estradiol dose is high)	33	↑ BL (↓ CL)	5, 6
Demethylation	Lower (especially when estradiol dose is high)	?	?	—

(continued)

Table 2–2.   Effects of oral contraceptives (OCs) and hormone
replacement therapy (HRT) *(continued)*

			Metabolism and elimination *(continued)*	
Variable	Findings in women vs. men	Percentage effect	Predicted impact on CL and/or BL in women	Reference
Glucuronidation	Higher	?	↓ BL	6
Renal elimination: creatinine clearance	Higher GFR with progesterone	15	↓ BL	7

Note. BL = blood level; CL = clearance; GFR = glomerular filtration rate.
References:
1. Wedmann et al. (1991) and Cruz et al. (1951).
2. Hutson et al. (1989) and limited data from Datz et al. (1987a), in which 2 of 15 females were on OCs.
3. Sakaguchi et al. (1991) and Cruz et al. (1951), who found that progesterone reduced total acid by 80%.
4. Gleichmann et al. (1973) and K. Wilson (1984). Percentage effect is estimated (e.g., from Jochemsen et al. [1982], where the protein unbound fraction for nitrazepam was 18% higher in women on OCs than in men).
5. Homeida et al. (1978) requires replication.
6. In Abernethy et al. (1984), absolute bioavailability increased by 63%. Dosage adjustment was recommended (i.e., reducing the dose by one-third). See also Jochemsen et al. (1982).
7. Christy and Shaver (1974), Dignam et al. (1956), and Attallah et al. (1988).

fect of OCs on liver volume, however, may be limited to compounds with higher doses of steroids. Studies using newer contraceptives with lower steroid dosages have not uniformly found changes (Abernethy et al. 1984).

Protein binding.   According to K. Wilson (1984), OCs decrease plasma albumin concentrations by 3%–12% (Gleichmann et al. 1973; Laurell et al. 1969; Song et al. 1970). It is well known that OCs can increase lipoproteins. Protein binding, however, does not necessarily change with chronic OC use, particularly at lower dosages (Abernethy et al. 1982a, 1984).

Metabolism and Elimination

Hepatic metabolism.   Cytochrome P450 responds to the synthetic estrogen commonly found in OCs, ethinyl estradiol, but not to the conjugated natural estrogens commonly found in postmenopausal HRT (Kok et al. 1986; MacKinnon et al. 1977); however, HRT increasingly uses combination pills (i.e., including a progestin). Marked effects of relatively high-dose exogenous progestins have been demonstrated on drug-metabolizing enzymes in vitro in animals (Juchau and Fouts 1966).[12] Competition between drugs and certain sex steroids for the same metabolic sites may explain some—but not all—of the decrease in metabolic rates in women (K. Wilson 1984).

Depending in part on the dose used, effects of estrogen are to inhibit or to induce hepatic enzymes. OCs generally inhibit oxidative pathways and facilitate conjugation (K. Wilson 1984). Oxidative changes can result in effects as large as about 30% (e.g., Abernethy et al. 1984). The conjugation rate is typically lower in women than in men, but estrogen-predominant OCs have been observed to increase CL for certain drugs eliminated by glucuronidation, perhaps by autoinduction of enzymes. In contrast to typical sex and OC effects on oxidative pathways, greater rates of conjugation will increase CL, suggesting the need for higher dosages over time.

Renal elimination.   Effects of estrogen on the kidney were reviewed by Christy and Shaver (1974), but findings are varied. As one example, Dignam et al. (1956) studied acute effects of intravenous estradiol (25–50 mg), finding a (nonsignificant) decrease in GFR, averaging 10%, in most women.[13] More recently, possible effects of progesterone on renal

---

[12] Treatment of rats with 50 mg/kg progesterone or norethynodrel inhibited side-chain oxidation of hexobarbital by about 40% and ring hydroxylation of zoxazolamine by 17%–38%. Because high doses were required for inhibition, it is unclear whether effects may be clinically relevant.

[13] Sharpey-Schafer and Schrire (1939) studied three menstruating and eight menopausal women (as well as several men) who received intramuscular estradiol benzoate (100,000 IBU [international benzoate units]) for 10 days. Subjects were maintained on a strictly *controlled diet,* and urine volume was found to be unresponsive to estrogen. A. L. Dean and colleagues (1945) studied renal function in four women on 4–6 mg of estradiol for 9–12 days, finding no change in GFR or renal

CL have been examined. Atallah et al. (1988) studied the effects of 200 mg intramuscular progesterone on renal function in premenopausal women at baseline and at 4 hours postinjection. Women were studied in the second half of the menstrual cycle. Acute treatment resulted in a significant, 15% increase in GFR. Possible effects of current OC and HRT preparations, delivered orally, are unknown.

Summary

OCs moderate some of the effects of sex (e.g., on gastric half-emptying, at least for liquids) and potentially either reverse (e.g., renal elimination) or heighten others (e.g., percentage of free versus bound drug). Due to predicted effects on these mechanisms, net bioavailability or active drug may increase in females overall. As we detail in next section, OCs also oppose certain effects of the menstrual cycle (e.g., on ECW); this is not surprising, given that OCs suppress the endogenous hormone fluctuations that help define the cycle. Drugs cleared by oxidation (e.g., hydroxylation) will likely show higher blood levels on OCs, although this effect may be opposed by elevated hepatic blood flow (i.e., when a drug has high hepatic extraction). Effects on hepatic metabolism will often be more important than those on absorption. Thus, the net effect of OCs will likely be to magnify the predicted sex difference in blood levels or CL—for example, with females on OCs showing even higher blood levels than are usual for females compared with males (e.g., imipramine, in Abernethy et al. 1984). We know much less about HRTs, but it may be important that some preparations have fewer effects than OCs on the liver. Even though some studies used older, higher dosages to demonstrate effects, there may be individual differences in sensitivity to exogenous hormones (i.e., such that some women may be sensitive to effects even at lower dosages). In contrast, for drugs that are not metabolized by the liver, OCs may induce or heighten the appearance of slight to

---

plasma volume. Dignam et al. (1956) studied acute effects of intravenous estradiol (25 or 50 mg) in women without intact ovarian function. Overall, there was not a significant effect on GFR. In seven of eight women, however, *GFR decreased by an average of about 10%* (with a range of 1%–25%); in the remaining subject, GFR increased by 10%. Thus, summary findings may be difficult to interpret due to interindividual variability.

moderate sex differences, albeit in a direction that is not typical of sex differences overall—that is, with females showing lower, rather than higher, blood levels—due to enhanced renal elimination.

Menstrual Cycle Effects

Physiological Basis for Menstrual Effects

Absorption and Bioavailability

Gastric emptying.   Eight studies have examined possible menstrual effects on gastric emptying (Davies et al. 1986; Gill et al. 1987; Horowitz et al. 1985; Jonderko 1989; I. MacDonald 1956; Notivol et al. 1984; Petring and Flachs 1990; Wald et al. 1981), with six showing positive results. Five groups found slower emptying (i.e., prolonged emptying time and/ or residual volume) premenstrually compared with the follicular phase (menses and postmenses before ovulation). Taken together, these findings suggest that the menstrual cycle does affect gastric emptying, with the preponderance of evidence showing a 28%–36% slower emptying premenstrually or menstrually, even in unselected, volunteer groups of women (for further details and assessment of the evidence, see Table 2–3).[14]

Small-intestinal transit time and indices of motility.   Because a large proportion of healthy women aged 18–45 years report loose stools with menses (Rees and Rhodes 1976), it has been suggested that (large-) intes-

---

[14] Gill et al. (1987) found slower emptying for solids but not liquids (comparing days 18–20 vs. days 8–10). Notivol et al. (1984) found significantly slower emptying for solids perimenstrually (days 19–28 and days 1–7) compared with midcycle (days 8–18). Petring and Flachs (1990) studied five healthy women aged 27–36 years at weekly intervals over 4 weeks and found an effect for semisolids, with slower gastric emptying premenstrually. Of the remaining three studies, only one found faster emptying for liquids premenstrually (I. MacDonald 1956). Another study found changes for solids that were consistent with the bulk of the studies, in terms of the *direction* of the effect (days 18–20 vs. days 8–10), although the magnitude of the effect did not reach statistical significance (Horowitz et al. 1985). The negative findings of Jonderko (1989) for semisolids are weak, given that women were not used as their own control subjects.

Table 2–3.   Effects of menstrual cycle-phase in pharmacokinetic parameters

	Absorption and bioavailability			
Variable	Findings in women vs. men	Percentage effect	Predicted impact on CL and/or BL in women	Reference
Gastric emptying time (S = solids; L = liquids)	Slower pre-menstrual phase (may lessen sex differences)	28–36 (S)	Less ↓ BL than with sex alone(?) in premenstrual phase	1
	Slower ± pre-menstrual phase	? (L)		
Small-intestinal transit time	Slower	29	↑ BL	2
Gastric acid secretion	Lower acid (increases gastric absorption of bases) in premenstrual phase	33–50	↑ BL (bases)	3

	Distribution			
Variable	Findings in women vs. men	Percentage effect	Predicted impact on CL and/or BL in women	Reference
Sodium retention and total body water	(Possible effects in women with premenstrual symptoms: weight gain)	?	↓ BL (dilutional effect) in premenstrual phase	4

	Metabolism and elimination			
Variable	Findings in women vs. men	Percentage effect	Predicted impact on CL and/or BL in women	Reference
Hepatic metabolism	(Increase inferred, but physio-logical basis is not well documented)	?	(Some show ↓ BL) in premenstrual phase	5

(continued)

Table 2–3.   Effects of menstrual cycle-phase in pharmacokinetic parameters *(continued)*

	Metabolism and elimination *(continued)*			
Variable	Findings in women vs. men	Percentage effect	Predicted impact on CL and/or BL in women	Reference
Renal elimination: creatinine clearance	Higher in premenstrual phase (in some women)	6–100 (usually 10–25)	↓ BL during premenstrual phase	6

Note. BL = blood level; CL = clearance. References:
1. Gill et al. (1987) and Petring and Flachs (1990).[14]
2. Wald et al. (1981).
3. I. MacDonald (1956) and Sakaguchi et al. (1991).
4. Janowsky et al. (1973) and Bunt et al. (1989).[18]
5. See Part II: Pharmacokinetics of Psychotropics.
6. Brochner-Mortensen et al. (1987), Davison and Noble (1981), and Paaby et al. (1987).[21]

tinal transit times may be rapid at this time in the cycle. However, Wald et al. (1981) found that GI transit time from mouth to *cecum* (i.e., including small-intestinal absorption) was prolonged by an average of 29% during the premenstrual (luteal) phase compared with the follicular phase, potentially allowing for greater absorption.[15] These data are particularly strong because a subgroup of four women were studied intensively, for three cycles each, and findings were highly consistent. The effect is further supported by Davies et al. (1986), who found an even greater (125%) increase in premenstrual transit times. It is unlikely that cycle phase–related changes in esophageal motility contribute to this effect (J. J. Hsu et al. 1993). Small-intestinal effects will likely outweigh those on gastric emptying, tending to result in higher blood levels premenstrually.

---

[15] Although Wald and colleagues reported a 25% effect, that value is actually rounded downward; reanalysis of the data showed a 29% effect.

Secretion of gastric acid.   Gastric acid secretion appears to decline by as much as 50% in the second half of the cycle (I. MacDonald 1956; Sakaguchi et al. 1991). If accurate, this result suggests higher blood levels of bases (e.g., TCAs) in females premenstrually compared with males.

A model drug index of absorption.   Fiset and LeBel (1990) used D-xylose, a model drug characterized by passive absorption and hydrosolubility, to study possible menstrual effects on intestinal absorption.[16] Overall there was little change, although C_{max} (μg/mL), an index of absorption, showed a significant 15% decrease for premenstrual (luteal) versus other comparisons.

Distribution

Body composition and fluids.   Some authors have suggested that sodium retention (Thorn et al. 1938), water content (Keats and Fitzgerald 1976), and urinary volume (Nowaczynski et al. 1962; Thorn et al. 1938) may vary across the normal menstrual cycle (Landau and Lugibihl 1961).[17] In general, however, significant changes in weight, body volume, percentage BF (Byrd and Thomas 1983), sodium retention, urinary volume, TBW, or plasma volume across the menstrual cycle probably do not occur in most women. In addition, studies using model drugs have not found significant changes in CL or apparent Vd during the cycle.

---

[16] Women ranged in age from 18–30 years, were within 10% of ideal body weight, and were nonsmokers. Indices were contrasted for follicular (days 2–7), ovulatory, and midluteal (days 20–25) absorption.

[17] Thorn et al. (1938) studied 50 unselected subjects, finding a premenstrual weight gain of at least 1 kilogram (2.2 pounds) in 48% and a *midcycle* increase in 76%. In a more intensive part of the study, in 2 of 4 nonpremenstrually symptomatic subjects on a *controlled diet,* a premenstrual decrease in urinary sodium output (i.e., sodium retention) and in urine volume was associated with weight gain. In a single, nonsymptomatic subject also maintained on a *controlled diet,* Nowaczynski et al. (1962) observed a decline in urinary volume at *midcycle.* Keats and Fitzgerald (1976) studied leg volume across the menstrual cycle, finding a rise in volume of 30–100 mL at *midcycle.* Thus, several groups have observed fluid changes at midcycle, with or without premenstrual changes. Several studies have shown that urinary aldosterone excretion (Katz and Romf 1972; Perrini and Piliego 1959; M. Reich 1962), plasma levels (Katz and Romf 1972; Sundsfjord and Aakvaag 1973), and aldosterone secretory rates (M. J. Gray et al. 1968) are higher in the second half of the normal menstrual cycle.

On the other hand, there may be individual differences in sensitivity to menstrual effects (e.g., Shader and Harmatz 1982). In particular, women who identify premenstrual symptoms of fluid retention constitute the group most likely to have premenstrual (specifically *late* luteal) phase changes in TBW, and in this group, the data are mixed. Of seven studies (Andersch et al. 1978; Bruce and Russell 1962; Bunt et al. 1989; Davison and Noble 1981; Faratian et al. 1984; Janowsky et al. 1973; Thorn et al. 1938), four found at least slight to moderate menstrual cycle–related changes in fluid volume in symptomatic women (for details and assessment of studies, see Table 2–3).[18] Importantly, in women with documented premenstrual weight gain, a significant premenstrual increase in TBW has been demonstrated (Bunt et al. 1989).[19] The implication is that for some women, a transient premenstrual increase in TBW or plasma water volume (Wong et al. 1972) may be associated with a decrease in blood levels of water-soluble drugs, presumably because of a dilutional effect (e.g., lithium). Increased plasma volume may also dilute plasma proteins, causing reduced colloid osmotic pressure. One group demonstrated a reduction in plasma colloid osmotic pressure during the premenstrual (luteal) phase of the cycle. The change in osmotic pressure was accompanied by mild weight gain (Tollan and Oian 1986).

In addition to potential changes in TBW (Deurenberg et al. 1988), there may also be shifts between compartments, especially in ECW

---

[18] Four studies found fluid or weight changes in women with premenstrual symptoms. The study by Janowsky et al. (1973) was especially well designed (i.e., with an adequate sample size and dietary controls); the Bruce and Russell (1962) study also controlled diet, but found ovulatory as well as premenstrual changes. Moreover, in women with documented premenstrual weight gain, a significant premenstrual increase in TBW (and percentage BF) has been demonstrated (Bunt et al. 1989). The Thorn et al. (1938) study included only two premenstrually symptomatic subjects in the intensive, clinical portion of the study. However, three other groups have not found fluid or weight changes in women with PMS (Andersch et al. 1978; Davison and Noble 1981; Faratian et al. 1984). All of the studies with negative findings used small samples and were poorly controlled. Ironically, even the well-controlled studies may have minimized effects, given that dietary habits may change in some symptomatic women such that sodium retention is increased, thus inflating small changes that have been observed in the bulk of studies.

[19] Indirectly or implicitly, premenstrual weight gain is also associated with an increase in percentage BF (e.g., see Byrd and Thomas 1983).

(Deurenberg et al. 1988; Gleichauf and Roe 1989; Lusseveld et al. 1993). The filtration of fluid through capillaries is dependent on the pressure gradient between vascular and extravascular space, as well as on capillary-wall integrity. Among women with premenstrual "bloating," the walls of small blood vessels appear to be more permeable premenstrually, as assessed by an electrocapacitance measure of capillary filtration coefficient (Wong et al. 1972).[20] Ostrow et al. (1982) found that red blood cell drug concentration rose and fell in phase with the menstrual cycle. Taken together, these results, while suggestive, are not conclusive.

Blood flow.   Women of reproductive age have lower plasma, as well as whole-blood, viscosity compared with prepubertal children, postmenopausal women, and comparably aged men (Mayer 1964). Because plasma viscosity increases after the cessation of menses, the hormonal milieu associated with menstrual (as opposed to menopausal) status may be related to viscosity and to sex differences in cerebral blood flow (Shaw et al. 1979).

Metabolism and Elimination

Hepatic metabolism.   Antipyrine is commonly used in kinetic studies as a model drug for assessing factors affecting phase II metabolism (e.g., hepatic enzyme activities). As summarized by K. Wilson (1984), a number of groups have failed to find sex differences in total metabolism of antipyrine. However, few studies have evaluated whether menstrual cycle phase influences antipyrine metabolism. One study found a large degree of variability in antipyrine metabolism; a modest decrease in metabolism across the menstrual cycle was interrupted by a slight rise on day 14, although this was not statistically significant (Riester et al. 1980). In this investigation, large day-to-day variability of antipyrine levels, perhaps due to the method of measurement used, may have obscured meaningful menstrual cycle–related changes in drug elimination. Additional studies are needed to evaluate clinically meaningful changes in this marker of metabolism by sex. Even if menstrual cycle effects on

---

[20] Petersen and Milles (1926) studied "blister time" and capillary permeability in relation to the menstrual cycle, finding that average capillary permeability varies maximally, by 7%, between menses and midcycle.

hepatic metabolism are not seen in most women, such effects may occur and be meaningful for a small subgroup of women.

Renal elimination.   Fiset and LeBel (1990) found 8% higher total D-xylose CL and 25% higher renal CL premenstrually (days 20–25) compared with early in the cycle (days 2–7). The menstrual effect is unlikely to result from effects on absorption, but, alternatively, may result from a premenstrual increase in GFR.

Variations in CL_{cr} across the menstrual cycle could potentially modify the elimination of psychotropic drugs. Six studies have reported on CL_{cr} by menstrual cycle phase (Brochner-Mortensen et al. 1987; Davison and Noble 1981; M. J. Gray et al. 1968; Harvey et al. 1966; Nafziger et al. 1989; Paaby et al. 1987). Three studies found a premenstrual or menstrual rise in CL_{cr}. Because studies made differing comparisons, however, it is difficult to generalize about the nature of the effect. Conservatively, one must view these data as mixed. In our view, however, the bulk and the weight of the evidence suggest that there may be a significant decline, usually of about 6%–25%, in CL_{cr} between premenstrual (luteal) and menstrual/early follicular (days 1–5) or menstrual to mid-follicular (days 6–12) cycle phases (for further details and assessment of studies, see Table 2–3).[21]

---

[21] Three studies found significantly higher CL_{cr} (mL/minute) in the second half of the cycle, and a fourth found changes in the same direction that failed to reach significance. Davison and Noble (1981), reporting data for two cycles, found 20% greater CL_{cr} during the late luteal phase (days 22–28) compared with the week of menses (days 1–7). Paaby et al. (1987) found 11% greater CL_{cr} (mL/minute × 1.73 m^2) in the midluteal (days 18–23) compared with the midfollicular phase (days 4–9). Brochner-Mortensen et al. (1987) found a 6% higher luteal phase (days 17–27) compared with follicular phase GFR (days 2–6) in young, healthy women. However, conflicting data exist. Three groups (M. J. Gray et al. 1968; Harvey et al. 1966; Nafziger et al. 1989) did not find a significant menstrual effect on CL_{cr}. M. J. Gray et al. (1968) studied 13 volunteers (sampled on days 7, 12, 19, and 25). There was a nonsignificant trend for CL_{cr} to be higher in the second half of the cycle. The Nafziger et al. (1989) study contrasted CL_{cr} by week of the cycle. There was an 8% decline between the late luteal (days 21–27) and the menstrual cycle phase (days 1–7). Harvey et al. (1966) studied only seven women, three of whom were taking OCs, and subjects were not used as their own control subjects. Thus, of the remaining four subjects, three were studied in the follicular cycle phase (days 6–8), with only one in a different cycle phase (day 16). The comparisons in Harvey et al.

Summary

Many of the effects of sex will be to increase blood levels or decrease CL in females; in contrast, certain effects correlated in timing with the premenstrual cycle phase will oppose the typical effects of sex: for example, dilutional effects may decrease bloods levels premenstrually, especially in a small subgroup of premenstrually symptomatic women. Thus, the effects of sex do not result solely from effects of the menstrual cycle.

Menopause or Age Changes

Effects of age and menopause are frequently confounded. Drug studies often use arbitrary cutoffs for defining age groups that are not physiologically based. For example, Raskin (1974) and D'Mello and McNeil (1990) used age 40 as the cutoff for defining groups. However, the median age of natural (nonsurgical) menopause is about 50 years, providing a more accurate physiologically based definition. Alternatively, if independent information were not available about menopausal status, it might be safest to use the following limits for defining groups: < 42 and > 58 years, since approximately 95% of natural menopause should occur between these age limits.[22] Studies of menopause are further confounded by failure to describe whether menopause is reached naturally or surgically and whether menopausal women are on HRT.[23]

(1966) therefore have little meaning, although the CL_{cr} at midcycle was 5% lower than the mean follicular CL_{cr}. In summary, four studies showed higher CL_{cr} in the second half of the cycle, with only one study showing a decline, and another being uninterpretable.

[22] Due to the wide age range for menopause, age and naturally reached menopausal status obviously could be unconfounded if groups were crossed on these variables, resulting in a 2×2 design (e.g., mean age 46 years and not menopausal, with normal cycling and hormonal profile; mean age 46 and menopausal; mean age 54 and not menopausal, with normal cycling and hormonal profile; mean age 54 years and menopausal).

[23] Additional questions of potential importance are 1) if menopause was reached surgically, the time period postsurgery (as this duration may affect the likelihood of observing various physiological changes); and 2) if HRT has ever been used, the type and duration of usage, and if it is no longer being used, the time period since discontinuation.

Physiological Basis for Menopausal Effects

Absorption and Bioavailability

Gastric emptying.   Hutson et al. (1989) found that postmenopausal women aged 46–68 years, on and off combination HRT (conjugated estrogen and medroxyprogesterone), had a 50%–62% slower gastric emptying of *liquids* compared with men. However, postmenopausal women *off HRT* had gastric emptying rates for *solids* similar to those of men— that is, 23%–40% faster than rates for women with higher circulating sex steroid hormones levels (i.e., premenopausal, menstruating women or postmenopausal women on HRT). This finding was supported by Wedmann et al. (1991) for fatty liquids.[24]

Secretion of gastric acid.   Even in premenopausally aged women, conjugated HRT (Premarin) decreases gastric acid secretion (Sakaguchi et al. 1991). Yamagata et al. (1975) found that sex differences in gastric acid secretion volume are greatest in the third and fifth decades, and stimulated acid secretion, in the third through fifth decades. The transition associated with the greatest change in secretion volume was between the fourth and fifth decades for women, suggesting a link to menopausal status.

Distribution

Blood flow.   The sex difference in cerebral blood flow declines in the fourth or fifth decade, and values are similar in males and females after the sixth decade (Shaw et al. 1979).

Protein binding.   In women aged 45–64 years, there is a variable pattern for the effects of menopause and HRT (with 21-day conjugated estrogen) on serum proteins (Hashimoto et al. 1991).

---

[24] Men in the Hutson et al. (1989) study ranged in age from 21 to 64 years, and the degree to which age and menopausal status confounded male-female comparisons is not clear. Datz et al. (1987b) also compared premenopausal women (aged 20–45 years) with postmenopausal women (46–68 years). The latter group had 25% faster gastric emptying.

Metabolism and Elimination

Renal elimination.   There is reduced renal tubular reabsorption of calcium postmenopausally (Nordin et al. 1991); little is known about menopausal effects per se that may be pertinent to pharmacokinetics.

Physiological Basis for Age Effects

Clinically important effects of age include 1) decreased serum albumin (increasing unbound, active drug), 2) decreased LBM (decreasing the Vd of water-soluble drugs and increasing the plasma concentration), 3) lower hepatic blood flow, 4) attenuated activity of selective metabolic enzymes (biotransformation by hydroxylation or conjugation), and 5) decreased renal excretion and elimination. Thus, mature women might appear to have even greater risk for reduced CL and increased half-life and blood levels of many commonly used drugs in comparison with younger women (i.e., *assuming that age changes are uniform by sex,* age will tend to heighten the typical effects of sex). Increased risk for toxicity has resulted in practice guidelines and quality assurance criteria recommending lowered dosages in individuals over 65 years of age by 50% (Ouslander 1981); the guidelines are notably blind to the issue of sex.

However, in theory, *age-related changes generally may not be as pronounced in women as in men* (M. D. Allen et al. 1980). D. J. Greenblatt et al. (1982) commented on sex-related differences in a review on drug disposition in old age. Women of any age group have a larger proportion of adipose tissue and Vd compared with men. There is a strong age-related decline in total drug CL in men, who tend to clear drugs faster when younger, such that with age they lose their more efficient disposition status relative to women (this may be an advantage or disadvantage, according to the situation); the effect of age in females is generally far less pronounced. Thus, changes in drug disposition with age appear to differ between the sexes. (As we shall see in Chapter 3, actual experiences with particular psychotropics do show varied age effects.)

Summary

Little is known about possible effects of menopause per se on pharmacokinetics. Effects of sex on absorption may be somewhat more important than effects of age (age has negligible effects on absorption); however, hepatic metabolism and renal CL are often relatively more important than absorption. Particularly for hepatically biotransformed drugs, if doses were advisedly decreased somewhat in young women compared with young men (an issue to be addressed in Part II), then there might be relatively little need to decrease dosages *further* in older women. Instead, it appears that age transforms the needs of older *men* (with slower CL than younger men) to more closely match those of younger *women* (also with slower CL than younger men).

Other Confounding Effects: Coadministration of Nonhormonal Drugs

The coadministration of a variety of drugs, including antidepressants and phenothiazines, can affect any or a variety of the stages of drug absorption, distribution, metabolism, or elimination. As one example, H_2 blockers such as cimetidine can alter gastric pH and the absorption of other compounds; they can also inhibit hepatic metabolism of coadministered medications. Compounds most likely to cause an interaction include cimetidine, ranitidine, metoclopramide, analgesics, anticonvulsants, oral hypoglycemics, sedatives, rifampin, ethanol, and cigarette smoking, although this is only a partial list (Sellers 1985). Alterations in pharmacokinetic parameters induced by coadministered drugs can potentially obscure (e.g., by suppression or masking) underlying sex differences in drug metabolism or elimination. Alternatively, when concurrent use of other compounds disproportionately occurs in one sex, the effect will be more pronounced in that sex. This is the case with alcohol and cigarette use, both of which are more prevalent in men. In this section we briefly consider the effects of cigarette smoking and alcohol consumption on the metabolism of psychotropic drugs.

Cigarette Smoking

A number of compounds in cigarette smoke may be responsible for enzyme induction in a variety of tissues (Conney et al. 1977). The best-studied compounds are the polycyclic aromatic hydrocarbons, which induce hepatic oxidizing enzymes (L. G. Miller 1990; Vestal and Wood 1983). Hypothetically, compounds whose metabolism is induced by cigarette smoke will have shortened half-lives, potentially resulting in decreased therapeutic efficacy.[25]

Smoking has historically been a gender-linked behavior (higher in males than in females), although the rates of women smokers are increasing. Goff et al. (1992) examined cigarette smoking and side effects in schizophrenic patients. Smokers were significantly more likely to be male than female. Although neuroleptic blood levels were not obtained, smokers were significantly less likely to have side effects. What appeared to have been an effect of sex was shown to be due to a sex-linked confounding variable (i.e., gender roles affect rates of smoking by sex). Thus, smoking can mimic sex differences.

---

[25] As reviewed by L. G. Miller (1990), benzodiazepine anxiolytics whose clinical efficacy may be decreased by cigarette smoking include chlordiazepoxide, clorazepate, oxazepam, and triazolam but not diazepam, lorazepam, or midazolam. Some authors have found that smoking decreases the efficacy of neuroleptics (Vinarova et al. 1984) and TCAs (Gex-Fabry et al. 1990; John et al. 1980; Perel et al. 1975a, 1975b), although others have failed to find any influence of cigarette smoke on the levels of TCAs (Ziegler and Biggs 1977). Perel and colleagues (1975b) found that smoking at least 15 cigarettes (or 6 cigars) per day lowered plasma steady-state levels of imipramine and desmethylimipramine to 45% of that expected in nonsmokers. Although the effect of smoking was reported to be especially large in men, comparative data were not presented by sex.

Given the multiple pathways of drug metabolism, some stages will be affected by cigarette smoke and some will not. In smokers, the activity of enzymes demethylating clomipramine are increased but the concentration of the desmethyl metabolites are equal (Gex-Fabry et al. 1990; John et al. 1980). On the other hand, hydroxylation of clomipramine is not affected by cigarette smoke. Because more males than females smoke, findings such as these point to the potential for a gender-smoking interaction. One model finds hydroxylation of clomipramine to be lower in females than in males, with no significant difference in rates of demethylation. In male smokers, both demethylation and hydroxylation would be higher, whereas one would expect that demethylation but not hydroxylation would be elevated in female smokers. Although the clinical significance of increased hydroxylated metabolites of clomipramine has not been determined, the effects of smoking on metabolites are potentially important for other hydroxylated metabolites such as hydroxynortriptyline; some authors suggest that clomipramine is associated with cardiotoxicity (Gex-Fabry et al. 1990; L. S. Schneider et al. 1988).

Alcohol Consumption

Alcohol dependence and abuse is seen more frequently in men (Robins et al. 1984), but women are more vulnerable to alcohol-related hepatic damage (e.g., Frezza et al. 1990). In nonalcoholic populations, the metabolizing enzyme responsible for the majority of the first-pass effect, gastric alcohol dehydrogenase, is less active in females than males (Frezza et al. 1990), with alcoholic women having the lowest alcohol dehydrogenase activity. Thus, for the latter group, larger amounts of alcohol will be absorbed and, if not detoxified by the liver, will be present to interact with coadministered medication.

The effect of concurrent alcohol ingestion on the pharmacokinetics of other drugs is dependent on the metabolic pathway of coadministered drugs and the pattern of alcohol use—that is, whether it is used occasionally or chronically. Alcohol's effect will also depend on whether alcohol is ingested before, concurrently with, or after another drug.[26] Pharmacology research generally has not assessed potential sex differences on the impact of concurrent alcohol use.[27] In pharmacoepidemiological studies, unassessed variations in alcohol use can lead to

---

[26] Earlier reviews summarized alcohol's effects on sedatives (Lane et al. 1985; Sellers and Holloway 1983).

[27] The acute administration of alcohol inhibits mixed-function oxidases and has been found to cause higher blood levels of some benzodiazepines (Lane et al. 1985). Over the long term, chronic alcohol use that has not caused hepatic damage will stimulate hepatic microsomal enzymes. Thus, chronic alcohol use has the opposite effect of acute, nonchronic use and leads to lower blood concentrations of concurrently administered medications in some instances (Lane et al. 1985). Chronic alcohol use, and hence lower blood levels, are more likely to occur with men, who show greater rates of alcohol abuse and dependence. Because women metabolize alcohol less efficiently and are less likely than men to be chronic users, they are less likely to be chronic users, and hence more likely to have higher blood levels. In severe alcohol abusers with cirrhosis, it is unlikely that gender effects will be important. The drug-metabolizing and -detoxifying capacity of these individuals is severely compromised.
  Alcohol use can affect serum levels of antidepressants. One study found that prior administration of alcohol led to a doubling of single-dose amitriptyline concentration (Dorian et al. 1983). On the other hand, demethylation of clomipramine was found to decrease in chronic alcohol users, probably secondary to alcoholic liver damage.

apparent sex differences in pharmacokinetics that are instead attributable to effects of a sex-linked confounding variable (i.e., gender roles affect rates of alcohol usage by sex).

Conclusion

Sex differences in pharmacology have been observed in animals and humans since at least the 1960s and have received commentary and review since at least the 1970s. Corroborative, though indirect, evidence for sex differences in pharmacology comes from studies of *physiological mechanisms* known to affect pharmacokinetics. Studies of the physiological basis for sex differences in pharmacokinetics accumulated from the 1930s through the present, and replicated data showing sex effects were available on many mechanisms by the 1970s (e.g., OC effects). Although age-related effects on pharmacokinetics received increasing clinical attention in the late 1970s and early 1980s, attention to sex differences has lagged considerably behind.

In this chapter we have carefully assessed both the quality and the quantity of the available data. We have sought to clarify what we do not know as well as what we do. Even the most conservative evaluation of these data would find evidence suggestive of sex-related differences and hormone effects on the physiological bases of a number of pharmacokinetic factors. Somewhat less conservatively, but still in keeping with our nuanced inspection of the data, we argue that considerable evidence now exists showing that OCs and menstrual cycle phase likely have pharmacokinetic effects that may be clinically meaningful in at least a subgroup of women. Thus, we recommend that factors related to possible sex differences and hormonal effects should be more often assessed in *basic science* studies of pharmacokinetics *in humans.* Data concerning the effects of menopausal status and HRT are scant, but limited evidence suggests that possible effects of pre-, peri-, and postmenopausal status, and of HRT use, deserve increasing consideration with regard to basic pharmacokinetic studies as well.

The observation of sex-related differences in the physiological substrate for pharmacokinetic effects may or may not be associated with significant differences in CL, plasma blood levels, or steady-state concentrations of certain psychotropic drugs. Even if effects are statistically significant, they may not be clinically meaningful. Moreover, effects of sex, hormonal and nonhormonal drugs, hormonal status, and age may be demonstrable in "pure" studies isolating each factor from the others, but may wash out in less controlled clinical trials. Thus, possible practice and public policy implications will rest on empirical findings to be discussed in Part II.

Sex Differences in Pharmacokinetics of Psychotropic Medications

Part II: Effects on Selected Psychotropics

Kimberly A. Yonkers, M.D.,
and Jean A. Hamilton, M.D.

This chapter is the second part of a two-part review of sex-related differences in pharmacokinetics. In Part I (Chapter 2), we examined the physiological bases for sex differences in pharmacokinetics generally. Here, in Part II, we more specifically examine what is known about possible sex-related effects on the pharmacokinetics of psychotropics per se.

Because of the proliferation of newly recognized psychotropic agents and the discovery of psychotropic uses for both old and new drugs, the present discussion is limited to selected examples from the five main classes of psychotropics: 1) antidepressants (including tricyclic antidepressants [TCAs], monoamine oxidase inhibitors [MAOIs], and newer atypical agents), 2) anxiolytics, 3) antipsychotics, 4) mood stabilizers, and 5) other hypnotics (Baldessarini 1979; Ballenger 1988; Gitlin and Weiss 1984; Lerer 1985; Schatzberg and Cole 1992). In this chapter we summarize the apparent sex differences for each of these five classes of psychotropic drugs and examine studies that specifically link pharmacokinetic effects to exogenous ovarian hormone treatment or endogenous hormonal fluctuations.

For an introduction to or overview of some of the important factors and concepts in pharmacokinetics, the reader is referred to Chapter 2. Several authors have hypothesized that apparent clearance (CL) and elimination half-life ($t_{1/2}$) are typically faster in males than in females (Fagan 1992; Hamilton 1991; K. Wilson 1984; Yonkers et al. 1992a). We discuss findings in terms of this hypothesis.

Sex Differences in Pharmacokinetics of Psychotropic Medications

Drugs in the same or similar classes, or even those with very similar chemical structures, may be absorbed, distributed, metabolized, or eliminated somewhat differently. Despite differences, most psycho-tropics share common features affecting pharmacokinetics. Here we compare the pharmacokinetic characteristics of TCAs, benzodiazepines, propranolol, phenothiazines, carbamazepine, phenytoin, lithium, and barbiturates. Characteristics of the selected psychotropics are summarized in Table 3–1 (Berkow 1982; Goodman and Gilman 1975; Moyer and Boeckx 1982; Sallee and Pollock 1990). A central purpose of this chapter is to provide a reference source for practitioners and researchers who are interested in learning about possible sex differences in psycho-pharmacology. (We realize that the material is presented in a rather dry manner, but we found it impossible to be comprehensive and analytical while simultaneously striving for a fine narrative style.)

Table 3–1.   Characteristics of selected psychotropics

Absorption and bioavailability

Variable	Antidepressant (tricyclic)	Antianxiety (benzodiazepine)	Sedative (propranolol)	Antipsychotic (phenothiazine)
Gastric acidity	Base	Base	?	Base
Completeness of oral absorption	95%	±	+	±
First-pass metabolism	++	±	+	?

Variable	Mood stabilizer (carbamazepine)	Possible mood stabilizer (phenytoin)	Mood stabilizer (lithium)	Other hypnotics (barbiturates)
Gastric acidity	(Base)	Acid	0(pk$_a$ = 8.3)	Acid
Completeness of oral absorption	70%	±	100%	±
First-pass metabolism	(+)	±	0	±

Distribution

Variable	Antidepressant (tricyclic)	Antianxiety (benzodiazepine)	Sedative (propranolol)	Antipsychotic (phenothiazine)
Lipophilic	+	Varies	+	(+)
Protein binding	73%–96%	99%	94%	94%
Vd (tissue binding)	10–83 L/kg	0.4–1.8 L/kg	39 L/kg	Large
Affected by protein change	No	Yes	(No)	No

Variable	Mood stabilizer (carbamazepine)	Possible mood stabilizer (phenytoin)	Mood stabilizer (lithium)	Other hypnotics (barbiturates)
Lipophilic	(+)	=	±	±
Protein binding	75%	75%–95%	0	Average 45%–50% (range: 5%–80%)
Vd (tissue binding)	Large	0.6 L/kg	Small	Large (only in TBW)
Affected by protein change	(No)	(No)	0	±

(continued)

Table 3–1.   Characteristics of selected psychotropics *(continued)*

Variable	Metabolism and elimination			
	Antidepressant (tricyclic)	Antianxiety (benzodiazepine)	Sedative (propranolol)	Antipsychotic (phenothiazine)
Primary hepatic biotrans- formation	Hydroxylation	2-keto:oxidation; 3-hydroxy: conjugation	Oxidation	Hydroxylation
Subsequent	Conjugation	Conjugation	Conjugation	Conjugation

Variable	Mood stabilizer (carbamaz- epine)	Possible mood stabilizer (phenytoin)	Mood stabilizer (lithium)	Other hypnotics (barbiturates)
Primary hepatic biotrans- formation	Hydroxylation	Hydroxylation	?	Oxidation
Subsequent	Conjugation	Conjugation	?	Conjugation

Note. TBW = total body water; Vd = volume of distribution.

Comparison of Selected Psychotropic Drugs

Pharmacokinetic Mechanisms Affected

Absorption and Bioavailability

Gastric emptying.   The rate of gastric emptying tends to affect drugs without complete oral absorption. Oral absorption is most complete for lithium, followed by the benzodiazepines and TCAs; it is also high for propranolol and carbamazepine. Gastric emptying may affect certain benzodiazepines, phenothiazines, and barbiturates.

First-pass metabolism affects bioavailability. First-pass effects are most prominent for TCAs and propranolol and are likely for carbamazepine; they are unimportant for lithium. Possible first-pass effects for benzodiazepines, phenothiazines, phenytoin, and barbiturates are less clear and depend greatly on the particular compound in the class in question.

Secretion of gastric acid. The psychotropics most affected by the sex difference in gastric acidity are the TCAs and phenothiazines (weak bases), carbamazepine (similar in structure to TCAs), and phenytoin and barbiturates (weak acids). Benzodiazepines and propranolol are unlikely to be affected, and lithium is unaffected.

Distribution

Body composition and fluids. The most lipophilic drugs are TCAs and propranolol, along with phenytoin. Some benzodiazepines are very lipophilic (e.g., diazepam) whereas others are less so (e.g., lorazepam). Phenothiazines and carbamazepine are at least moderately lipophilic. Lithium storage is variable, as is storage for barbiturates.

Volume of distribution (Vd) is related to tissue binding. The Vd for amitriptyline is 83 L/kg, and that for imipramine is 10–20 L/kg. Propranolol has a Vd of 39 L/kg, and phenothiazines also have a large Vd (Bressler 1982). Vd is expected to be large for carbamazepine and barbiturates. The Vd for phenytoin is only moderate to small (0.6 L/kg), and the Vd for benzodiazepines varies greatly. Although most benzodiazepines have a Vd around 1.1 L/kg in women, chlordiazepoxide has a lower (0.4 L/kg) and diazepam a higher Vd (0.96–1.87 L/kg). Vd for lithium is relatively low because it is restricted to total body water (TBW).

Protein binding. Protein binding is greatest overall for the benzodiazepines, which are 99% bound. Other highly bound psychotropics include TCAs (73%–96%), propranolol and phenothiazines (94%), and phenytoin (70%–95%). Carbamazepine has an intermediate level of binding, at 75%. Barbiturates are typically less protein bound (45%–50%), but binding level varies among specific compounds. Lithium is unbound.

Considering both protein binding and Vd, the drugs most likely to be affected by changes in proteins are the benzodiazepines, which are highly bound and have variable Vd. Barbiturates differ greatly in degree of binding; those that are highly bound might be sensitive to protein changes because barbiturates have a low therapeutic index (TI).

Metabolism and Elimination

Hepatic metabolism.   All of these drugs except lithium and certain 3-hydroxy benzodiazepines are dependent on nonsynthetic hepatic biotransformation. Those most dependent on oxidation are the barbiturates and 2-keto–like benzodiazepines such as diazepam; those dependent on hydroxylation are the TCAs, the phenothiazines, phenytoin, and probably carbamazepine.

After hydroxylation, the phenothiazines, carbamazepine, phenytoin, and the barbiturates are conjugated. 3-hydroxy benzodiazepines, such as oxazepam and lorazepam, are primarily metabolized by conjugation. Propranolol is metabolized by various pathways.

Antidepressants

In animals and humans, imipramine is metabolized by liver N-demethylation to desmethylimipramine, and amitriptyline is similarly metabolized to nortriptyline.

Animal studies.   Liver metabolism of imipramine is more rapid overall in male than in female rodents (Skett et al. 1980). In rodents, chronic administration of imipramine leads to the accumulation of that its major metabolite, desmethylimipramine, in the brain. There are significant sex differences in rates of demethylation, with males showing 66% lower desmethylimipramine accumulation in the brain and 69% *lower concentrations in serum* (M. A. Wilson and Roy 1986). In contrast, evidence exists that hydroxylation occurs at rates two- to threefold lower in females than in males (Roskos and Boudinot 1990).

Human studies.   In this chapter, imipramine is used as a model drug for TCAs. Hamilton (unpublished review, November 1993) recently completed the first comprehensive review of sex differences in the pharmacokinetics of antidepressants, with a focus on imipramine (this study is summarized in Hamilton and Grant 1993, Hamilton 1995, and Hamilton, Grant, and Jensvold [Chapter 12, this volume]). Briefly, only 12 published studies of imipramine plasma levels allow examination of possible sex-related differences in plasma concentrations of imipramine and desmethylimipramine. As shown in Table 3–2, without adjustment

Table 3–2.   Sex-related effects on imipramine plasma concentrations (ng/mL)

	Imipramine		Desmethylimipramine		Total	
	Female	Male	Female	Male	Female	Male
Mean	110	93	191	171	278	253
SD	53	65	114	98	156	143

Source. Data from Hamilton and Grant 1993.

for dose or weight, steady-state plasma concentrations of imipramine and desmethylimipramine are significantly higher in women than in men.

This finding remains significant when adjusted for *dose alone,* but not when adjusted for *dose* and *weight.* The fact that dose *and weight* adjustment eliminates the sex differences suggests that the apparent effect of sex may be trivial; that is, blood levels could be standardized across sex in research studies by using a dose that was adjusted by the subject's body weight. Nonetheless, the effects of sex of blood levels may be *clinically meaningful,* even if mediated (in large part) by sex-linked differences in weight. This follows because it is unclear whether clinicians adequately individualize dosages by weight. Even to the extent that dose-adjusted differences exist by sex, however, careful analysis further reveals that age may be an important factor. That is, *only older-aged females* have higher dose-adjusted plasma concentrations of imipramine and desmethylimipramine (reanalysis of Moody et al. 1967; Sutfin et al. 1988, in Hamilton and Grant 1993).

As shown in Table 3–3, only one published study has reported CL, $t^1/_2$, and Vd by sex for imipramine (Gram and Christiansen 1975). All subjects were 50 years of age or less, but unfortunately there were only two male or female subjects in each group. Direct assessment of bioavailability found it to be 28% higher on average in women than in men. Similarly, $t^1/_2$ was 13% higher in women, and CL was 38% lower.

These effects are seemingly consistent with the global hypothesis that a tendency exists for CL to be lower in women. Again, however, close inspection revealed that the effect was entirely due to oral contraceptive (OC) use (ethinyl estradiol + norethisterone) in one woman. This subject had the most extreme value on each of these measures. In contrast,

Table 3–3. Sex-related effects on tricyclic antidepressant pharmacokinetics

	Clearance (CL [L/minute])		Elimination half-life ($t^{1}/_{2}$ [hour])		Volume of distribution (Vd)		Bioavailability (f [%])	
	Female	Male	Female	Male	Female	Male	Female	Male
Imipramine, oral administration (Gram and Christiansen 1975)								
Mean	0.8	1.3	13.5	12.0	—	—	35.0	41.5
SD	0.1	0.6	0.7	5.7	—	—	33.9	9.2
Clomipramine, oral administration (Nagy and Johansson 1977)								
Mean	—	—	35.8	17.1	—	—	—	—
SD	—	—	—	3.8	—	—	—	—
N	—	—	1	4	—	—	—	—
Clomipramine, intramuscular administration (Nagy and Johansson 1977)								
Mean	0.35	0.33	39.6	24.7	19.8	11.9	—	—
SD	—	0.06	—	8.4	—	4.8	—	—
N	1	4	1	4	1	4	—	—

Source. Data from Hamilton and Grant 1993.

the other female subject had lower bioavailability than either of the male subjects and similar values on other measures (corroborative data on OC effects are from Abernethy et al. 1984, as discussed in a later section).

Preskorn and Mac (1985) found that increasing age and female sex were associated with higher amitriptyline plasma levels. The amitriptyline/nortriptyline ratios averaged 0.76 in women and 1.3 in men taking amitriptyline (Edelbroek et al. 1986). This finding suggests the occurrence of relatively high nortriptyline concentrations in females. J. L. Cramer et al. (1969) speculated that demethylation is more extensive in women than in men, resulting in lower ratios of parent drug to its demethylated metabolite. This hypothesis is plausible, given that the P450 enzyme IIIA3/4 is more active in women than in men (Hunt et al. 1992). A comprehensive review has not been undertaken for amitriptyline in terms of either outcome or pharmacokinetics by sex.

Shown in Table 3–3 are findings from a study of clomipramine administered orally and intramuscularly. Nagy and Johansson (1977) studied four men and one woman, all younger than age 50. They reported only one parameter for oral administration, $t\frac{1}{2}$. As predicted, the woman's $t\frac{1}{2}$ after oral administration was the highest value, at 35.8, compared with a range among the men of 11.6–20.0 hours. Importantly, the authors specified that the woman was *not* taking OCs. After intramuscular administration, $t\frac{1}{2}$ for the woman was 39.6 hours, and the men's average was 24.7 hours. Intramuscular administration is potentially of interest because it bypasses gastrointestinal absorption and first-pass metabolism.

In other studies, women were found to have higher plasma levels of clomipramine (Gex-Fabry et al. 1990), although data are mixed (Vazquez Rodriquez et al. 1991). In addition, Gex-Fabry et al. (1990) suggested that younger women have slower apparent CL for hydroxylation metabolites. A comprehensive review has not been undertaken for clomipramine pharmacokinetics by sex.

Although TCAs are lipophilic, their storage in the brain is fourfold higher compared with that in adipose tissue (Sallee and Pollock 1990). No significant relationship has been found between body weight and imipramine CL (Ereshefsky et al. 1988). Thus, it is unlikely that clinically important variation in TCA plasma levels will be observed in women who undergo cycles of weight loss and gain ("yo-yo" dieting). However, some effects of obesity may reflect other alterations in drug disposition, such as Vd rather than CL.

Reduced CL of a newer heterocyclic antidepressant, trazodone, has been reported for elderly men, suggesting an age-sex effect opposite to that globally predicted (D. J. Greenblatt et al. 1987). The effect was attributed to a greater Vd for women and elderly individuals.

There does not appear to be a sex difference in kinetics for the novel monocyclic bupropion (Findlay et al. 1981). Bupropion metabolites, however, have not been studied with methods that allow assessment of possible sex differences (Golden et al. 1988).

Van Harten (1993) has reviewed pharmacokinetics for selective serotonin reuptake inhibitors (SSRIs). Protein binding does not seem to be clinically important. No convincing relationship exists between plasma levels and clinical efficacy. Plasma concentrations of sertraline were found to be higher in young women compared with young men, but this effect is not believed to require adjustments in dosage by sex (Warrington 1991).

Anxiolytics

Sex differences have been observed for some antianxiety agents (Yonkers and Ellison, Chapter 13, this volume; Yonkers et al. 1992b).

Benzodiazepines.   Potential sex-related differences in the profile of benzodiazepines have been investigated for a number of compounds. As with other studies, findings are limited by possible confounders such as concurrent cigarette smoking or OC use. In addition, there is a lack of pharmacokinetic data describing bioactive metabolites of the experimental drug. On the other hand, several well-designed studies have specifically assessed the effects of concurrent exogenous hormone use.

The evidence regarding sex effects on CL of diazepam given intravenously is conflicting. D. J. Greenblatt et al. (1980a) and Ochs et al. (1981) found evidence that the rate of apparent diazepam CL and $t_{1/2}$ is higher in women, whereas another group reported opposite results for CL (MacLeod et al. 1979). In a regression analysis, sex was a greater determining factor than age for diazepam's $t\frac{1}{2}$ and CL (D. J. Greenblatt et al. 1980a). Cigarette smoking was also significant, and the rate of smoking in men was more than twice that in women. This should have preferentially increased CL among the males in the cohort. Summary data for selected benzodiazepines are shown in Table 3–4.

According to Yonkers and Ellison (Chapter 13, this volume), it appears that prazepam and clonazepam show no evidence of sex effects on CL, despite CL *via* oxidative and nitroreductive pathways, respectively. For chlordiazepoxide delivered intravenously, CL may be somewhat slower in women than in men (Roberts et al. 1979), although conflicting data exist (D. J. Greenblatt et al. 1977, 1989).

Oxazepam, lorazepam, and temazepam are biotransformed by glucuronide conjugation. Consistent with our generalization, the $t\frac{1}{2}$ of oral oxazepam appears to be 24% longer and the unbound clearance (CL_u) 28% slower in women than in men (D. J. Greenblatt et al. 1980b). The $t\frac{1}{2}$ of temazepam administered orally appears to be 27% longer and the CL_u 18% slower in young women compared with men (Divoll et al. 1981), although this finding was not replicated in a subsequent study by the same group (R. B. Smith et al. 1983).

Nitrazepam is biotransformed by nitroreduction, and kinetics probably do not differ by sex (D. J. Greenblatt et al. 1985; Jochemsen et al. 1982). If there are differences for triazolam, it may be unusual, in that the direction of the effect is for *lower* CL in elderly men (R. B. Smith et al. 1983).

Compared with TCAs, benzodiazepines are more likely to show variable plasma levels in women who undergo extreme and rapid cycles of weight loss and gain (yo-yo dieting). Although speculative, this possibility deserves follow-up.

Alprazolam.   Alprazolam is structurally related to the TCAs; however, unexpected directions of effects of sex have been reported. One group has found alprazolam's $t\frac{1}{2}$ in men to be 126% *greater* than it is in women, whereas its oral CL in men was 74% *less* than that in women (Kristansson and Thorsteinsson 1991). However, other researchers have not supported any sex-related differences. Peak serum concentrations are higher in women than in men, but this relationship is due to differences in weight (Kirkwood et al. 1991).

Table 3–4. Sex-related effects on benzodiazepine pharmacokinetics

Study	Clearance: unbound (CLu [mL/minute/kg])		Elimination half-life (t $^1/_2$ [hour])		Volume of distribution (Vd [L/kg])	
	Female	Male	Female	Male	Female	Male
Chlordiazepoxide, intravenous administration						
D. J. Greenblatt et al. 1977 (n = 11 F and 11 M)						
Mean	0.37	0.59	13.6	7.9	0.84	0.34
SD	0.07	0.14	3.5	1.1	0.04	0.25
Roberts et al. 1979 (n = 7 F and 7 M)						
Mean	0.35[a]	0.43	14.8[*]	8.9[*]	0.40	0.33
SD	0.17	0.12	5.9	2.5	0.14	0.12

Study	Clearance: unbound (CLu [mL/minute/kg])		Elimination half-life (t $^1/_2$ [hour])		Unbound volume of distribution (Vd [L])	
	Female	Male	Female	Male	Female	Male
Diazepam						
D. J. Greenblatt et al. 1980a (n = 11 F and 11 M)						
Mean	43.6[**]	29.9[**]	42.4[**]	36[**]	145.2	87.3
SD	19.3	11.5	13.5	14.5	33.6	37.2
Ochs et al. 1981 (n = 13 F and 10 M)						
Mean	60[**]	40.2[**]	37.1	34.4	179[**]	103[**]

Temazepam

Divoll et al. 1981 (n = 7 F and 7 M)

Mean	46.8	57.2	16.2	12.8	1.4	1.53
SD	18.4	19.3	6.1	4.9	—	—

Oxazepam, oral administration

D. J. Greenblatt et al. 1980b (n = 20 F and 18 M)

Mean	19.6**	27.6**	9.7**	7.8**	15.0	17.4
SD	8.5	13.6	1.8	3.2	4.6	6.4

Note. This table includes a secondary analysis of published data.   F = females; M = males.
[a] Unbound clearance was lower in females (8.7 vs. 15.6).
* Significant to at least $P < .05$.
** Significant to at least $P = .05$.

Propranolol.   Women have serum levels of propranolol that average 80% higher than those of men after taking the same oral dose, a difference that persists after correction for weight (Walle et al. 1985). Serum levels are not strongly related to propranolol's antihypertensive efficacy, nor is it clear whether antianxiety effects are dose related. In view of the overall 10- to 50-fold interpatient variability, a dosage adjustment for women is probably not required as a clinical practice guideline.

Buspirone.   The pharmacokinetics of buspirone (BuSpar) may not be influenced by sex. Although its $t_{1/2}$ was longer in men in one study, the effect failed to reach significance (Gammans et al. 1986).

Antipsychotics

Few studies have compared antipsychotic blood levels in men and women. In several cases, women had higher serum concentrations than men. CL of thiothixene (Ereshefsky et al. 1991) was 55% slower in women than in men, a finding unrelated to weight. Fluphenazine decanoate blood levels in women were higher than those of men, typically by about one-third, a finding unrelated to weight or to dose adjusted by weight (G. M. Simpson et al. 1990). Young (1986) failed to observe a sex difference in plasma levels of chlorpromazine.

According to Szymanski (Chapter 14, this volume), female schizophrenic patients have shown higher plasma levels of clozapine (Haring et al. 1989). Clozapine plasma concentrations were 45% higher in women, apparently even after correction for dose and body weight (Dawkins and Potter 1991).

Mood Stabilizers

Lithium.   Given the differences in creatinine CL between men and women, it is expected that the rate of lithium CL would differ by sex. Schou et al. (1986) found that lithium CL was significantly higher in men (23%) than in women. However, when they corrected CL by dividing dosage by body surface, sex was no longer significant. Nonetheless, the need to consider female sex when prescribing lithium is underscored by the work of several groups (Lesar et al. 1985; Zetin et al. 1983) who developed formulas for predicting optimal lithium dosages. As with creatinine CL, correcting the dose downward for female patients is required even though weight is considered. One study suggested that dosage estimates for overweight women should rely on ideal body weight rather than actual weight, to avoid overestimating doses (Kook et al. 1985).

Antiseizure/anticonvulsant agents.   Carbamazepine and other anti-scizure/anticonvulsant drugs are increasingly used to treat severe de-pressions, especially those occurring episodically (Ballenger 1988); thus, this agent has been considered a mood stabilizer. Sex differences in car-bamazepine plasma levels have been found in pediatric populations (Furlanut et al. 1985; Summers and Summers 1989). This effect may depend more on age than on sex, given that other authors have not found significant differences in carbamazepine levels of men compared with women (Froscher et al. 1988).

Other Hypnotics

Mephobarbital shows a stereoselective sex difference (Dawkins and Pot-ter 1991). R-mephobarbital had a greater total body CL and $t_{1/2}$ in young men than in comparable-aged women (Hooper and Quing 1990). It is unclear whether there are primary effects of sex on drugs such as meth-aqualone; however, this drug is rarely, if ever, used in the United States.

Summary

Although scant, some evidence exists for sex differences among phar-macokinetic variables for certain psychotropics. Many effects appear to be small (to perhaps moderate) in size, and it is unclear whether they are clinically meaningful. The strongest findings are for certain ben-zodiazepines, fluphenazine decanoate, clozapine, and lithium—that is, with effects having an order of magnitude of about 20%. However, the paucity of available data should be noted. Pharmacokinetic studies are typically conducted early in drug development, and, given the exclusion of women from these investigations (Kinney et al. 1981), the research necessary to detect sex differences does not exist for a large number of medications.

When sex differences have been observed, women have tended to show greater bioavailability and slower apparent clearance compared with men. This finding supports hypotheses put forth by others (Fagan 1990; Hamilton 1991; K. Wilson 1984; Yonkers et al. 1992a). In some cases, a difference between sexes may be due to only one factor, such as weight. Alternatively, sex differences can be due to a combination of factors, such as differences in hepatic metabolism and weight. In the latter condition, sex differences in plasma levels persist even when dosages are given on a mg/kg basis or when blood levels are adjusted for weight (Ereshefsky et al. 1991; Haring et al. 1989; G. M. Simpson et al. 1990; Walle et al. 1985).[1,2]

Effects of sex will be of little clinical importance for drugs with a wide TI or for medication for which there is a low correlation between plasma concentrations and efficacy or side effects. Although psychotropics tend to have a wide TI, plasma concentrations of certain antidepressants and antiseizure/anticonvulsants are correlated with outcome and side effects. In such instances, blood levels are used to guide treatment. For these psychotropics in particular, sex differences may be clinically meaningful.

---

[1] Examples of drugs thought to show sex differences include acetaminophen, alcohol (which is cross-tolerant with benzodiazepines), amitriptyline, chlordiazepoxide, clozapine (Haring et al. 1989), desmethyldiazepam, diazepam, ethosuximide, flurazepam, fluphenazine decanoate (G. M. Simpson et al. 1990), imipramine (in older populations; Hamilton and Yonkers, Chapter 2, this volume), lidocaine, lorazepam, oxazepam, piroxicam (a nonsteroidal antiinflammatory) in the elderly (Richardson et al. 1985), propranolol (in younger populations), temazepam, and thiothixene (Ereshefsky et al. 1991). Imipramine in younger populations may be an exception to the rule (Gram and Christiansen 1975).

[2] Although data are not definitive, it may be of interest that 79% (15/19) of drugs believed to be affected by sex are psychotropics. In comparison, only 40% (19/48) of drugs included in a major review of age-related effects were psychotropics (Ouslander 1981). These proportions raise the question of whether psychotropics are especially likely, compared with other drugs classes, to show effects of sex or age. If so, the disproportionate and high representation of psychotropics may be, in part, due to pharmacodynamic as well as pharmacokinetic effects.

The evidence, while not conclusive, is at least suggestive that when sex differences in bioavailability and CL occur, optimal dosages based on dose-ranging studies in males may be relatively high in females. Unless adequate dosage adjustments are made, the implication is that females may be placed at increased risk for drug side effects, including toxicity (Hamilton 1995), and may receive less benefit from treatment (Hamilton, in press a). In fact, it appears that women generally experience drug side effects about twice as often as men (Bottiger et al. 1979; Domecq et al. 1980; Hamilton and Parry 1983; Hurwitz 1969; U. Klein et al. 1976; Seidl et al. 1966, Zilleruelo et al. 1987). More specifically, data also suggest that females have an excess of side effects in response to treatment with psychotropics compared with males. As examples, a female excess in type, number, or severity of side effects has been reported for antidepressants (e.g., D. J. Goldstein, personal communication: gender analyses of fluoxetine versus placebo in major depressive disorder [efficacy, reasons for discontinuation, adverse events, statistical methods], Lilly Research Laboratories, Lilly Corporate Center, Indianapolis, IN, November 16, 1993; Mindham et al. 1973; Raskin 1974; Rickels et al. 1967; L. G. Schmidt et al. 1986; Schulterbrandt et al. 1974; Steiner et al. 1993; however, for a more complete review, see Hamilton 1995), a monoamine oxidase (MAO)–inhibiting antidepressant (Hamilton et al. 1984a; Middlefell et al. 1960) and antipsychotics (J. M. Kane and Smith 1982; Tepper and Haas 1979). As reviewed by Hamilton (1986), the higher rate of tardive dyskinesia in women is probably not the single result of differences in absolute or relative dosage, length of drug use, or polypharmacy (Odejide 1980; G. M. Simpson et al. 1978; Yassa et al. 1983). An excess of extrapyramidal side effects in women has also been observed for metoclopramide, an antiulcer drug that increases gastric emptying and has dopamine-antagonizing properties (J. M. Simpson et al. 1987).

Observed Effects of Synthetic and Conjugated Hormones on Psychotropics

Comparisons of pharmacokinetic parameters in men and women would not be complete without an additional consideration of the effects of endogenous and exogenous hormones. In this section we specifically address these effects.

In general, OCs tend to reduce CL for some drugs metabolized by oxidative mechanisms (e.g., caffeine, chlordiazepoxide, diazepam [Giles et al. 1981], and perhaps nitrazepam). Concomitantly, OCs tend to increase CL for selected drugs metabolized by conjugation (e.g., to some extent, nitrazepam).

Antidepressants

Abernethy et al. (1984) found that when imipramine was used in combination with OCs, absolute bioavailability increased by 63%. For chronic long-term OC users, these authors recommended that imipramine dosages be decreased by one-third to reduce risk for toxicity. The clinical relevance of this recommendation is supported by several case studies. Gram and Christiansen (1975) found markedly higher bioavailability and lower first-pass metabolism (166% and 208%, respectively) and lower apparent CL (22%) of imipramine in a woman on OCs compared with another not on OCs. On the other hand, conjugated estrogen did not alter blood levels of imipramine (Shapiro et al. 1985).

Anxiolytics

There are substantial data suggesting that OCs affect diazepam pharmacokinetics. Ellinwood et al. (1983) assessed diazepam-related performance effects on a psychomotor and a cognitive encoding task in women taking 21-day OCs and in men. Cycle-phase effects on impairment were demonstrated. Women experienced greater acute performance impairment during their 7-day menstrual pause (i.e., on 21-day preparations). This effect did not appear to be due to differing plasma levels or to alterations in plasma protein binding of diazepam. The variable most likely to account for the effects was differences in rates of absorption. This study was notable because it demonstrated OC effects with the new lower-dose OCs (e.g., Brevicon). The dosage and behavior changes associated with impairment are meaningful, since the performance was measured with a tracking task controlled by an automobile steering wheel. Importantly, the cyclic difference was found only for *high-pro-gestin* OCs.

The metabolism of diazepam and chlordiazepoxide seem to be impaired by OCs. For diazepam, CL was reduced to between 40% and 50% of control values in OC users, while the drug's $t\frac{1}{2}$ was extended by 47%–83% (Abernethy et al. 1982a; Giles et al. 1981). Similar results have been reported for chlordiazepoxide. As shown in Table 3–5, CL in OC users is decreased to 40%–84% of non-OC users' values, while $t\frac{1}{2}$ is increased by 56%–61% (Patwardhan et al. 1983; Roberts et al. 1979).

OCs may reduce alprazolam's CL and increase its $t\frac{1}{2}$ (Huybrechts 1991). The elimination-rate constant of this compound is significantly different in OC users than in nonusers, but CL in OC users increased only by a nonsignificant 12% (Stoehr et al. 1984).

Treatment with ethinyl estradiol (0.05 mg/day) specifically *decreased* CL of propranolol through *side-chain* oxidation by 31% and *increased* CL through *ring* oxidation and *glucuronidation* by 82% and 69%, respectively. Changes with OCs (also containing 1.0 mg/day norethindrone) were similar but less marked (Fagan et al. 1993). In males, there is a significant positive correlation between testosterone administration and *side-chain* CL (Wallé et al. 1992).

Although it appears that higher-estrogen-dose OCs may accelerate CL of conjugatively metabolized benzodiazepines (Patwardhan et al. 1983), other groups have failed to find statistically significant differences in the metabolism of lorazepam (Abernethy et al. 1983; Stoehr et al. 1984) or oxazepam in women taking low-estrogen OCs (Abernethy et al. 1983). Lorazepam CL in women on OCs is increased 17%–21% (Abernethy et al. 1983; Stoehr et al. 1984). Although not significant, this effect is expected, since estrogen is an inducer of conjugation. In one study, the elimination-rate constant of lorazepam was significantly greater for women on OCs (Stoehr et al. 1984).

Antipsychotics

Effects of OCs per se are unknown. Although estrogen has been given to postmenopausal women as a treatment for tardive dyskinesia, effects on antipsychotic blood levels were not reported (Bedard et al. 1977; Gordon 1980; Villeneuve et al. 1983).

Mood Stabilizers

Possible effects are unknown.

Other Hypnotics

Despite the fact that methaqualone has primarily oxidative metabolism, its CL has been shown to be *increased* by OCs instead of decreased. The oxidative effect may diminish the usual midcycle increase in the rate of methaqualone metabolism (K. Wilson 1984).

Summary

As summarized in Table 3–5, OCs exert the bulk of their effects on drugs metabolized by oxidative pathways. For example, ethinyl estradiol can decrease P450 cytochrome oxidase. OC-related effects on oxidative pathways tend to further decrease CL and to elevate plasma levels of drugs.

In contrast, effects on conjugative pathways oppose the typical (hypothesized) sex-related effect, tending to increase CL and to lower drug levels. Autoinduction also may occur (mainly for conjugative pathways), leading to further increases in CL (Edelbroek et al. 1984) and suggesting the need for higher dosages for some women over time.

Hormone replacement therapy (HRT) with conjugated estrogen does not affect drugs with oxidative metabolism (Kok et al. 1986), although it may affect absorption. However, combined preparations are increasingly used for HRT, so clinicians may need to pay attention to the precise preparation an individual is using.

Menstrual Cycle Effects

Above we noted a general tendency for medications to have greater bioavailability and slower CL in women, except for selected compounds, when they are given in conjunction with OCs. Medication levels can also fluctuate across the menstrual cycle, and in some women levels decline

Table 3–5.   Anxiolytics and oral contraceptives (OCs)

Study	Clearance: bound and unbound (CL [mL/minute])		Elimination half-life ($t \frac{1}{2}$ [hour])		Volume of distribution (Vd)	
	(−)OCs	(+)OCs	(−)OCs	(+)OCs	(−)OCs	(+)OCs
Chlordiazepoxide						
Patwardhan et al. 1983 (n = 6 F and 6 M)						
Mean	33.22*	13.41*	14*	6.0*	26.4	21.4
SD	12.37	46.9	6.2	3.1	7.5	4.8
Roberts et al. 1979 (n = 11 F and 7 M)						
Mean	22.05	18.7	14.8	24.3	25.2*	34.1*
SD	10.71	7.56	5.9	12.0	8.8	12.6
Diazepam						
Giles et al. 1981 (n = 10[−]OCs and 5[+]OCs)						
Mean	0.52	0.21	40.3	73.8	1.69	1.44
SD	0.17	0.07	11.9	49.3	0.28	0.92
Abernethy et al. 1982a (n = 8[−]OCs and 8[+]OCs)						
Mean	0.45*	0.27*	47.0*	69.0*	1.57	1.73
SD	0.11	0.06	11.3	25.5	0.56	0.28

Note. This table includes a secondary analysis of published data. F = females; M = males; (+)OCs/(−)OCs = subjects taking (+)/not taking (−) OCs.
*Significantly different to at least $P = .05$.

during the premenstruum. Although this effect is opposite to what has been proposed above, it is consistent with dilutional effects and with the conjugative enzyme–inducing properties of some OCs.

Antidepressants

For some women, plasma levels of antidepressants are lower during the late luteal phase of the menstrual cycle. Reports of lower antidepressant levels have appeared for women treated with desipramine and trazodone (Kimmel et al. 1992) and with nortriptyline (Jensvold et al. 1992). The steady-state plasma levels of these drugs have dropped by as much as 53% (Kimmel et al. 1992). Menstrual effects are pronounced in the subgroup having premenstrual dysphoric symptoms.

Wirz-Justice and Chappuis-Arndt (1976) demonstrated an influence of cycle phase on neuroendocrine responses to clomipramine, but possible kinetic effects and clinical implications are unclear.

MAOIs.   Some authors have shown that *platelet* MAO activity varies in relation to endogenous sex steroid changes. Lower levels of platelet MAO activity were observed in women around midcycle or premenstrually (Belmaker et al. 1974), although data on *plasma* MAO are conflicting (Rapkin et al. 1988). It is not known whether the concentration of MAOIs changes across the menstrual cycle.

Anxiolytics

Benzodiazepines.   Jochemsen et al. (1982) found that nitrazepam kinetics were not significantly affected by the menstrual cycle. However, as noted by K. Wilson (1984), several trends were seen that deserved attention. Jochemsen and colleagues' study found a slower average absorption rate, a lower mean peak plasma concentration, a longer plasma $t\frac{1}{2}$, and higher average CL in the *follicular* phase (days 1–5) than in the early luteal and premenstrual phases (days 14–19). The direction of such effects is contrary to those noted above for antidepressants.

Alprazolam.   Although alprazolam is structurally related to TCAs, no effect of the menstrual cycle was observed by Kirkwood et al. (1991).

Propranolol.   In a woman with premenstrual migraines, the onset of menses was associated with an average 54% decrease in propranolol concentration (Abdu-Aguye et al. 1986; Gengo et al. 1984). However, in seven non–(premenstrually) symptomatic women, significant effects of the menstrual cycle on propranolol CL and hepatic metabolism were not observed, although CL was 13% lower in the follicular cycle-phase than menstrually or premenstrually (Fagan 1992). Moreover, there is no correlation between CL of propranolol and endogenous estradiol in females, although there is a positive correlation with testosterone (Walle et al. 1992). The latter finding is of interest because it is known that endogenous testosterone and other androgens fluctuate across the normal human menstrual cycle (G. E. Abraham 1974; Persky 1974; Ribeiro et al. 1974; Vermeulen and Verdonck 1976), with an increase at midcycle.

Buspirone. Effects for buspirone, a novel anxiolytic with antidepressant properties, are more likely to be paradoxical (e.g., increased restlessness) if therapy is initiated in the midluteal as opposed to the midfollicular cycle phase. Buspirone has a novel structure (related to piperazines) and a moderate effect for dopamine type 2 (D_2) receptors, but its mechanism of action is not yet well established. Aside from the possibly higher side effect rates for treatments initiated in the luteal phase, the incidence of buspirone-induced restlessness is about 2%. Although these reports are anecdotal, clinical observations such as these should stimulate follow-up studies.

Antipsychotics

A case report by Stevens (1973) involved a woman treated with high doses of phenothiazines who nonetheless experienced premenstrual exacerbations of her illness. Although plasma levels were not obtained, this case raises the possibility of a menstrual-related decline in efficacy that may be related to a drop in plasma levels.

Mood Stabilizers

Lithium. Recurrent premenstrual deterioration occurred in an adolescent with manic-depressive illness. This clinical decompensation was related to a fall in serum lithium levels premenstrually, even though the patient's dose remained constant throughout the cycle. Use of higher dosages premenstrually resulted in better clinical management (Conrad and Hamilton 1986). The effect appears to be complicated, because the direction of change in lithium levels is unclear: both a premenstrual increase (Kukopulos et al. 1985) and a decrease (Conrad and Hamilton 1986) have been observed. It is likely that most women will not show menstrual cycle fluctuations in lithium levels (Chamberlain et al. 1990), but cyclic changes in clinical status may warrant closer investigation of menstrual cycle effects for some.

Antiseizure/anticonvulsants.   It is not known whether phenytoin functions as an effective mood stabilizer as well as an anticonvulsant, but it is a compound frequently used for psychiatric patients. Some women with premenstrual ("catamenial") seizures have been found to have a marked menstrual decrease in phenytoin levels compared with age-matched control subjects (Kumar et al. 1988) or women with epilepsy unrelated to the menstrual cycle (Shavit et al. 1984). Although carbamazepine blood levels do not generally vary across the menstrual cycle, high coefficients of variation (22% and 32%) were observed in two menstrual cycles in two women with epilepsy; a third woman showed a significant positive correlation ($r = .40$) between estradiol and carbamazepine in one of two cycles, with menstrual-linked variations in estradiol accounting for 16% of the variability in carbamazepine blood levels across that cycle (Bäckström and Jorpes 1979).

Other Hypnotics

Methaqualone has a 29% shorter $t\frac{1}{2}$ and 86% higher CL at midcycle than postmenstrually (K. Wilson et al. 1982). Menstrual effects on other sedative-hypnotics are unclear.

Summary

Menstrual effects on distribution, metabolism, and elimination appear to exceed those on absorption. Some effects of endogenous steroid hormone fluctuations appear to be small or moderate in magnitude (e.g., desipramine, trazodone, and methaqualone, with effects of 30%–50%) and some effects may apply only to a small subgroup of women (e.g., propranolol for some women with premenstrual migraines; lithium for some women with premenstrual worsening of bipolar disorder). At least some effects appear to be clinically meaningful (e.g., resulting in recommended dosage adjustments) (Conrad and Hamilton 1986; Jensvold et al. 1992). When unrecognized, menstrual effects on pharmacokinetics will generally contribute to decreased efficacy of treatment for a small—but perhaps clinically significant—group of women. Data at present are especially strong and consistent for effects on TCAs.

Although speculative, there is some evidence to suggest that women with premenstrually occurring symptoms may compose a subgroup vulnerable to menstrual cycle–related effects on drug disposition. For example, in Part I we reviewed the physiological basis of effects, demonstrating that these may be highest among women who are premenstrually symptomatic; elsewhere, it has been estimated that perhaps 5%–10% of the female population have substantial premenstrual symptoms (e.g., Hamilton and Gallant 1993). Individual differences in use of alternative metabolic pathways, or in endogenous levels of sex steroid hormones or sensitivity to their effects, may explain why some women show menstrual cycle–related effects and others do not.

Patterns of recreational drug use may also vary across the cycle. In a study by Mello and Mendelsohn (1985), 5 of 15 women increased marijuana use premenstrually. Only women who were dysphoric premenstrually used more marijuana premenstrually. Drug use did not covary with the menstrual cycle if there were no premenstrual symptoms. Case reports and findings such as these are of potential importance clinically and deserve efforts aimed at replication.

Menopause or Age Changes

Little is known about pharmacokinetic changes occurring with menopause. As in young women, pharmacokinetic parameters in postmenopausal women may or may not be affected by concurrent treatment with exogenous hormones (see above).

Antidepressants

For imipramine, *postmenopausal* women show higher plasma concentrations of imipramine and desmethylimipramine compared with men (20% and 32%, respectively, based on a reanalysis of Moody et al. [1967]). Data comparing plasma levels of imipramine for older and younger women are conflicting: Moody et al. (1967) observed a 13% decrease in levels with increasing age, and Sutfin et al. (1988), a 92% increase. Data from a study comparing plasma levels of desmethylimipramine in older and younger women showed a 39% increase in des-methylimipramine levels (Moody et al. 1967).[3] One study evaluating predictors for variability in amitriptyline levels found age and sex to be significant factors for total TCA levels (Preskorn and Mac 1985). Men more than 50 years of age achieved levels that were 87% of those in comparably aged women. After partialing out the total concentration to individual amitriptyline and nortriptyline levels, findings were no longer significant, although concentrations remained higher in older women. Summary data on TCAs from another group showed higher levels in women of all ages and in older men and women (Ziegler and Biggs 1977). Separate analyses were not presented for older women.

Gex-Fabry et al. (1990) found that clomipramine is metabolized less slowly in older women than in men. They also noted a significant reduction of hydroxylation, demethylation, and renal excretion with increasing age.

Anxiolytics

As with other medications, data for anxiolytics demonstrate that CL of several benzodiazepines is less in postmenopausal than in younger women. As shown in Table 3–6, a reduction in CL was not found among postmenopausal women in a study by MacLeod et al. (1979), but inspection of the data reveals unusually high CL in one individual—a finding that skewed the data. In contrast, other studies have found that both age and sex contributed to lower CL and longer $t\frac{1}{2}$ of this drug in postmenopausal women (D. J. Greenblatt et al. 1989; Ochs et al. 1981).

Temazepam, which is conjugated and excreted, has a 73% longer half-life in older women than in younger women. Another report indicates a significant increase in $t\frac{1}{2}$ and decrease in CL among older women when these parameters are compared with those of comparably aged men or younger women (R. B. Smith et al. 1983).

Not all benzodiazepines are differentially metabolized in postmenopausal women, however. For example, there were no differences

---

[3] Women studied by Bjerre et al. (1981) were also postmenopausally aged (68–78 years).

Table 3–6.   Pre- versus postmenopausal pharmacokinetics of benzodiazepines

Study	Clearance: bound and unbound (CL [mL/minute/kg]) Pre-	Post-	Elimination half-life ($t\,{}^{1}\!/_{2}$ [hour]) Pre-	Post-	Volume of distribution (Vd [L/kg]) Pre-	Post-
Diazepam						
MacLeod et al. 1979 ($n = 5[-]$OCs and $5[+]$OCs)						
Mean	0.372	0.422	43.9	56.6	1.28	1.89
SD	0.11	0.32	11.47	14.7	0.21	1.1
D. J. Greenblatt et al. 1980a ($n = 11[-]$OCs and $11[+]$OCs)[a]						
Mean	0.51	0.48	42.4	71.8	1.73	2.64
SD	0.18	0.19	13.5	44.1	2.8	0.91
Temazepam						
Divoll et al. 1981 ($n = 7$ pre- and 10 post-)						
Mean	1.1	0.97	16.2	17.2	1.4	1.39
SD	0.29	0.20	6.1	8.3	—	—
R. B. Smith et al. 1983 ($n = 5$ pre- and 5 post-)						
Mean	1.36	0.74	11.5	18.4	1.33	1.11
Nitrazepam						
D. J. Greenblatt et al. 1985 ($n = 12$ pre- and 9 post-)						
Mean	1.09	1.19	27	28	14.4	13.6
SD	1.72	0.9	4.8	5.7	3.46	2.4

Note. This table includes a secondary analysis of published data. OCs = oral contraceptives; $(+)$OCs/$(-)$OCs = subjects taking $(+)$/not taking $(-)$ OCs; pre-/post- = premenopausal/postmenopausal subjects.
[a]Unbound clearance differed significantly between pre- and postmenopausal women (29.9 vs. 43.6).

in the pharmacokinetic parameters of nitrazepam for postmenopausal women compared with either men or young women (D. J. Greenblatt et al. 1985).

Mood Stabilizers

Possible effects are unknown.

Summary of Effects of Aging

A number of medications show decreased CL and increased plasma levels among postmenopausal women (Table 3–6). Medications reviewed include imipramine, clomipramine, lithium, diazepam, and temazepam. In many instances, the decrease in the CL of older women was significantly different from the CL of either similarly aged men or younger women. However, older men were also likely to show this effect and, in some drugs (trazodone), this diminution in metabolism in older men was more profound than that seen in women.

Conclusion

Animal research in drug metabolism documents substantial sex differences in metabolism and elimination. Research in humans on physiological processes that affect pharmacokinetics (see Part I) also suggests the likelihood of such differences. In this chapter we have presented an updated and semiquantitative review of the pharmacokinetic profile of a number of psychotropic agents. Overall, the hypothesis that CL is slower in women finds some support. When effects exist, they are most pronounced in older women and are perhaps greatest for women on OCs. However, the effects appear to be small to moderate in magnitude, and it often remains unclear whether effects are clinically meaningful. It is possible that they are meaningful only for a relatively small subgroup of females. To document that effects are meaningful, it will be necessary to demonstrate not only that pharmacokinetic effects exist but also that effects are associated with sex-related differences in outcome in response to treatment—for example, in efficacy, dropout rates, side effects, or speed of recovery (for detailed reviews on antidepressants, see Hamilton 1995, in press a; Hamilton, Grant, and Jensvold, Chapter 12, this volume).

It is unfortunate that more is not known about potential sex differences in the absorption, distribution, metabolism, and elimination of psychotropic agents. Similarly, there is a paucity of information on the ways in which pharmacokinetic parameters are affected by exogenous hormones and advanced age. It is hoped that new U.S. Food and Drug Administration (FDA) guidelines, which encourage pharmacokinetic testing in women and in older individuals (J. C. Bennett 1993; Merkatz et al. 1993a), will increase available information on this topic. With the help of such research, we can be better assured that we are offering optimal and safe treatment for all of our patients.

Sex Differences in Brain Morphology and Pharmacodynamics

Maria Dorota Majewska, Ph.D.

The brain, like the body, is intrinsically female.

Simon LeVay

Then his chapter delineates some neuromorphological, neurochemical, and physiological differences between the sexes that may contribute to the distinct occurrence, severity, and outcome of some neuropsychiatric disorders and that may affect pharmacological treatment. These factors have implications for gender-sensitive pharmacotherapies.

Gender Differences in Brain Morphology and Function

It is surprising that most biomedical research has been conducted with males, although in sexually dimorphic animals the intrinsic pattern of sexual development is female. The male path of development is determined by a switching mechanism located in mammals in specific gene(s) on the Y chromosome (Koopman et al. 1991), resulting in the formation of testes from the indifferent genital ridge early in embryonic development. Further diversion from the default female pathway to the male path depends on organizational and activational actions of fetal testosterone. Because androgens ultimately reprogram fetal development in the male direction, the morphological and psychological differences between the sexes can be fluid, and there are naturally occurring sex variants and orientations. In addition to the prevalent heterosexuals, there are intersexuals, homosexuals, bisexuals, and transsexuals, which may result from exposure to different levels of, or sensitivity to, androgens during fetal/postnatal development. Fetal androgen levels, metabolism, and receptivity depend on both genetic and environmental factors, such as maternal stress, which has been hypothesized to influence the occurrence of male homosexuality (LeVay 1993).

Perinatal exposure to sex steroids is responsible for development of dimorphic brain morphology and function. Although explicit determinism of sex differences in brain architecture is lacking, certain anatomical and functional differences have been observed. In mammals, including humans, females typically have larger brains in proportion to their bodies and larger gross brain measurements relative to brain weight than males (de Lacoste et al. 1990; Juraska 1991). The neocortex is sexually dimorphic. Women usually have larger corpora callosa and anterior commissures relative to brain size than do men (L. A. Allen et al. 1991; de Lacoste et al. 1990; Fausto-Sterling 1992). Also, in homosexual men the anterior commissure was found to be larger on average than in heterosexual men (L. S. Allen and Gorski 1992).

The male brain shows greater hemispheric asymmetry, with right-side advantage, whereas left-side advantage is typical for the female brain (LeVay 1993). Hemispheric lateralization is also observable in males of other species; in rats, the right hemisphere is measurably thicker than the left one (M. C. Diamond 1991). The male-typical hemispheric laterality is determined by actions of testosterone aromatized to estrogens in fetal/neonatal brain, and that laterality was reversed in male rats who were postnatally castrated or prenatally exposed to stress, resulting in increased thickness of the left cortex (M. C. Diamond 1991; Fleming et al. 1986). Other studies showed that perinatal exposure of animals to estrogens reduced the thickness of the cerebral cortex, while exposure to progesterone increased it (M. C. Diamond 1991; Menzies et al. 1982).

The limbic system, including the hippocampus, is also sexually dimorphic (Madeira and Lieberman 1995). Differences were found in patterns and densities of dendrites of CA3 pyramidal neurons (Gould et al. 1991; Juraska 1991), in numbers of dentate gyrus granule cells, and in the size of neuronal cell bodies in the medial septum (Westland-Danielsson et al. 1991). Sex difference in hippocampal plasticity was also observed: female rats responded to enriched environments by greater sprouting of dendritic trees than did males, apparently due to suppression of the plasticity by testosterone (Juraska 1991). Sex hormones also support adult hippocampal morphology and function; peripubertal increase of dendritic spine density in CA1 pyramidal neurons was shown to depend on androgens in male rats and on ovarian hormones in female rats (G. Meyer et al. 1978).

The hypothalamus, which is involved in regulation of sexual behaviors, is gender dimorphic (LeVay 1993). In the medial preoptic area, which plays a role in male-typical sexual behavior, there is at least one nucleus that is larger in male than in female rats (Gorski et al. 1980). Also, two nuclei that are on average bigger in males than in females were found in the human preoptic area (L. S. Allen et al. 1989). One of these nuclei—implicated in sexual orientation and gender identity—was found to be smaller in homosexual men than in heterosexual men (LeVay 1991). Other sex differences in the hypothalamus have also been found, such as distribution of neurotransmitters, shape of the suprachiasmatic nucleus, and shape of synapses (LeVay 1993).

Sexual dimorphism also exists in brain functioning. For example, larger amplitudes and shorter latencies of cerebral cortical event–evoked potentials were measured in women than in men (Josiassen et al. 1990). Positron-emission tomography (PET) study showed about

15% greater global cerebral cortical blood flow and glucose metabolism in women than in men (R. E. Gur and R. C. Gur 1990), while more recent investigations have revealed sex differences in regional glucose metabolism both at rest and during certain mental activities. Compared with men, women at rest had higher metabolic activities at the cingulate gyrus, a recently evolved and cytoarchitecturally intricate part of the limbic system; whereas men had higher metabolic activities than women in temporolimbic regions and in the cerebellum, more ancient and primitive regions of the limbic system (R. C. Gur et al. 1995). Functional magnetic resonance study, measuring brain activities during linguistic tasks, revealed that during phonological processing (rhyming), women engaged both left and right sides of the inferior frontal gyrus, whereas men activated only the left side of this area (Shaywitz et al. 1995). Although studies comparing the brain functions of women and men are still in preliminary stages, clear differences have been demonstrated in the processing of certain cognitive tasks and emotions; in the processing of emotions, women appear to engage the more evolved brain parts— those capable of symbolic processing of emotions—whereas men activate the more primitive parts of their limbic systems—those involved in direct actions. Globally, the emerging proof of architectural and neurochemical differences between female and male brains and the evidence that brains of homosexual men have many female-like features suggest that definition of gender based on sexual organs may be misleading. It may perhaps be more appropriate to determine sexual identity by gender-specific brain organization.

Pharmacodynamics and Brain Gender-Dimorphism

Steroids and Gamma-Aminobutyric Acid (GABA)

Gonadal hormones determine male or female patterns of development and influence physiology via both genomic and membranous mechanisms. Sex hormones affect neuronal functions by regulating the synthesis and activity of enzymes, neurotransmitters, receptors, and effectors. Steroids are potent bimodal modulators of the $GABA_A$ receptor

(Majewska 1992), which regulates chloride conductance in neurons and which is a target for several psychotropic drugs. The GABA$_A$ receptor's function is enhanced by anxiolytics, hypnotics, anticonvulsants, and anesthetics but is reduced by convulsants. Because the GABA$_A$ receptor governs neuronal excitability, its regulation has profound physiological and pharmacological consequences. We were the first to discover that metabolites of progesterone (3α-5α-tetrahydroprogesterone; THP) and deoxycorticosterone (3α-5α-tetrahydrodeoxycorticosterone; THDOC) are allosteric agonists of the GABA$_A$ receptor (Majewska et al. 1986), whereas pregnenolone sulfate (PS) and dehydroepiandrosterone sulfate (DHEAS) are antagonists (Majewska and Schwartz 1987; Majewska et al. 1990).

The brain content and distribution of the GABA-ergic steroids—which can have both central and peripheral origin—is sexually dimorphic in many species, including humans (Baulieu et al. 1987). The brain levels of GABA-ergic steroids undergo physiological changes and they profoundly influence brain functions. PS and DHEAS may act as endogenous analeptics, memory enhancers, and antidepressants (Majewska 1995; Majewska et al. 1989). THP, whose plasma and brain level is increased during the luteal phase and in pregnancy, acts as a sedative, anxiolytic, anticonvulsant, and proanesthetic (Majewska 1992; Majewska et al. 1989). It is possible that progesterone and THP withdrawal before menstruation or postpartum provokes anxiety or depression, similar to that observed during withdrawal from chronic use of benzodiazepines and barbiturates. Progesterone withdrawal and its deficiency accompanied by hyperestrogenism have been also implicated in the etiology of catamenial epilepsy (Narbone et al. 1990). In addition, estrogens have been shown to upregulate the GABA$_A$ receptors (Maggi and Perez 1986). Hence, fluctuations of progesterone, THP, and estrogens during the menstrual cycle may contribute to plasticity of mood and cognition in some women, and diurnal changes of PS, DHEAS, and THDOC may help regulate sleep-wake cycles, mood, and learning.

Sex Steroids and Dopamine

In humans and other mammals, the brain dopamine systems are sexually dimorphic (Konradi et al. 1992). Receptors for progesterone and estrogens exist in dopamine-rich areas (McEwen and Parsons 1982). Fluctuations of biogenic amines in the rat brain, associated with the estrous cycle, were first reported by Fludder and Tonge (1975). Next, activity of dopamine neurons in the rat's nigrostriatal and mesolimbic areas and dopamine turnover were shown to change during the ovarian cycle (Fernandez-Ruiz et al. 1991) and after treatment with estradiol and progesterone (Fernandez-Ruiz et al. 1990). Also, amphetamine-stimulated striatal dopamine release in rats was found to be greater during estrous than diestrus (Becker and Cha 1989), due to actions of both estrogen—which increased dopamine content, release, and rotational behavior (Becker 1990)—and progesterone—which potentiated dopamine release (Dluzen and Ramirez 1989). Estradiol treatment also produced changes in the sensitivity and density of dopamine receptors in the striatum (Hruska et al. 1982).

Modulation of dopamine functions by sex hormones includes their effects on monoamine oxidase (MAO); estrogen inhibits MAO-A but stimulates MAO-B activity, and progesterone increases MAO-A activity (Chevillard et al. 1981; Luine and Rhodes 1983). Treatment of female rats with estrogen reduced locomotion and apomorphine-induced stereotypy, and increased haloperidol-induced catalepsy, whereas progesterone decreased stereotypy and catalepsy (Palermo-Neto and Dorce 1990), suggesting antidopaminergic activity of estrogens. Apparent conflicts in data about the effects of estrogens on dopamine functions may result from different times/doses of hormone exposure, underscoring the complexity of these interactions.

Gender Dimorphism in Other Neurotransmitter Systems

The brain serotonin (5-HT) system in mammals is sexually dimorphic. Higher levels of brain tryptophan—5-hydroxytryptamine (5-HT) and 5-hydroxyindoleacetic acid (5-HIAA)—were found in women than in men (Carlsson and Carlsson 1988), concomitant with greater density and more pronounced right-hemispheric dominance of imipramine binding sites in the orbital cortex (Arato et al. 1991). The sex difference in sensitivity to 5-HT stimulation (Clarke and Maayani 1990) may lie at the basis of differences in sexual behaviors, aggressiveness, mood regulation, impulsivity, and some mental disorders. Sex differences in the cholinergic systems are evident across many species. Females were reported to have higher levels of acetylcholine, choline acetyltransferase (ChAT), and muscarinic receptors in several brain regions (J. C. Miller 1983). This could, in part, be determined by the sex hormones because estrogens were shown to increase the activity of ChAT (Luine 1985).

The brain glutamatergic system is sexually dimorphic. Fluctuations of glutamate in the hypothalamus were observed during the estrous cycle in rats (Loscher et al. 1992). Estradiol was shown to increase glutamate-mediated neuronal excitability (S. S. Smith 1989) and to increase density of the N-methyl-D-aspartate (NMDA) receptors (Weiland 1992) and of excitatory synapses in the hippocampus (Woolley et al. 1990), whereas progesterone attenuated glutamate responses (S. S. Smith 1991). Interactions between the sex hormones and the glutamatergic system, mediated via both intra- and extracellular receptors, play a role in learning and memory.

Sexually dimorphic opiate peptide systems underlie reproductive behaviors. Estrogen and progesterone receptors are co-localized with β-endorphin or enkephalin in the hypothalamus of the female brain (Olster and Blaustein 1990), where estrogen stimulates the expression of proenkephalin mRNA (Romano et al. 1990). It is possible that sex hormones also interact with opiate peptides in other brain regions, thereby influencing neurophysiology or psychopathology.

Sex Differences in Brain Pathology and Neuropsychophysiology

Morphological-functional brain dimorphism may lie at the basis of predispositions to some illnesses or conditions. Some of these are described in this section.

Brain Injury and Neurodegeneration

Aging-related progression of brain atrophy seems to be slower in women than in men (Hatazawa et al. 1982). Also, women usually develop fewer complications and permanent neurological deficits after brain trauma—due, in part, to better interhemispheric connection, which allows for a more effective compensation of neurological losses than in men. Reproductive-age women may derive additional protection from sex hormones, as suggested by a study showing that female rats had much less cerebral edema after head trauma than did male rats; this finding was attributed to the neuroprotective effect of progesterone (Roof et al. 1993). Also, Parkinson's disease is more frequent and severe in men than in women (Mayeux et al. 1992).

Cognitive Functions and Learning Disabilities

Gender-typical cognitive differences—such as women's superiority, on average, in verbal and perceptual skills and men's superiority in visuospatial aptitudes—may be influenced by architectural brain dimorphisms resulting from differential perinatal exposure to sex steroids. Prenatal exposure to high levels of progesterone feminizes the brain and has been shown to increase cortical thickness (Menzies et al. 1982) and intelligence of girls and boys (Dalton 1968). Also, some studies have shown that changes of sex hormones in women influence cognitive performance (Sanders and Reinish 1985). In the follicular phase, automatized memory tasks (speed of reading/talking) were facilitated, whereas in the luteal phase, these tasks were impaired. The reverse was true for perceptual-reconstructive tasks—those linked to artistic/scientific creativity.

Androgens have a complex effect on cognition. During development, androgens may retard growth of the cerebral cortex, slow cortical maturation, and impair learning (Bachevalier and Hagger 1991; Steward and Kolb 1988). After puberty, a curvilinear relationship exists between testosterone and spatial/mathematical abilities: lower levels of testosterone seem beneficial for men's mental performance, while higher levels are beneficial for women's (Gouchie and Kimura 1991). Consistently, androgynous types have been reported to show cognitive and artistic abilities superior to those of individuals with more typical sex features (Hassler 1991).

Developmental errors that cause learning/language disabilities are more common in males (Hier 1979), possibly as a result of abnormal testosterone/estrogen exposure or sensitivity during prenatal development, resulting in delayed or defective cerebral cortical maturation (Geschwind and Galaburda 1985a). Indeed, children with aberrant sex chromosome complements have very high rates of language and speech disorders (Tallal 1991).

Schizophrenic Disorders

Women usually develop schizophrenia later in life, are better responders to treatment, and have a better outlook for recovery than men, who develop schizophrenia at an earlier age and have more neurological impairments and poorer outcomes (Bardenstein and McGlashan 1990). Some authors also have found that more men than women are diagnosed with schizophrenia (Lewine et al. 1984).

Maturational neuropathology has been suggested as a factor responsible for schizophrenia. Lewine et al. (1990) observed that brains of male schizophrenic patients had more deviance in morphology than brains of female patients. Schizophrenic brains show cerebral cortical atrophy and frontal/temporal cortical hypometabolism, particularly in the left hemisphere (Wolkin et al. 1985), which is more often defective in men than in women (DeLisi et al. 1989; Geschwind and Galaburda 1985b). Also, pathology in the basal ganglia and limbic system, especially in the hippocampus (Bogerts et al. 1985; Schiebel and Kovelman 1981), may be more pronounced in schizophrenic men than in schizophrenic women. Differences in hormonal milieu may contribute to the distinct courses of schizophrenia in women and men. During fetal life, greater exposure to ovarian hormones may protect females against perinatal hypoxia/trauma, and during reproductive years, estrogens may protect women from excessive dopamine activity (Seeman and Lang 1990). This view is supported by findings of increased incidence of psychoses premenstrually, postpartum, and postmenopausally and decreased incidence during pregnancy (J. Glick and Steward 1980), and by the fact that women in reproductive years require lower doses of neuroleptics (Seeman and Lang 1990; see also Szymanski, Chapter 14, this volume).

Tardive Dyskinesia

Tardive dyskinesia (TD) is a crippling, usually permanent movement disorder induced in some patients by chronic treatment with neuroleptics. Older women show a higher incidence of TD than do men or younger women (J. M. Smith et al. 1978; Yassa and Jeste 1992). The reason for this difference is unknown, but factors such as treatment of women with larger doses of neuroleptics and longer duration of treatment have been considered along with overrepresentation of older women in surveys. Seeman and Lang (1990) proposed that premenopausal women could be protected from TD by estrogens. Animal studies have suggested that neuroleptic-induced movement disorder may be caused by a reduction of nigral GABA neurotransmission due to atrophy of GABA-ergic striatal neurons (Gunne et al. 1988). Given that GABA neurotransmission is enhanced by female sex hormones, young women may be better protected from developing TD than older women.

Brain dimorphisms may also account, in part, for sex differences in affective and anxiety disorders and drug addictions, although further research is needed.

Conclusion

Dimorphism of brain morphology and function contributes to a distinct predisposition, occurrence, and outcome of various neurological and mental disorders that differentiate women and men.

Since female sex hormones modulate the functions of major neurotransmitters, it is reasonable to expect that physiologically changing levels of these hormones influence pharmacodynamics of major classes of psychotropic drugs. More studies are needed to evaluate sex differences in pharmacodynamics of psychotropic drugs. For example, based on the preclinical and limited clinical data, one can predict that women exposed to high levels of endogenous progesterone (during the midluteal phase and in pregnancy) would require lower doses of antiepileptic agents, anxiolytics, hypnotics, or general anesthetics to achieve therapeutic effects, due to synergistic actions with progesterone metabolites.

In many cases it may be difficult to determine the relative contributions of pharmacokinetic and pharmacodynamic factors accounting for sex differences in drugs. Pharmacokinetic factors (e.g., concentrations of drugs in plasma, drug metabolism) may be affected by hormonal milieu (Galeazzi 1985). Pharmacodynamic studies may be additionally confounded by the phenomena of neuroadaptation, involving either tolerance or sensitization, which may also be affected by hormonal milieu. Despite intrinsic difficulties in interpretation of such data, knowledge of sex differences in drug sensitivity is an essential element of rational and humanistic pharmacotherapy.

Association Among Ovarian Hormones, Other Hormones, Emotional Disorders, and Neurotransmitters

David S. Janowsky, M.D., Uriel Halbreich, M.D., and Jeffrey Rausch, M.D.

A variety of studies (recently reviewed by Rausch and Parry [1993]) suggest gender differences in the prevalence of affective and other psychiatric disorders. For example, the lifetime risk of developing depression is increased in women, especially in women with unipolar depression, in those with the depressive subtype of bipolar illness, and in those with cyclical forms of affective illness such as seasonal affective disorder or rapidly cycling bipolar disorder. Also, specific phases of the menstrual cycle and some states in female reproductive life are associated with repeated or cyclic affective changes as well as other psychological changes. Examples include depression, irritability, and anxiety associated with the late luteal and perimenstrual phases of the menstrual cycle, the ingestion of oral contraceptives, the postpartum period, and the menopause (Dalton 1964; Halbreich 1987; Hamilton et al. 1988; Janowsky and Rausch 1985).

The brain is recognized as a target tissue for complex effects of gonadal steroid hormones. The gonadal steroids can affect hormone-sensitive steroid receptor–containing areas of the brain, both through nuclear receptor-mediated gene expression of enzymes, neurotransmitters, and neurotransmitter receptors (genomic effects) and through membrane-mediated effects of a more rapidly occurring nature (nongenomic effects). Newer insights into intracellular receptors of steroid hormones, which bind the steroids and carry them to nuclear receptors for genomic action, have supported the long-held view that these compounds act not as direct stimuli affecting behavior but rather as modulatory influences on the excitability of critical central nervous system (CNS) mechanisms (B. W. O'Malley and Means 1993). However, some evidence suggests that certain steroid metabolites may have direct membrane sites of action that may directly influence brain excitability (French-Mullen and Spence 1991).

The more rapidly occurring effects of the gonadal steroids appear to be mediated primarily by nongenomic mechanisms, whereas the longer latency effects are represented by nongenomic mechanisms mediated through the nucleus. The complexity of gonadal steroids' effects on the CNS is illustrated by the example that 24 hours after estrogen treatment, in addition to changes in neurotransmitter receptors, there are changes in progesterone receptors and changes in synaptic density in discrete areas of the brain, such as brain regions in the steroid-sensitive ventromedial nuclei of the hypothalamus (McEwen et al. 1987). For example, estradiol treatment has been shown to increase dendritic spine density in rats, and the numbers of these spines have been shown to increase and decrease during the estrus cycle of rats (McEwen 1991; Segarra et al. 1991). Thus, among other effects of the gonadal steroids, there is evidence that these steroids may indeed influence synaptic structure and number.

Fluctuations in the hypothalamic pituitary gonadal axis have been repeatedly shown to produce perturbations in neurochemistry that are potentially capable of inducing behavioral changes. Likewise, the results of several experiments indicate that gender and hormonal milieu are important variables in determining the experimental and clinical responses to psychotropic drugs. For example, changes in brain monoamine levels (e.g., norepinephrine, dopamine) have been found to occur cyclically throughout the estrus cycle in rats, providing a theoretical basis to suggest that such alterations in neurotransmitter function may be linked to behavioral changes associated with hypothalamic pituitary gonadal fluctuations (Janowsky et al. 1971). Such changes have also been found more recently in humans (review—Halbreich et al. 1988).

In this chapter we provide a brief overview of the role of gonadal steroids and other hormones that might be associated with or influenced by the reproductive system in regulating various psychiatric and psychological syndromes. The effects of these substances on mood and behavior and their relationship to syndromes putatively associated with ovarian hormones are reviewed first. A review of the interactions of reproductive and other hormones with central neurotransmitters and neuromodulators then follows.

Premenstrual Dysphoric Syndromes

As reviewed by Rausch et al. (1982), Janowsky and Rausch (1985), Halbreich et al. (1988), and Rausch and Parry (1993), between 20% and 80% of women (depending on the study cited) report some degree of cyclic mood, cognitive, or neurovegetative disturbances associated with the premenstrual/menstrual phases of their menstrual cycles. Furthermore, the percentage of women who report severe premenstrual and menstrual symptoms to a degree that impairs social or occupational functioning is estimated at 5% (Hamilton et al. 1984b). Overall, premenstrual mood and behavioral symptoms are very diversified (Halbreich et al. 1982) and include primarily anxiety, depression, irritability, and cognitive impairment, as well as changes in sleep, energy, appetite, and impulsivity. More severe syndromes have been reported to include psychosis, mania, and suicidal ideation in some women (Dalton 1964).

Whereas some authors suggest that premenstrual dysphoric syndromes are derivatives of expectation and prejudice, others propose psychobiological causes (Halbreich et al. 1988). The most obvious etiological hypothesis for premenstrual syndromes involves fluctuations in the ovarian hormones. Premenstrual symptoms are generally most severe during the late luteal phase, when estrogen and progesterone withdrawal is occurring. Imbalances in these hormones (i.e., relatively high estrogen levels compared with rapidly falling progesterone levels) have been postulated as being responsible for cyclic psychological symptoms. However, the fact that most women do not experience such symptoms during the late follicular and preovulatory phases, at the time when estrogen levels are elevated, suggests the presence of a more complex phenomenon than simple estrogen excess and/or estrogen withdrawal.

Rapidly falling levels of progesterone or low progesterone have also been proposed as etiological of premenstrual syndromes. Supportive of this possibility, affective symptoms have been observed to occur after withdrawal of exogenous progesterone, and some investigators have found progesterone to be lower (or low relative to estrogen) in patients with premenstrual dysphoric syndromes. However, this finding has not been noted in all studies.

An association between the ratio of change of gonadal hormones and the severity of premenstrual dysphoric syndromes has been reported. It has been suggested that differential rapid change over time in levels of gonadal hormones and other related factors might trigger impaired homeostasis and the occurrence of symptoms in vulnerable women (Halbreich et al. 1988).

Fluctuations in the renin-angiotensin-aldosterone system have also been proposed as etiological of premenstrual dysphoric syndromes. Studies of women without menstrually related dysphoric symptoms suggest that fluctuations of aldosterone and angiotensin II parallel the emotional changes occurring during the menstrual cycle. In addition, sodium-potassium ratios in urine fluctuate in parallel with negative affect during the menstrual cycle, and this concordance has been postulated to reflect aldosterone-angiotensin effects (see review by Janowsky et al. 1973; Rausch et al. 1982). However, patients with premenstrual dysphoric syndrome have not been shown to have significantly different serum aldosterone levels when compared with asymptomatic control subjects, although there is some evidence that the aldosterone antagonist spirolactone is useful in treating some premenstrual syndromes (Rausch et al. 1982).

Prolactin has also been implicated in the etiology of premenstrual dysphoric syndromes (see review by Rausch and Parry 1993). Several investigations indicate that prolactin levels do indeed vary during the menstrual cycle, with peaks occurring at ovulation and during the mid- and late luteal phases. Several studies have reported increases in prolactin levels to the high normal range in women with premenstrual dysphoric syndromes compared with nonsymptomatic control subjects (Halbreich et al. 1976). However, the findings of several other studies were not consistent with those of Halbreich and co-workers, especially with respect to evidence suggesting that patients with premenstrual dysphoric syndromes have higher absolute prolactin levels than do control subjects (O'Brien et al. 1979). Nevertheless, bromocriptine, a specific dopamine agonist that suppresses prolactin, has been reported effective in treating some premenstrual symptoms (especially mastalgia) in some, but not all patients (Green 1982).

Psychological Changes Induced by Oral Contraceptives

Earlier studies have indicated that up to 50% of women reported depression as a side effect of estrogen/progestogen–containing oral contraceptives (F. J. Kane et al. 1969). In 1981, Slap reviewed the literature on side effects in clinical studies of oral contraceptives in adults. In this review, nine studies indicating depression in 16%–56% of women using oral contraceptives were considered. Three studies indicated no association between oral contraceptive use and depression or other mood disorders.

Emotional symptoms induced by oral contraceptives may be linked to the content or ratio of ovarian steroids in the pills. For instance, women with a history of premenstrual irritability who took progesterone-dominant pills had a significantly lower incidence of adverse mental changes than did those who took estrogen-dominant pills. The incidence of depression associated with oral contraceptive use may now be lower, given that the newer formulations contain estrogens and progestogens in lower doses (Kay 1984). This supposition is in accord with

Cullberg (1972), who reviewed three studies suggesting that increased depressive symptoms were associated with oral contraceptives high in progesterone. It should be noted that side effects of oral contraceptives cannot be generalized. They depend on the specific synthetic steroids used; on differences in half-life, combinations, and dosages; and on the use of a sequential as compared with a steady formula.

Postpartum Changes and Psychiatric Illness

Up to 50% of postpartum mothers have been found to have at least mild affective symptoms. These usually remit spontaneously within 2 weeks of delivery and include mild depression, affective lability, anxiety, crying, sleep difficulties, and mild cognitive problems. Postpartum blues usually are apparent by the third or fourth postpartum day (Garvey and Tollefson 1984) and peak during the fifth postpartum day (R. E. Kendell et al. 1981).

In a minority of women, these postpartum changes can be precursors to the development of more severe emotional upsets, including major depression, mania, and schizophreniform psychosis. Such psychopathology often follows prominent postnatal depression and emotional lability and occurs most often in women with a history of affective illness. Estimates of the incidence of severe depression occurring in the postpartum period range from 3% to 12% of women. Patients with a history of depression, especially previous postpartum depression, as well as those with a history of severe premenstrual dysphoric syndrome, have a much higher chance of developing a subsequent postpartum depression. In one study, such patients were prospectively identified with an antepartum mood scale (Garvey and Tollefson 1984; Garvey et al. 1983).

Earlier studies evaluating aberrations in gonadal hormone levels in patients with postpartum emotional upsets have generally not yielded theoretically promising results. For example, a study of 27 healthy pregnant women failed to produce data indicating that prepartum progesterone levels, the rate of progesterone decline, or estrogen-progesterone ratios were different in symptomatic mothers (Nott et al. 1976). However, Nott et al. (1976) did note that predelivery estrogen levels were weakly correlated with irritability after delivery, and that decreases in progesterone levels were associated with depression. Another study found that those women who experienced postpartum blues had higher concentrations of salivary progesterone and estradiol when compared with symptom-free control subjects (Feksi et al. 1984). In still another study of mothers 2–5 days postpartum, no significant correlations were found between the incidence of postpartum blues and plasma concentrations of follicle-stimulating hormone (FSH), prolactin, estrone, estradiol, cortisol, or progesterone (Kuevi et al. 1983).

Several recent studies have reported an association between high prolactin levels and postpartum hostility and depression. In one investigation, postpartum women with increased prolactin levels were significantly more hostile than women in a control group. Also, the prolactin-suppressant bromocriptine was found to reduce hostility, depression, and anxiety in postpartum women, and these changes paralleled a decrease in prolactin levels (Kellner et al. 1984).

Recently, there have been several reports (Kumar et al. 1988) that postpartum depression and psychosis might be related to the rapid withdrawal of gonadal hormones. Treatment trials with estrogens have been quite promising and might support that hypothesis.

Psychological Sequelae of Menopause

Menopausal symptoms have been reported to include several features common to depression and related affective symptoms—for example, depressed affect, fatigue, sleep disturbance, irritability, and other related mood changes and mood lability. In a study of Swedish women by Hammar et al. (1984), 75% of the women reported menopausal symptoms, and 33% experienced periods of depression more often than they did premenopausally.

With respect to timing, the World Health Organization in 1981 reported that an increased incidence of psychological symptoms occurs 1–2 years before the cessation of menses. These symptoms decreased in frequency over the 1–2 years after menopause. A survey of 539 women from a general population indicated that increased psychiatric morbidity occurred before the menopause. This increased morbidity was found to last until about 1 year after menstrual periods had ended (Ballinger 1975).

The symptoms of menopause have also been found to be associated with surgical menopause by ovariectomy. Depression, decreased libido, anxiety, sleep disturbances, and associated vasomotor symptoms occur in ovariectomized women. In 100 women evaluated after bilateral ovariectomy, the most frequent symptoms at the time of interview were depression, insomnia, loss of libido, and dyspareunia, as well as vasomotor symptoms (Chakravarti et al. 1977). In another study of 49 women who had previously undergone hysterectomy and bilateral ovariectomy, the predominant emotional symptom was found to be anxiety rather than depression (Dennerstein et al. 1979). As with "natural" menopause, these symptoms responded to administration of exogenous ovarian hormones, especially estrogen, as did symptoms of severe, persistent depression in women in general (Klaiber et al. 1979; Oppenheim 1986).

Neurotransmitter/Neuromodulator Changes in Disorders Putatively Linked to Ovarian Hormones

Cumulative evidence suggests that emotional disorders are moderated by changes in central neurotransmitters and neuromodulators. Changes in catecholamines such as norepinephrine, serotonin, and dopamine have been implicated in the etiologies of affective, anxiety, and psychotic disorders. Changes in endogenous opioids, serotonin, acetylcholine, gamma-aminobutyric acid (GABA), and oxytocin/vasopressin have also been noted in a variety of emotional disorders. In this section we review evidence indicating that these hormones—which vary during the menstrual cycle, change during menopause, and are the major components of oral contraceptives—perturb various central neurotransmitter and neuromodulator systems. Thus, it may be that hormonal-neurotransmitter linkages underlie the emotional disorders associated with menstruation, parturition, menopause, and the ingestion of oral contraceptives.

Serotonin

Considerable evidence indicates that altered central serotonergic activity may underlie mood disorders, at least in some patients. Both hypofunction and hyperfunction of serotonin (5-hydroxytryptophan, or 5-HT) neurotransmission have been proposed to be associated with depression. Tryptophan, the precursor of 5-HT, is reduced in the cerebrospinal fluid (CSF) of depressed patients, as is the principal metabolite of 5-HT, 5-hydroxyindoleacetic acid (5-HIAA). Similarly, the brains of suicide victims with a history of depression show decreased 5-HT activity, and 5-HT receptor numbers have been reported to be increased in depressed persons, a finding consistent with upregulation due to low 5-HT levels. Thus, 5-HT binding is increased in the brains of suicide victims, in the brains of depressed individuals obtained postmortem, and in the platelets of depressed individuals. Many clinically effective antidepressants perturb the 5-HT system. Administration of most chronic antidepressant therapies normalizes aberrant serotonergic binding. Furthermore, certain newer antidepressants show selectivity for 5-HT receptors in vitro.

It appears that 5-HT is clearly implicated in the regulation of gonadotropin release. Serotonergic neurons in the dorsal raphe appear to exert a stimulatory influence on gonadotropin release by acting on 5-HT receptors through projections to the median eminence. Likewise, serotoninergic axons have been shown to terminate on luteinizing hormone (LH)–releasing neurons in the preoptic area (D. C. Meyer et al. 1992; Tanaka et al. 1993; Tillet et al. 1993).

5-HT appears to be important in the expression and development of sexual behavior, at least in animals. Reduction of 5-HT activity by the serotonin-depleting drug P-cholorophenylalanine (PCPA) enhances masculine sexual behavior in male rats and potentiates the observed defeminizing effect of exogenous testosterone in female rats (Janowsky et al. 1973). In another study, 5-HT levels in the preoptic area of the brain were found to be correlated with increases in the percentage of male rats that were observed to not mount or intromit (Segarra et al. 1991). Low doses of 5-HT_{1A} agonists in the presence of estrogen appear to facilitate sexual receptivity in female rats, specifically if progesterone is absent (S. D. Mendelson and Gorzalka 1986). When progesterone is present in combination with estrogen, the 5-HT$_{1A}$ agonists (ipsapirone, gepirone, and buspirone) inhibit rather than facilitate sexual receptivity (S. D. Mendelson and Gorzalka 1986).

There are nonsexual differences in 5-HT sensitivity that depend on sex and hormonal state. Compared with female rats, male rats appear subsensitive to a serotonergic pargyline/tryptophan combination with respect to provocation of the 5-HT behavioral syndrome. Similarly, male rats appear to be less sensitive to 5-HT$_{1A}$ receptor–mediated effects in other nonsexual ways. The hypothermic effects of the 5-HT agonist 8-hydroxy-2-{di-n-propylamino} tetralin (8-OH-DPAT) appear to be more pronounced in female than in male mice. The hypothermic effects of 8-OH-DPAT are attenuated by ovariectomy or testosterone and are enhanced by estradiol or orchiectomy (Matsuda et al. 1991).

Consistent with the observation that gender differences in 5-HT sensitivity exist, several effects of gonadal steroids on 5-HT levels as such have been noted. Gonadectomy and chronic steroid replacement therapy appear to alter brain monoamine metabolism in a regional and sex-dependent manner. Orchiectomy increases central levels of 5-HIAA and decreases 5-HT levels, a phenomenon reversible with testosterone or estrogen (Bitar et al. 1991). Progesterone treatment appears to decrease the accumulation of 5-HT in the ventromedial hypothalamus, the pars lateralis, and the dorsal midbrain central gray matter (Krey and Luine 1987). 5-HIAA concentrations have been found to be elevated in the dorsal raphe of estradiol-treated rats, and, consistent with this observation, estrogen treatment has also been noted to increase monoamine oxidase A (MAO-A) activity (McEwen et al. 1987).

In conjunction with observations that sex steroids may influence 5-HT levels as such, there is also evidence that ovarian steroids may influence 5-HT receptors. Estrogen seems to have a rapid and direct effect on brain membranes that modifies 5-HT receptor availability while exerting a slower change on the same receptors via interactions with intracellular estrogen receptors. Indeed, estrogen appears to exert a biphasic effect on the density of 5-HT receptors in the brains of female rats. After estrogen exposure, an acute reduction in 5-HT receptor density throughout the brain occurs after 48–72 hours, as shown by a selective increase of 5-HT in those brain regions known to contain estrogen receptors (e.g., hypothalamus, preoptic area, amygdala). Moreover, an acute reduction in 5-HT receptor density has been mimicked in vitro by estradiol administration (Biegon and McEwen 1982).

The ovarian steroids prompt distinct changes in the different subtypes of 5-HT receptors. Estrogen treatment of ovariectomized female rats results in an initial decrease in 5-HT$_1$ receptors with a concomitant increase in 5-HT$_2$ receptors. Progesterone alone may cause similar effects, albeit with a smaller increase in 5-HT$_2$ receptors. When given with estrogen, progesterone blocks the estrogen effect on 5-HT receptors but does not appear to inhibit the estrogen-mediated decrease in 5-HT$_1$ receptors (Biegon et al. 1983). In addition, estrogen enhances 5-HT$_{1A}$ responses in hippocampal slices (Clarke and Goldfarb 1989), and progesterone may modulate the sensitivity of the 5-HT$_{1A}$ responses (S. D. Mendelson and Gorzalka 1986).

Thus, there is evidence from animal studies that, in rich and complex ways, 5-HT may be influenced by the gonadal steroids and vice versa. These hormones may influence the expression and development of sexual behavior as modulated through their effects on 5-HT receptors, 5-HT levels, and 5-HT metabolism. Depending on the timing and appearance of the ovarian hormones, quite different effects on 5-HT sensitivity can be orchestrated.

With respect to studies in humans, it has been hypothesized that menstrually related changes in mood and behavior might be due to changes in the 5-HT function. For example, the responsivity of prolactin and cortisol to serotonergic agonists is relatively blunted during the late luteal phase (as reviewed in Halbreich and Tworek 1993). As reviewed by Rausch and Parry (1993) and Halbreich and Tworek (1993), and with respect to other human studies suggesting ovarian hormone linkages with 5-HT, low plasma-free tryptophan levels were shown to be significantly associated with postpartum depression and weeping. Furthermore, it has been shown that during the second to fifth postpartum days, plasma-free tryptophan concentrations tended to rise and to positively correlate with positive mood states. An absence of this rise has been significantly associated with the presence of severe postpartum blues and with depression at 6 months postpartum. However, exogenous L-tryptophan did not reduce postpartum blues in comparison with placebo.

Current biochemical research suggests that the progestogen-based oral contraceptives decrease tryptophan oxygenase and cause a pyridoxine deficiency in some women. Such changes as are induced by oral contraceptive steroids on tryptophan metabolism have been correlated with depression in women taking these agents (Shaarawy et al. 1985). Finally, oral pyridoxine has been reported in some, but not all, studies to relieve symptoms of depression in oral contraceptive users.

It is reasonable to expect that if low levels of serotonergic activity contribute to the pathophysiology of menstrually related changes, serotonergic agonists should work to alleviate symptoms. The 5-HT$_{1A}$ agonist and antianxiety/antidepressant drug buspirone was given to women with premenstrual dysphoric syndromes. Many of the women discontinued medication within 2–3 days after initiation of treatment, reporting intolerable anxiety and other premenstrual symptoms. The efficacy of the drug for premenstrual dysphoric symptoms was doubtful, even when the dosage was increased to 30 mg/day in divided doses during the late luteal phase (see Halbreich and Tworek 1993). It should be noted that these results differ from a more positive report by Rickels and colleagues (1989). It is tempting to hypothesize that the anxiogenic response to buspirone when initiated during the midluteal phase is due to the existence of upregulated receptor hypersensitivity associated with decreased serotonergic levels and activity.

In contrast to results in controlled trials with buspirone, the relatively specific serotonin reuptake blocker fluoxetine appears effective in the treatment of dysphoric premenstrual syndrome. Fluoxetine has been shown to be superior to placebo when given in a steady dosage of 20 mg/day during the luteal phase (Stone et al. 1990). In a possibly related finding, it has been noted that the serotonergic agonist d-fenfluramine reduced food cravings and increased appetite associated with premenstrual symptoms, but its influence on dysphoric symptoms was less pronounced.

Catecholamines

The catecholamine hypothesis of affective disorders proposes that depression results from a deficiency—and mania results from a relative excess—of norepinephrine impacting on central receptors. A variation of this hypothesis proposes that dysfunction of catecholamine receptors and/or second messengers is associated with affective disorders (Maas 1975).

The catecholamine hypothesis arose initially from the insightful observations that 1) MAO inhibitors (MAOIs) improved mood when these drugs were administered for the treatment of tuberculosis, and 2) MAOIs also increase brain catecholamine levels. Subsequent studies showed that many drugs that deplete brain catecholamines, such as the antihypertensive drug reserpine, produce depressive episodes that are clinically indistinguishable from major depressive disorder. Furthermore, administration of reserpine-like drugs to animals produces behavioral changes that appear analogous to depression in humans.

The catecholamine hypothesis also has received support from the observation that structurally diverse drugs that have antidepressant activity have all been noted to share the ability to block the reuptake of norepinephrine and therefore to increase the central availability of this catecholamine. Conversely, tricyclic antidepressants and MAOIs can trigger mania in predisposed individuals.

As with 5-HT, ovarian steroid hormones affect several catecholamine neurotransmitters and catecholamine receptors that are relevant to the affective disorders. As earlier reviewed by Janowsky et al. (1971), ovarian steroids might influence catecholamine function at a number of points, including catecholamine synthesis, release, uptake, metabolism, and receptor activation. Some catecholaminergic neurons in the diencephalon contain a co-localization of estrogen and progestin receptors, as well as tyrosine hydroxylase, the rate-limiting enzyme in the synthesis of catecholamines. Estradiol decreases MAO and tyrosine hydroxylase activity in some diencephalic nuclei, which suggests that it can differentially regulate catecholamine synthesis and degradation. Estrogen-induced increases in norepinephrine turnover and content have been reported in some diencephalic nuclei, and blockade of labeled norepinephrine uptake into synaptosomes also suggests an overall stimulation of norepinephrine activity by estrogen.

In vitro, estrogen has been found to cause the outflow of dopamine and norepinephrine from cultured rat hypothalamus (Paul et al. 1979) and to decrease dopamine release into hypophyseal portal blood (O. M. Cramer et al. 1979). Estrogen also generally enhances central norepinephrine availability (Paul et al. 1979) and causes a bidirectional sensitization of dopamine receptors (Chiodo and Caggiula 1983). Chronic estrogen treatment has also been shown to reduce β-adrenergic receptors in rat cortex (H. R. Wagner et al. 1979).

In other studies, chronic estrogen has been reported to downregulate dopamine (D_2) receptors in the anterior pituitary of the rat (Munemura et al. 1989). This may be how estrogen reverses the inhibition of prolactin release by dopamine (Munemura et al. 1989). In addition, estradiol has also been shown to directly affect D_2 receptors in the striatum. However, the precise mechanism and physiological significance of this effect is unclear (Roy et al. 1990).

In human studies, estrogen alters α_2-adrenergic binding in platelets, and variations in platelet binding have been reported during the menstrual cycle (reviewed in Best et al. 1992). In postmenopausal women treated with estradiol, a decrease in the norepinephrine metabolite plasma 3-methoxy-4-hydroxyphenylglycol (MHPG)—but no change in platelet yohimbine binding—was reported (Best et al. 1992).

Significant postpartum changes in catecholamine function may also be associated with mood disturbances. Women who experienced postpartum blues were found to have significantly lower levels of circulating norepinephrine and epinephrine compared with levels of preceding or following days, when they felt psychologically better (Kuevi et al. 1983). Furthermore, platelet MAO activity has been positively correlated with postpartum depressive symptoms. Like the premenstrual-menstrual increases in platelet α_2-receptors noted by S. B. Jones et al. (1983), women who had episodes of postpartum blues have been shown to have significantly higher platelet α_2-adrenoreceptor capacity than women without such episodes. The physiological role of α_2-adrenoreceptors after delivery is still unsettled because, in general, the number of platelet α_2-adrenoceptors decrease after childbirth, corresponding to the fall in the circulating levels of estrogen and progesterone (Metz et al. 1983).

Gamma-Aminobutyric Acid

GABA is an amino acid that serves as a ubiquitous inhibitory neurotransmitter within the CNS. A number of studies have demonstrated low levels of GABA in the blood and CSF of depressed patients. Other studies have shown that depressed individuals have low levels of glutamic acid decarboxylase, the rate-limiting enzyme in the synthesis of GABA. Most clinically effective antidepressants increase binding of GABA to the GABA receptor, and drugs that enhance GABA function often alleviate the symptoms of depression. Decreases in GABA levels in CSF have been associated with clinical depression (Gold et al. 1980; K. G. Lloyd et al. 1989).

Rapid progress in understanding the mechanism of action of GABA has followed the cloning of $_c$DNA for its receptor. The GABA receptor is coupled to a chloride channel and has binding sites for benzodiazepines, barbiturates, and—most relevant to this chapter—progestins. Benzodiazepines and barbiturates presumably exert their anxiolytic action by altering the permeability of the chloride channel and thereby the excitability of the neuron.

The GABA$_A$/benzodiazepine receptor chloride channel complex is a member of the ligand-gated ion superfamily. To understand the molecular mechanisms by which steroid hormones modulate the GABA$_A$ receptor, one must conceptualize the GABA$_A$ receptor as a macromolecular complex that may adopt different conformations and whose subunit composition may vary. Gonadal steroids may have direct effects on the conformation of the GABA$_A$ receptor complex as it changes between active and inactive states. Also, given the observed heterogeneity of GABA$_A$ receptor binding within the brain, it has been postulated that steroid hormones, acting at the genomic level, could change the expression of the receptor for different subunits of the receptor complex (Schumacher et al. 1989b).

LH-releasing hormone (LHRH) and GABA neurons in the medial preoptic area are synaptic targets of dopamine axons, originating in the anterior periventricular area (Horvath et al. 1993). Activation of GABA$_B$ receptors in the anterior pituitary inhibits LH secretion (Lux-Lantos et al. 1992), whereas under conditions of basal LH release, activation of GABA$_A$ receptors in the anterior pituitary can enhance LH secretion (Brann et al. 1992). Consistent with these observations is the finding that the GABA agonists clonazepam and diazepam increase LH concentrations (Mannisto et al. 1992).

With respect to the GABA$_A$ receptor itself, it appears that ovarian steroids may have differing effects on receptor regulation. Estrogen and progesterone appear to exert opposite effects on the GABA$_A$ receptor within certain brain nuclei (Schumacher et al. 1989a, 1989b). Estrogen has been shown to increase nuclear progesterone receptors in GABA neurons in the primate hypothalamus (Leranth et al. 1991). It has been hypothesized that estrogen itself may not only increase the efficacy of facilitative neurotransmitters but also reduce the efficacy of inhibitory transmitters (McEwen et al. 1987). Estrogen treatment decreases GABA$_A$ receptors in the ventromedial nucleus, arcuate nucleus, and midbrain central gray matter (Schumacher et al. 1989a, 1989b) but increases receptors in the CA1 field of the hippocampus (Schumacher et al. 1989b). Progesterone appears to have effects on the affinity and density of the brain GABA-binding sites, which are also region-specific. Thus, progesterone may reduce the affinity of specific [^{3}H]-muscimol (i.e., GABA) binding in the hippocampus and enhance it in the medulla (Jussofie 1993).

Estrogen-induced upregulation of GABA receptors can be blocked by the estrogen receptor antagonist tamoxifen and requires an intact transcriptional system, suggesting a genomic effect of estrogen (O'Connor et al. 1988). In contrast, progesterone and its metabolites have been shown to modulate the binding affinity of GABA$_A$ receptors via nongenomic effects on the receptor complex (Gee 1988).

Recent work has suggested that there are natural progesterone metabolites with sedative-hypnotic properties that bind specifically to the GABA$_A$/benzodiazepine receptor–chloride ionophore complex and open the chloride channel. Significant anxiolytic behavior and anticonvulsant activity have been detected in rats upon administration of progesterone, and there is some evidence that these effects are associated with an increased sensitivity of GABA$_A$ receptor function. These CNS effects of progesterone are thought to be due to the bioconversion of progesterone to allopregnanolone, which may augment GABA$_A$ receptor–mediated function (see Majewska, Chapter 4, this volume).

In humans, some synthetic progestins, given in high doses, induce soporific effects comparable to those observed with the administration of barbiturates and benzodiazepines. The dose of progestin needed to induce an anxiolytic response is comparable to that required to induce estrus behavior in animals, suggesting that this behavioral effect of progestins may have a physiological role, at least in rodents. Withdrawal of progesterone or progestogens could be expected to have opposite results.

Acetylcholine

The central cholinergic nervous system has been implicated in the pathophysiology of mood disorders (Janowsky et al. 1972). Cholinesterase inhibitors, cholinergic agonists, and acetylcholine precursors such as choline and lecithin can cause depressed moods both in women without histories of affective disorder and in euthymic affective-disorder patients. Furthermore, these agents antagonize manic symptoms. Conversely, many of the antiadrenergic drugs that influence mood— such as methyldopa and reserpine—also have central cholinomimetic properties.

In addition, there is a growing body of evidence suggesting that cholinergic receptors may be supersensitive in the mood disorders. Supersensitivity to muscarinic cholinergic agonists has been noted in bipolar patients and patients with major depressive disorders with respect to rapid eye movement (REM) sleep parameters, pupillary constriction, and release of adrenocorticotropic hormone (ACTH) and β-endorphin, as well as with respect to behavioral variables such as depression and anergia (Dilsaver and Coffman 1989; Janowsky et al. 1972).

Ovarian hormones have a number of effects on acetylcholine and its receptors. In general, estrogen augments cholinergic neurotransmission. Estrogen augments the electrical firing of neurons in hypothalamic slices that occurs after administration of acetylcholine. In addition, in ovariectomized rats, muscarinic acetylcholinergic receptors have been shown to exist in increased numbers in the ventromedial and anterior hypothalamic nuclei 72 hours after estradiol administration (Rainbow et al. 1980). In contrast, progesterone has been found to inhibit nicotinic acetylcholine receptors (Valera et al. 1992).

Also, with respect to animal behavior, cholinergic muscarinic stimulation by the cholinesterase inhibitor physostigmine via cannulation of the anterior hypothalamus, the mesencephalic reticular formation, or the lateral ventricle has been shown to facilitate lordosis, a scopolamine and atropine–reversible sexual behavior in the rat (Clemens et al. 1989).

This effect was found to be especially robust in rats primed by estrogen and progesterone (Clemens et al. 1989).

In a somewhat parallel study in humans that used growth-hormone changes as an outcome variable, plasma progesterone and estradiol values were significantly correlated with growth-hormone responsivity to pyridostigmine, a cholinergic agonist (O'Keane and Dinan 1992). Thus, ovarian hormones, especially estrogen, appear to activate cholinergic neurotransmission and/or effectiveness. Finally, when levels of estrogen or progesterone decrease, such as during the premenstrual phase, muscarinic receptors may theoretically become unmasked, leading to exaggerated cholinergic hypersensitivity.

Ovarian hormones, therefore, appear to activate cholinergic neurotransmission, a phenomenon that may parallel presumed changes in depression. Finally, falling levels of estrogen or progesterone can be presumed to unmask upregulated muscarinic receptors, leading to hypersensitivity.

Endogenous Opiates

Endogenous opiates, such as β-endorphin, are naturally occurring central neuropeptides—produced in the brain, pituitary, and elsewhere—that have narcotic-like activity. The psychological and psychiatric effects of opiates were well known even before the discovery of endorphins. Indeed, for a time in the 1970s and before, opiates were hypothesized to be etiological of the affective disorders. Although changes in endogenous opioids are not generally thought to be a major cause of depression or other psychopathology, they have been considered important in the pathophysiology of self-destructive behavior, eating disorders, and possibly other psychiatric disorders such as schizophrenia.

Many studies have demonstrated the sensitivity of hypothalamic and circulating endogenous opioid peptides to gonadal steroids and vice versa. For the most part, these studies have examined the effect of gonadal steroids on the endorphins' modulation of gonadotropin regulation and on the effects of opioids and opiate antagonists on mating behavior. Although there are some inconsistencies in the findings, chronic estrogen administration generally appears to decrease endorphin levels in areas such as the mediobasal hypothalamus of rats, an effect that seems to be mediated by a subset of neurons in the hypothalamus that contain estrogen receptors and that synthesize β-endorphin. It also appears that this decrease in endorphin is mediated by estrogens' ability to decrease hypothalamic pro-opiomelanocortin (POMC).

Indeed, the symptoms occurring in premenstrual dysphoric syndromes have been hypothesized to involve endogenous opioid withdrawal by several investigators (Halbreich and Endicott 1981; Reid and Yen 1981). Similarly, β-endorphin levels appear to decrease at menopause (Schurz et al. 1988). Of further interest, β-endorphin facilitates the release of prolactin (as does naloxone) and inhibits the secretion of oxytocin and vasopressin (Laatikainen 1991). Gonadotropin-releasing hormone (GnRH), in contrast, stimulates the release of β-endorphin.

With respect to emotional disorders associated with pregnancy, naloxone-binding density (i.e., opiate binding) and β-endorphin content in the preoptic area of the hypothalamus were found to be increased during pregnancy in animals. The lowest levels were noted during lactation, with intermediate levels in castrated rats that had received hormonal replacement therapy. In a related study, Genazzani et al. (1987, 1990) demonstrated that progesterone increased β-endorphin levels in a number of brain sites.

Conversely, endorphins consistently decrease LH release, probably via suppression of GnRH due to the inhibition of catecholamine release. Opiate antagonists increase LH release at those times in the reproductive cycle when estrogen and progesterone are present. Significantly, endorphins and opiates decrease sexual activity and sexual desire in humans and the analogs of these behaviors in animals. Probably related to the inhibition of LH release by endorphins and to a decrease in sexual behavior, serum β-endorphin levels are increased in the luteal phase, at the time when estrogen and progesterone levels are elevated.

Prolactin-Induced Changes in Neurotransmitter Function

As mentioned earlier, fluctuations in prolactin may be related to ovarian hormone–linked emotional disorders. There is also some evidence that prolactin interacts with several neurotransmitters that have been linked to affective disorders and other related disturbances. Mansky et al. (1982) have demonstrated that norepinephrine turnover is correlated with prolactin levels in estrogen-pretreated, ovariectomized animals. In addition, prolactin increases dopamine turnover in the median eminence's nucleus accumbens (Fuxe et al. 1977) and decreases such turnover in certain other areas of the brain. Conversely, dopamine is a potent inhibitor of prolactin release, and prolactin increases the density of dopamine receptors and potentiates dopamine-enhanced stereotyped behaviors.

Prolactin has been demonstrated to cause several animal behavioral effects, including maternal behavior, feeding behavior, enhancement of grooming behavior (quite likely a dopaminergic effect involving the nigrostriatal dopamine system), facilitated acquisition of active avoidance (also proposed to be due to selected dopaminergic transmission), and reduced responsiveness to electrical foot shock (Drago et al. 1981). Significantly, several of these behavioral effects also appear related to opioid neurotransmission, in that they are reversed by the opiate antagonists naltrexone and naloxone. Furthermore, in animals, heroin self-administration is decreased by prolactin, and the development of tolerance to morphine and morphine-induced analgesia is facilitated by prolactin, effects reversed by antiprolactin serum (Drago and Scapagnini 1986).

Oxytocin

Several animal behavioral studies have indicated that oxytocin plays a role in maternal and sexual behavior. There is evidence that the sequential actions of estrogen and progesterone may bring this neuropeptide and its receptors into a state that enhances oxytocin's behavioral effects (McEwen 1991). It has been demonstrated that estrogen treatment induces a four- to fivefold increase in the number of oxytocin receptors in the ventromedial nucleus, and that progesterone, given after estrogen, will cause oxytocin-containing neurons outside the ventromedial nucleus to expand laterally so that they come into contact with the oxytocin receptors (Schumacher et al. 1989a). In the latter study, infusion of oxy-

tocin into the ventromedial hypothalamus increased the display of lordosis behavior only in female rats primed with both estradiol and progesterone.

Discussion

In considering the association between ovarian hormones and emotional states, it must be emphasized that changes in various hormones
are but one of many interwoven variables that influence human behavior. The significance of interpersonal, cultural, social, psychodynamic,
stress-related, and characterological determinants in the regulation of
sexual and emotional activity is of obvious significance in determining
the extent and direction of behavioral patterns.

The information presented in this chapter has indicated that emotional fluctuations and certain animal behaviors might be correlated
with fluctuations in ovarian and other hormones. At present, not
enough information exists to define which hormone or combination of
hormones cause specific ovarian hormone–linked behavioral changes.
However, in general, elevated or rapidly falling levels of estrogen, progesterone, prolactin, aldosterone, and angiotensin—such as occur in the
third trimester of pregnancy, postpartum, during or after ingestion of
progestins, and in the late luteal and perimenstrual phases of the menstrual cycle—seem to promote emotional instability. On the other hand,
although the above assertion seems to be almost self-evident, Dalton
(1964) has noted that postmenopausal and oophorectomized women
may either develop de novo or intensify preexisting cyclic emotional
changes, which then occur at the same intervals as they did when the
women had menstrual periods. This assertion, however, has not been
confirmed. In addition, it is not clear whether these "cycles" were caused
by estrogen-progesterone replacement therapy. However, it is possible
that the ovarian hormone–linked disorders are caused by other parallel
brain function changes that are actually temporally or even physiologically associated but not necessarily causally linked to ovarian hormone
alterations as such.

A central focus of this chapter has been the idea that hormones that
fluctuate throughout women's life cycles are associated with emotional

disorders and are involved in the regulation of normal and abnormal sexual and other behaviors in women. These hormones might alter neurotransmitters and neuromodulators in the brain; it is through those central chemicals that emotional and sexual behavior changes are likely to occur. Regarding this point, it is important to note that none of the neurotransmitter hypotheses of mental illness have been proven, and all await further direct studies. Similarly, although much evidence exists indicating that neurotransmitters and neuromodulators are affected by the hormones previously considered, the actual occurrence of these changes in women under physiological conditions is far from certain and is largely based on indirect evidence and animal studies. In addition, it is obvious from this review that most neurotransmitters interact with and perturb each other, leading to downstream phenomena, as do almost all mental illness treatment modalities—which, even if they appear to alter mostly one neurotransmitter, actually may perturb many. Thus, although it is likely that the behavioral changes described in this chapter are meaningful in causing ovarian cycle– and hormone-linked emotional disorders, the true significance of these changes awaits further elaboration.

Despite the existence of a number of unanswered questions, alternative possibilities, and conflicting facts and paradoxes, it seems reasonable to conclude that the proposed etiological relationship of endocrine-induced neurotransmitter/neuromodulator alterations to ovarian hormone–linked emotional and sexual behavioral changes remains a strong hypothetical possibility—one worthy of continued investigation.

Molecular Approaches to Sex Differences in Brain Functions, Including Motivation and Libido

Donald W. Pfaff, Ph.D.,
and Sally K. Severino, M.D.

S ex differences in brain morphology have been heralded widely, although in most cases links to behavioral functions have been obscure. In this chapter we concentrate on molecular mechanisms in brains of experimental animals and argue that these molecular mechanisms can be related to basic instincts toward reproduction. In the terms of experimental analysis of behavior, such instincts would come under the heading of motivation, while in the history of psychiatry and psychoanalysis, they would be related to the concept of libido, a drive concept that has straddled the border of mental life and physiological mechanism.

In at least two cases, it is easy to illustrate strong sex differences in the regulation of gene expression in the forebrain. In addition, prominent sex differences exist in reactions to medically useful psychotropic drugs. Furthermore, experimental demonstrations in animals show a more rapid recovery from cerebral cortical damage by genetic females than by males.

Basic Theory

During the past few years, much of the overwhelming interest in brain research has had to do with natural or experimentally controlled alterations in brain function and behavior. Thus, a tremendous amount of attention has centered on mechanisms of learning and memory, processes of neuronal development, promotion of rapid repair after brain injury, and processes of brain degeneration and declining mental ability during normal aging or Alzheimer's disease. The umbrella concept under which all of these areas are grouped is "neural plasticity," which refers to any well-organized change in nerve cell circuit structure or function.

At the end of the day, however, a thorough molecular understanding of neural plasticity will depend absolutely on the prior demonstration of the exact neuronal and molecular mechanisms by which normal behavioral responses are elicited. That is, all "plastic changes" are built on preexisting mechanisms that must be elucidated for their alterations to make any sense. The highly evolved molecular mechanisms and hardwired neuronal circuitry that underlie instinctive behaviors are of great practical interest. Such instinctive behaviors include the normal performance of and sex differences in reproductive behaviors, parental behaviors, aggression in its normal and pathological aspects, and feeding behavior.

All of these instinctive behaviors, necessary for survival and potentially disruptive or socially devastating when disordered, are characterized not only by their possibilities for alteration (as emphasized in recent years) but also by the normal biological limits on their performance. For example, the limits—the biologically sensible constraints—on sex behavior and the sex differences therein can be formulated according to the following perspective.

In the absence of a comprehensive quantitative theory of brain function and behavior, a safe approach that is intellectually orderly and makes great evolutionary sense is the axiomatic approach. Working deductively backward from the existence of living animals and humans, the requirements for all living beings include reproduction. In turn, successful reproduction requires not only hormone actions on the brain—as will be emphasized from a molecular point of view in this chapter—but also the proximity of a mating partner; adequate nutrition, water, and salt; permissive conditions of temperature and daylight; nesting material; and a relative absence of stress. Thus, even in relatively simple experimental animals, reproduction requires complex, highly integrated social behaviors. One of the effects of sex steroid hormones on the brain is to drive estrogen- and androgen-dependent communicative behaviors using several sensory modalities, to provide for a "hormone-dependent behavioral funnel" by which a reproductively competent male and female of the same species, and only they, may get together (Floody and Pfaff 1977). In the normal case, the male and female meet effectively only if all of the constraints on reproduction listed above have been satisfied. For a simple, female-typical reproductive behavior in quadrupeds—lordosis—the neuronal circuit and some of the cellular mechanisms have been determined (Pfaff 1980).

Several principles have been derived from that area of neurobiological work that focuses on sex differences in brain morphology and function, including 1) the universality across vertebrates of certain sex steroid hormone–concentrating neuronal groups in the brain, and 2) the conservation of molecular endocrine mechanisms outside the central nervous system for use in the modulation of brain function; in addition, research on reproductive behavioral mechanisms has demonstrated that it is possible to determine the neuronal circuit for a vertebrate behavior (Pfaff et al. 1994). Lordosis is the primary reproductive behavior by which the vertebrate female permits fertilization. Obvious in the neuronal circuitry for lordosis behavior are modules at different levels of the neuraxis by which the behavior is controlled. Estrogens and progestins most powerfully control the circuit via hypothalamic and preoptic neurons.

Knowledge of the circuit for a hormone-dependent reproductive behavior constituted a launching platform for molecular investigations that remain ongoing. The molecular investigations discussed in this chapter will be illustrated by experiments on the gene for the progesterone receptor and the gene for preproenkephalin, the precursor for the opioid peptide enkephalin. Nevertheless, it is already apparent that even for a simple behavior in an experimental animal, we are not dealing with a one hormone–one gene–one behavior situation. In this context, for example, it appears extremely unlikely that anyone should extrapolate from the correlations between genetic polymorphisms, or differences in chromosomal deoxyribonucleic acid (DNA), on the X chromosome (Hamer et al. 1993) and male homosexuality to discuss, in any serious way, "a gene for determining sexual preference."

In summary, we must ask how the rapid progress in the cellular and molecular analyses of instinctive behaviors, including reproduction, can be placed in our current views of the plasticity of brain function. Clearly, the most elementary form of plasticity is the alteration of state from an animal in which no response occurs to the state in which a well-defined response occurs. The very change in neuronal function from zero activity to the performance of the instinctive response of interest is itself the most fundamental form of neuronal plasticity. In the history of American behavioral analysis, therefore, molecular investigations that explain this change of state would be explaining a manifestation of "motivation" (Pfaff 1982). In the history of psychoanalysis, the instinct toward reproduction may be related to "libido," a central drive concept.

Molecular Assays

Two genes, each related to the performance of reproductive behavior by female rats, have proven especially fortunate for analysis: the gene for the progesterone receptor and the gene for preproenkephalin. The gene for the progesterone receptor is important because, in a variety of experimental animals, progesterone supplements estrogenic action on the brain to foster courtship and copulatory responses. The gene for preproenkephalin is related to reproductive behavior in that enkephalin action, operating through delta enkephalin receptors, can permit more frequent lordosis behavior, perhaps by reducing antagonistic responses—that is, behavioral responses through which the male is rejected (Pfaus and Gorzalka 1987a, 1987b; Pfaus and Pfaff 1992).

Progesterone Receptor Gene

Using in situ hybridization—a technique in which labeled DNA is used to recognize a specific RNA in its cellular context—Romano et al. (1988) discovered hypothalamic neurons expressing the gene for the progesterone receptor. The progesterone receptor is itself a transcription factor—that is, a protein that facilitates synthesis of ribonucleic acid (RNA) from DNA. The distribution in the hypothalamus of cells expressing the gene for the progesterone receptor matched what would have been predicted from progesterone binding, thus constituting one form of validation of the in situ hybridization method.

Another validation of the in situ hybridization method for locating cells expressing certain genes comes from the difference in regulation between the progesterone receptor gene and the gene for the estrogen receptor (Lauber et al. 1990b, 1991). To date, the most striking alteration in progesterone receptor-gene expression in the hypothalamus has come from pretreatment with estradiol benzoate (Romano et al. 1989). Estrogen treatment recruited ventromedial hypothalamic neurons to express the progesterone receptor gene such that the number of such cells after estrogen treatment was four times greater than that in the ovariectomized control animals (Romano et al. 1989). Especially striking was the fact that the same estrogen treatment administered to genetic females and effective in inducing progesterone receptor-gene induction was absolutely ineffective in castrated males (Lauber et al. 1991).

Moreover, these molecular responses are tissue-specific within the brain. The same estrogen treatment that induced the progesterone receptor gene in female rat hypothalamic neurons was ineffective in the amygdala. Thus, at least three features of the progesterone receptor gene as expressed in brain stand out: its induction by hormones, its brain region specificity, and the sex difference in its regulation. These characteristics should be explained by further molecular analysis.

Electrophoretic mobility shift assay.   This assay, also called "gel shifts," is a method of separating compounds on the basis on their rates of migration in an electrical field. The electrophoretic mobility shift assay detects proteins binding to certain DNA sequences. If indeed estrogenic hormones attached to their estrogenic receptor protein in the cell nucleus can bind to the promoter (a genetic regulatory region, a segment of DNA that serves as a recognition signal for RNA polymerase and that marks the initiation of transcription) or other regions of the progesterone receptor gene to effect an induction of gene transcription (the process by which a single-stranded RNA sequence complementary to one strand of double-stranded DNA is synthesized), then in the electrophoretic mobility shift assay it should be possible to detect bands that demonstrate estrogen receptor binding to presumed estrogen response elements in this gene. Such DNA elements have been proven to mediate estrogen's control over transcription. These studies have yielded an intriguing configuration of results. Even under conditions in the gel shift assay that demonstrate conventional estrogen receptor binding to a consensus estrogen response element in the uterus and the brain, the characteristics of binding of the estrogen receptor to the presumed estrogen response element on the progesterone receptor gene are different (A. H. Lauber, D. W. Pfaff, I. Alroy, "Hypothalamic Estrogen Receptor Binding to a Consensus ERE and a Putative ERE From a Progesterone Receptor Gene" [unpublished study], December 1993). In the same series of investigations, we noticed that a DNA binding element called AP-1, which could bind the nuclear proteins fos and jun and bind fos-related antigens, overlapped the presumed estrogen response element. In turn, even though nuclear proteins from hypothalamic neurons exhibited orthodox characteristics of binding in gel-shift assays to a consensus AP-1 DNA sequence, the characteristics of binding to the presumed AP-1 element as part of the compound progesterone receptor DNA sequence element were different—they did not have the characteristics of conventional AP-1 binding. Thus, it seems plausible at this time to envision that in the actual control of the progesterone receptor gene, estrogen receptor binding to the requisite DNA sequence is influenced by the binding of fos-related and jun-related nuclear proteins that can signal that synaptic input has occurred. Such interactions would provide for the integration of hormonal and synaptic inputs as they affect gene expression by individual, behaviorally relevant hypothalamic neurons.

Antisense DNA.   Do alterations in gene expression make any difference in reproductive behavior? The most direct approach to this question is to block progesterone receptor messenger RNA (mRNA) function by antisense DNA treatment. mRNA carries the information encoded in a DNA sequence to the site of translation, or protein synthesis; it specifies the order of amino acid residues. Antisense DNA contains a sequence complementary to a specific mRNA and can disrupt that RNA's function. We microinjected 15-mers antisense (DNA containing 15 nucleotides) to the progesterone receptor mRNA in the region spanning the translation start site, directly amongst ventromedial hypothalamic neurons in estrogen-primed female rats. The control condition was to use the same 15 nucleotide bases but to scramble them so that they would not carry genetic information—thus, the chemical constituents were held constant while the genetic information was destroyed in the controlled condition (Ogawa et al. 1994). Under these conditions, with a timing specifically related to the time of onset of estrogen treatment, the antisense DNA treatment significantly reduced lordosis behavior performance. More impressive, the courtship behaviors of the female rat, which are exquisitely progesterone-sensitive, were reduced by 80%. In parallel with the behavioral studies, it was shown that progesterone immunoreactive neurons in the basal medial hypothalamus near the site of antisense microinjection were, as predicted, reduced in number.

The concatenation of experimental results presented above makes it possible, for the first time, to directly relate the synthesis of a transcription factor to the performance of a specific behavior. First, the progesterone receptor is itself a transcription factor. Estrogen leads to an increase in the progesterone receptor's gene expression and to female rat reproductive behavior. In turn, the mRNA for the progesterone receptor is required for estrogen-stimulated reproductive behavior. In this simple example in female rats, therefore, molecular and behavioral results are in perfect registration.

Preproenkephalin Gene Expression

The gene for preproenkephalin is expressed in a diverse set of brain regions (Harlan et al. 1987). In situ hybridization technology permits study of the gene's regulation (Romano et al. 1987). In a robust fashion, estrogen treatment leads to an induction of preproenkephalin mRNA in ventromedial hypothalamic neurons, but not in the amygdala or the caudate (Romano et al. 1988). This induction is rapid—occurring within 1 hour—and can be potentiated by progesterone (Romano et al. 1989).

Most interesting was the fact that the same estrogen treatment that could induce preproenkephalin gene expression in genetic females was ineffective in the hypothalamus of genetic males (Romano et al. 1990). This lack of effect was not attributable to an inability of the genetic male ventromedial hypothalamic neuron to express the gene, since basal levels were just as high as in genetic females. Nor was it the case that the genetic male simply required testosterone, because that sex hormone had no effect either. Thus, three features of preproenkephalin gene expression remain to be explained by further molecular analysis: tissue specificity of basal expression, strong estrogen regulation, and the prominent sex difference in that regulation.

Relation to behavior.   In a comprehensive dose-response experiment, there was an orderly relationship between the amount of estrogen given subcutaneously to ovariectomized female rats and the amount of preproenkephalin gene expression in the ventromedial hypothalamus (Lauber et al. 1990a). That dose-response relation was specific, since it did not obtain for preoptic-area neurons. Every rat used in the study was measured for the frequency of reproductive behavior responses before sacrifice for molecular assays. Female rats demonstrated an orderly ascending curve of reproductive behavior frequency as a function of the amount of preproenkephalin mRNA in the ventromedial hypothalamus (Lauber et al. 1990a). Moreover, there was an apparent "threshold level" for the amount of preproenkephalin mRNA: above that level, virtually all female rats displayed lordosis behavior, whereas below that level, virtually none did. The connections of opioid peptide gene expression to behavior are not merely correlational: delta opioid receptor agonists injected into the lateral ventricle of female rats can actually promote female-typical reproductive behavior (Pfaus and Gorzalka 1987b; Pfaus and Pfaff 1992), perhaps by reduction of rejection and other antagonistic responses by the female toward the male (H. E. Brown, unpublished observations, June 1993).

Molecular mechanisms.   In part, the tissue specificity of preproen-kephalin gene expression in the rat brain may be accounted for by differential methylation of the promoter. However, in no sense does the degree of DNA methylation line up perfectly with the intensity of transcription, nor do we expect it to explain hormonal regulation (Funabashi et al. 1993a, 1993b). We noted that the first intron, or noncoding intervening sequence in a gene, of the rat preproenkephalin gene was completed unmethylated.

DNAse hypersensitivity assays (assays that reveal points on the DNA susceptible to cleavage by the DNAse enzyme) might be expected to pinpoint areas of the preproenkephalin promoter that are accessible to transcription factors. In such studies (Funabashi et al. 1993a, 1993b), a major DNAse hypersensitivity site was revealed about 1,800 nucleotide bases upstream of the transcription start site, while a hypersensitivity site present in brain but not in liver tissue was revealed about 200 bases upstream. Most interesting were minor sites of DNAse hypersensitivity that appeared somewhat affected by estrogen treatment in ovariectomized female rats and that showed a sex difference—detectable in females but not in males. It was intriguing that these sites were discovered in the first intron, a DNA sequence that does not code for protein but that might be of regulatory importance.

The orthodox hypothesis for explaining the estrogen effect would devolve upon a possible estrogen response element 365 nucleotide bases upstream from the conventional preproenkephalin start site. Indeed, recent studies in our laboratory (Zhu et al. 1994), using gel shifts, have revealed specific binding by the estrogen receptor to this sequence in the preproenkephalin promoter. The binding is weaker than that to a consensus estrogen response element but nevertheless has characteristics that would allow effects of estrogen on preproenkephalin gene transcription. This is not the only means by which the hormone could affect gene expression, however. Unexpectedly, Brooks et al. (1993) found an intronic (noncoding) sequence—present in a significant number of neurons in the basal forebrain, thalamus, and hypothalamus—that might reflect an alternative transcription start site for the rat preproenkephalin gene. Moreover, estrogen effects are revealed by probes directed toward a particular intron, the first intron in a particular location, 3-prime (downstream) of this potential alternative transcription start site but not 5-prime (upstream). At least some hypothalamic cells revealing surprisingly high amounts of this intronic sequence are different from those that generate the conventional preproenkephalin mRNA (Brooks et al. 1993).

Gene transfer into adult brain tissue.   Foreign DNA may be introduced into a host cell by a viral vector consisting of a viral chromosome into whose genome a fragment of foreign DNA has been inserted. A novel viral vector for expressing foreign genes in the brain is helping to define the requirements for basal transcription and hormone-regulated transcription of preproenkephalin in the rat brain. This vector uses an origin of replication and a cleavage packaging sequence from the gene called herpes simplex-1 viral genome in a manner pioneered by N. Frankel and A. Kwong (reviewed in Kaplitt et al. 1993) and has been applied successfully for expression of a foreign gene in the adult rat brain (Kaplitt et al. 1991). Different fragments of the preproenkephalin promoter (a regulatory segment of DNA marking the initiation site of transcription), when attached to the reporter gene β-galactosidase (a gene whose phenotype is relatively easy to monitor and that may be attached to promoter regions of interest; β-galactosidase is easily assessed by enzymatic histochemical stain), provide for in vivo promoter analysis and show that in some forebrain regions, an enhancer between 1,431 bases and 2,700 bases upstream of the conventional start site is required for basal expression (Kaplitt et al. 1994). Moreover, this 2,700-base fragment of the preproenkephalin promoter apparently permits an estrogen effect in hypothalamic neurons (Yin et al. 1994).

In summary, the molecular analysis of a prominent sex difference in the regulation of gene expression for an opioid peptide is presently expected to rest on the differences in proteins binding within the first 2,700 bases of the preproenkephalin promoter, with possible additional participation by proteins binding within the first intron. Sex differences in these basic molecular aspects of brain function within the hypothalamus make it clear that psychoactive drugs promoted as helpful in the treatment of emotional disorders must be tested in females as well as males.

Some Other Medically Relevant Neurochemical Sex Differences in Rat Brain and Behavior

If there were no differences between the sexes in responses to psychoactive drugs, then the careful inclusion of women in drug trials would not be so thoroughly justified, because of the risks of an unrecognized pregnancy and because of the statistical complications of dealing with possible variations throughout the menstrual cycle. However, such sex differences are easy to illustrate. For example, it has been established that repeated administrations of amphetamine lead to enhanced behavioral responses—a sensitization (increased rapidity or amplitude of response) to subsequent applications (Robinson et al. 1982). Impressively, the magnitude of the sensitization to amphetamine, as displayed by changes in rotational behavior, was greater in females than in males. The increase in the number of rotations was actually twice as large in female as in male rats (Robinson et al. 1982). Stereotyped responses fostered by amphetamine injections were sensitized at a high rate in both normal females and ovariectomized control females (Camp and Robinson 1988b); but in genetic males, presence of testes was responsible for the lower rate of amphetamine sensitization. The authors suggested that a sex difference exists in the responsiveness of brain dopaminergic systems to repetitive activation. The male animals tended to be more variable in their responses to amphetamine treatment because their results fell naturally into two groups based on both neurochemistry and behavior (Camp and Robinson 1988a). Overall, the conclusions of this important series of studies indicate obvious sex differences even for simple behavioral responses to a psychoactive drug in lower animals.

In the field of experimental determination of factors governing responses to brain injury, there are likewise sex differences. Rats were given frontal cortex aspiration lesions, and their performance on delayed spatial alternation learning (in which rats must remember their last spatial response for a defined interval) was compared across hormonal groups (Attella et al. 1987). Those female rats who were subjected to the cortical damage while pseudopregnant had less impairment than did normally cycling females. Because high levels of circulating progesterone are a prominent feature of pseudopregnancy, it was thought that progesterone as it affects brain edema might be the link to improved behavioral recovery from brain injury. Subsequently, therefore, Roof et al. (1992) subjected male and female rats to a cortical contusion injury and rats were injected with progesterone or an oil vehicle after the experimental damage. Progesterone-treated rats, both male and female, had much less edema after cortical injury (Roof et al. 1992). When males, proestrus females (in the phase preceding the estrus phase of heightened sexual activity), and pseudopregnant females were directly compared for the percentage increase in water content of brain-tissue samples from injured areas compared with noninjured distal areas, the males showed by far the greatest increase (Roof et al. 1993). It appears, therefore, that progesterone, as secreted in females, can have a protective effect after injury to the brain and thus represents another possibly clinically important neurochemical difference between the sexes.

In summary, both molecular and neuropharmacological data support the necessity of including significant numbers of female subjects in clinical trials of psychoactive drugs.

Relationship of Molecular Data to Motivational Concepts: Drive Systems for Libido and Aggression

Since, under the influence of estrogen, female rats will not only perform chains of instinctive reproductive responses but will also learn arbitrary responses for the opportunity to reproduce, these behaviors have the characteristic of sexual motivation (reviewed in Pfaff 1982). Thus, when a series of cellular and molecular studies as summarized above explains the occurrence of these hormone-driven behaviors, one may question whether a "drive"—a particular form of sexual motivation—is being explained as well. Especially because the parts of the hypothalamus, basal forebrain, and brain stem that govern these reproductive behavior responses have changed much less during evolution toward the human brain than would be true, for example, of the cerebral cortex and thalamus, one is left to wonder whether biologically crucial motivational tendencies as manifested in animal behavior might lie at the base of the most primitive human psychological motivations. The psychoanalytic concept that comes closest to filling the bill is that of drives, an idea that has always straddled the border between psychology and physiology in psychoanalytic thinking.

Drive, conceptualized theoretically by Freud (1920/1955) as the origin of unconscious psychic conflict and the determinant of character structure, is still considered an important component of mental functioning in psychoanalytic circles despite arguments to replace it with other theories, such as attachment theory, object relations theory, affect theory, cognitive theory, and relationship theory. Freud (1915/1957) described drives (sexual and aggressive) as originating in physiology but linked to mental life by thoughts and affects.

Kernberg (1992) provided a contemporary description of the origin and structure of libido and aggression as motivational forces:

> *Affects* link the series of *undifferentiated self/object representations* so that gradually a complex world of *internalized object relations,* some pleasurably tinged, others unpleasurably tinged, is constructed. But even while affects are linking internalized object relations in two parallel series of *gratifying* and *frustrating* experiences, *"good"* and *"bad"* internalized object relations are themselves being transformed. The predominant affect of *love* or *hate* of the two series of internalized object relations is enriched and modulated and becomes increasingly complex. . . . Love and hate thus become stable intrapsychic structures in the sense of two dynamically determined internally consistent, stable frames for organizing psychic experience and behavioral control in *genetic continuity* through various *developmental stages.* By that very continuity, they consolidate into *libido* and *aggression.* Libido and aggression, in turn, become *hierarchically supraordinate motivational systems,* expressed in a multitude of differentiated affect dispositions under different circumstances. *Affects* are the building blocks, or constituents, of drives; they eventually acquire a signal function for the activation of drives. . . . *Drives* are manifest not simply by affects but by the activation of a specific object relation, which includes an affect and in which the drive is represented by a specific desire or wish. . . . The *wish* derives from the drive and is more precise than the affect state. (pp. 19–20, italics added).

If we assume that particular object relations reflect, as Kernberg says, activation of specific desires and wishes and hence drives, even the very complicated mental life of human beings may allow basic neurobiological investigation to shed light on how motivational states contribute to intrapsychic organization. Neuroendocrine and neurobiological differences (at the molecular level) between men and women provide one potential type of insight. Understanding how these molecular phenomena in limbic and hypothalamic neurons are elaborated into libido and aggression in the adult human represents a considerable challenge for modern brain research.

Conclusion

Clear molecular differences between the sexes in the regulation of gene expression in hypothalamic neurons of rats may explain not only sex-typed instinctive responses, including certain reproductive behaviors, but also motivational phenomena. All such sex differences in neurochemistry, mood, and behaviors mandate that females as well as males be included in the testing of potentially therapeutic psychoactive drugs. Finally, although drive theory permits clear inferences from neurobiological data in animals to the foundations of libido and aggression in humans, these extrapolations remain, at present, at the theoretical level.

Gender and Ethnic Differences in the Pharmacogenetics of Psychotropics

Michael Smith, M.D.,
and Keh-Ming Lin, M.D., M.P.H.

Considerable interindividual variations exist in medication responses, dosage requirements, and side-effect profiles for a large number of drugs, including the majority of psychotropics (Kalow 1991). Ethnicity and gender have been identified as important determinants of these variabilities. Multiple biological, psychological, and sociocultural factors contribute to

From the Research Center on the Psychobiology of Ethnicity and the Department of Psychiatry, Harbor–UCLA Medical Center. Supported in part by Research Center on the Psychobiology of Ethnicity Grant MH47193.

121

these variations in a complex and interactive manner, much of which remains little understood. Of these factors, issues relevant to pharmacogenetics—the study of genetic control of drug metabolism—have been most extensively studied; these issues will be the primary focus of this chapter.

The metabolism of the majority of pharmacoactive agents has long been known to be under strong genetic control (Kalow 1982; Nebert and Weber 1990). Recently, a number of genetically determined polymorphisms in drug metabolism have been identified. Drug-metabolizing enzymes that are polymorphic show bimodal distribution of their activities in a given population, such that its members can be classified as extensive metabolizers (EMs) and poor metabolizers (PMs) (Gonzalez and Nebert 1990; Kalow 1991; U. A. Meyer et al. 1990; Wilkinson et al. 1989; A. J. Wood and Zhou 1991). Enzyme systems that are polymorphic in nature include some of the major cytochrome P450 isozymes, such as debrisoquin hydroxylase (CYP2D6) and mephenytoin hydroxylase (CYP_{mp}), as well as N-acetyltransferase, alcohol dehydrogenase, and aldehyde dehydrogenase. In addition, genetic influences are substantial both in controlling the rate of glucuronidation and in the polymorphism of α_1-acid glycoprotein, an important drug-binding plasma protein. In this chapter we review the relevance of these influences to ethnicity and gender (Agarwal and Goedde 1990; Dawkins and Potter 1991; Eichelbaum et al. 1982; Kalow 1982; Nebert and Weber 1990; Yonkers et al. 1992a).

The P450 Enzyme System

Many pharmacologically active agents are relatively nonpolar and require two metabolic steps—functionalization (i.e., oxidation or hydroxylation) and conjugation—to be rendered sufficiently water soluble for excretion. Phase I of the process, involving the addition of a functional group into the substrate, is predominantly carried out by the cytochrome P450 isozymes (W. G. Clark et al. 1988; Shen and Lin 1990). Phase II involves the conjugation of these agents via glucuronidation and sulfation.

Two of the human P450 isozymes—CYP2D6 and CYP_{mp}—have been found to be polymorphic. Subsequent molecular genetic studies have revealed that such differences in the enzyme activities are genetically controlled: the enzymes are defective in PMs because of mutations in the nucleic acid sequence in the DNA and, consequently, alterations in its corresponding amino acid structure in the enzyme.

Studies involving these two enzymes may be of particular significance for psychiatry, because they are responsible for the metabolism of many commonly used psychotropics. Drugs that are metabolized by CYP2D6 include tricyclic antidepressants (Bertilsson and Aberg-Wistedt 1983; Bertilsson et al. 1980; Mellstrom et al. 1983; Skjelbo et al. 1991), neuroleptics (Dahl-Puustinen et al. 1989), benzodiazepines (Bertilsson et al. 1989; Wilkinson et al. 1989), barbiturates (Kupfer and Preisig 1984) and propranolol (Shaheen et al. 1989; Ward et al. 1989) (Table 7–1). In contrast, the enzyme CYP_{mp} is involved in the N-demethylation of diazepam (Bertilsson et al. 1989), the demethylation of imipramine (Skjelbo et al. 1991), as well as the side-chain oxidation of propranolol (Ward et al. 1989).

In addition, recent studies have also reported that the PM phenotype of CYP2D6 may be related to higher incidence of Parkinsonism

Table 7–1.   Drugs subject to CYP2D6 P450 enzyme metabolism

Alprenolol	Methoxyphenamine
Amiflamine	Metiamide
Amitriptyline	Metoprolol
Bufralol	Nortriptyline
CGP 15210G	Perhexilene
Chlorpromazine	Perphenazine
Clomipramine	Phenacetin
Codeine	Phenformin
Desipramine	Propafenone
Dextromethorphan	Proplalamin
Encainide	Propranolol
Flecainide	Sparteine
Guanoxan	Thioridazine
Imipramine	Timolol
Indoramin	Tomoxetine
Methoxyamphetamine	

(Barbeau et al. 1985; Otton et al. 1983) and to unique personality traits (Bertilsson et al. 1989), suggesting that the functional variation of this enzyme may not be limited only to the liver, but may be present in the brain as well.

Ethnicity and the Cytochrome P450 Isozymes

Substantial cross-ethnic differences exist in the frequency of the PM phenotype with these enzymes. As can be seen from Table 7–2, the frequency of poor metabolizing of CYP2D6 varies from less than 3% in Cuna Amerindians (Arias et al. 1988; Jorge et al. 1990), Egyptians (Mahgoub et al. 1979), Saudi Arabians (Islam et al. 1980), and several Asian subgroups including Chinese (Du and Lou 1990; Lee et al. 1988; Lou et al. 1987; Xu and Jiang 1990), Japanese (Horai et al. 1990; Ishizaki et al. 1987; Nakamura et al. 1985), Malayans (Lee et al. 1988), and Thai (Wanwimolruk et al. 1990), to 3%–10% in Caucasians and Hispanics in Europe and North America. A wider range of frequencies is found in Black Africans, with 0%–8% of Saharan Africans, 4% of Venda in South Africa, 1.9% of African Americans, and 19% of Sans Bushmen being classified as PMs.

CYP$_{mp}$ hydroxylation displays a phenotypy discrete from that of CYP2D6 (Table 7–3). In contrast to findings that poor metabolizing of CYP2D6 is more frequent in Caucasians than Asians, PMs of CYP$_{mp}$ are more prevalent in Asian populations, with approximately 20% of Japanese being classified as PMs (Horai et al. 1989; Jurima et al. 1985; Nakamura et al. 1985). Chinese in their native land also demonstrate a high frequency of PMs (Horai et al. 1989), while Chinese in Canada display a much lower frequency (Jurima et al. 1985) similar to that of Caucasians (Drohse et al. 1989; Inaba et al. 1984; Jacqz et al. 1988; Jurima et al. 1985; Nakamura et al. 1985; Sanz et al. 1989; Wedlund et al. 1984). African Americans demonstrate a rate of 18.5%, similar to that in Asians (Pollock et al. 1991).

Gender and the Cytochrome P450 Isozymes

Information on gender variation in the expression of cytochrome P450 isozymes is mostly limited to animal studies. This research has identified several sex-specific P450 enzyme systems in rats and mice. Sex and pi-

Table 7–2. Debrisoquin (CYP2D6)/dextromethorphan/sparteine oxidation

Authors	Country	Sample size	No. (%) poor metabolizers	Drug
Studies in Africans and African Americans				
African Americans				
Relling et al. 1991	U.S.	106	2 (1.9)	DM
Sub-Saharan Africans				
Eichelbaum et al. 1982	Ghana	154	0 (0)	SP
Iyun et al. 1986	Nigeria	137	0 (0)	DB
Mbanefo et al. 1980	Nigeria	123	10 (8.1)	DB
Woolhouse et al. 1979	Ghana	80	5 (6.3)	DB
Sans bushmen				
Sommers et al. 1988	South Africa	96	18 (19)	DB
Venda				
Sommers et al. 1989	South Africa	98	4 (4.1)	DB
Sommers et al. 1991	South Africa	97	0 (0)	SP
Studies in Amerindians and Hispanics				
Cuna				
Arias et al. 1988	Panama	170	0 (0)	SP
Jorge et al. 1990	Panama	89	0 (0)	DB
Hispanics				
Lam et al. 1991	U.S.	22	1 (4.5)	DM
Ngawbe Guaymi				
Arias et al. 1988	Panama	97	5 (5.2)	SP
Studies in Asians				
Chinese				
Du and Lou 1990	China (Han)	140	2 (1.4)	DB
Inaba et al. 1981	China	19	6 (32)	DB
Kalow et al. 1980	Canada	13	4 (31)	DB
Lee et al. 1988	Singapore	97	0 (0)	DB
Lou et al. 1987	China	269	2 (0.7)	DB
Xu and Jiang 1990	China	220	3 (1.4)	DB
Japanese				
Horai et al. 1990	Japan	55	1 (1.8)	DB & SP
Ishizaki et al. 1987	Japan	84	2 (2.4)	SP
Nakamura et al. 1985	Japan	100	0 (0)	DB
Malayans				
Lee et al. 1988	Malaya	95	2 (2.1)	DB
Thai				
Wanwimolruk et al. 1990	Thailand	173	2 (1.2)	DB

(continued)

Table 7–2.   Debrisoquin (CYP2D6)/dextromethorphan/sparteine
oxidation *(continued)*

Authors	Country	Sample size	No. (%) poor metabolizers	Drug
Studies in Caucasians				
Arvela et al. 1988	Finland			DB
	(Finns)	155	5 (3.2)	
	(Lapps)	70	6 (8.6)	
Benitez et al. 1988	Spain	377	25 (6.6)	DB
Drohse et al. 1989	Denmark	358	33 (9.2)	SP
D. A. Evans et al. 1980	Britain	258	23 (8.9)	DB
Inaba et al. 1983	Canada	80	6 (7.5)	DB
Inaba et al. 1983	Canada	48	4 (8.3)	SP
Inaba et al. 1984	Canada	83	6 (7.2)	SP
Ishizaki et al. 1987	Germany	52	3 (5.8)	SP
Jacqz et al. 1988	France	132	4 (3)	DM
Kalow et al. 1980	Canada	38	2 (5)	DB
Lam et al. 1991	U.S.	30	2 (6.7)	DM
Leclercq et al. 1987	Belgium	167	12 (7.2)	DB
Mahgoub et al. 1977 (race not stated)	Britain	94	3 (3.2)	DB
Nakamura et al. 1985	U.S.	183	16 (8.7)	DB
Peart et al. 1986	Australia	100	6 (6)	DB
Relling et al. 1991	U.S.	480	37 (7.7)	DM
Sanz et al. 1989	Sweden	205	18 (8.9)	DB
Schmid et al. 1985	Switzerland	268	23 (8.6)	DM
E. Steiner et al. 1988	Sweden	757	41 (5.4)	DB
Syvalahti et al. 1986	Finland	107	6 (5.6)	DB
Szorady and Santa 1987	Hungary	100	8 (8)	DB
Veronese and McLean 1991	Australia	152	13 (8.6)	DB
Wedlund et al. 1984	U.S.	156	11 (7.0)	DB
Studies in Egyptians				
Mahgoub et al. 1979	Egypt and Britain	72	1 (1.4)	DB
Studies in Saudi Arabians				
Islam et al. 1980	Saudi Arabia	102	1 (1)	DB

Note. DB = debrisoquin (CYP2D6); DM = dextromethorphan; SP = sparteine.

Table 7–3. Mephenytoin (CYPmp) oxidation phenotypes

Authors	Country	Sample size	No. (%) poor metabolizers
Studies in East Indians			
Doshi et al. 1990	India	48	10 (20.8)
Studies in Amerindians			
Inaba et al. 1988	Panama	90	0 (0)
Studies in Asians			
Chinese			
Horai et al. 1989	China	98	7 (17.4)
Jurima et al. 1985	Canada	39	2 (5)
Japanese			
Horai et al. 1989	Japan	200	45 (22)
Jurima et al. 1985	Canada	31	7 (23)
Nakamura et al. 1985	Japan	100	18 (18)
Studies in Caucasians			
Pollock et al. 1991	U.S.	123	5 (4.1)
Drohse et al. 1989	Denmark	358	9 (2.5)
Inaba et al. 1984	Canada	83	2 (2.4)
Jacqz et al. 1988	France	132	8 (6)
Jurima et al. 1985	Canada	118	5 (4.2)
Kupfer and Preisig 1984	Switzerland	–	– (5)
Lam et al. 1991	U.S.	30	2 (6.7)
Nakamura et al. 1985	U.S.	183	5 (2.7)
Sanz et al. 1989	Sweden	253	7 (2.8)
Wedlund et al. 1984	U.S.	156	4 (2.6)
Studies in Hispanics			
Lam et al. 1991	U.S.	22	1 (4.8)
Studies in African Americans			
Pollock et al. 1991	U.S.	27	5 (18.5)

tuitary hormones appear to be involved in the modulation of these enzymes (Gonzalez 1988; Gonzalez and Nebert 1990). Exposure to testosterone in the neonatal period is critical to the expression of the male-specific P450h isozyme (Dannan et al. 1986). Castration of a neonate completely abolishes its expression, while castration of an adult results in only a partial reduction; full expression can be restored by supplementation with testosterone (Gonzalez 1988; Gonzalez and Nebert 1990).

The female-specific P450i isozyme, although present in both sexes, displays a differential response to testosterone exposure during puberty; in females testosterone exposure results in expression, whereas in males it results in suppression (Dannan et al. 1986).

These sex-specific P450 isozymes (Mode et al. 1981; E. T. Morgan et al. 1985, 1986) are highly dependent on gender-specific patterns of growth hormone secretion—patterns determined by neonatal and adult exposure to androgens. These include the pulsatile configuration seen in males and the constant-excretion pattern of growth hormone seen in females (Jansson et al. 1985). The expression of the female-specific P450i isozyme's activities disappears in hypophysectomized female rats but was restored by continuous infusion of growth hormone (Kato et al. 1986). Similarly, in hypophysectomized male rats, the resultant decrease in P450h expression was reversed by periodic injection of growth hormone (E. T. Morgan et al. 1985, 1986).

Similar degrees of gender difference in the expression of cytochrome P450 have not been reported in humans. However, indirect evidence suggests that lesser degrees of difference do exist. Studies have reported that both propranolol and diazepam exhibit decreased clearance in women compared with men (MacLeod et al. 1979; Walle et al. 1992). The reduced clearance of propranolol in women was specifically linked to a decrease in the side-chain oxidation for which CYP_{mp} is responsible (Walle et al. 1992). Walle and colleagues (1992) noted that the administration of testosterone to women resulted in increased clearance, whereas the administration of ethinyl estradiol produced opposite results. Fagan et al. (1993) observed that the CYP_{mp}-dependent side-chain oxidation of propranolol increased in women who were also given estradiol. The results of the two studies not only demonstrate that human P450 isozymes are under hormonal control but also suggest that different metabolic patterns may exist for each sex (i.e., women would tend to favor metabolism via hydroxylation through the CYP2D6 system, whereas the CYP_{mp} system would predominate in men). Because the hydroxy metabolites of most tricyclic antidepressants (TCAs) are associated with more side effects than are the demethylated metabolites, this differential pattern of drug metabolism may have important clinical implications. For example, although the overall pharmacokinetics of TCAs such as imipramine have been shown to be similar in women and men, the efficacy and side-effect profiles of these TCAs could still be significantly influenced by sex—that is, women could have more hydroxyimipramine, which is associated with more side effects than desipramine (hydroxyimipramine and desipramine are metabolites of imipramine). In addition, given that substantial ethnic differences in the phenotypes of these enzymes also exist, a gender-ethnicity interaction may occur, leading to an even more exaggerated gender variation in the efficacy and side-effect profiles in certain ethnic groups.

Glucuronidation

As a major metabolic process in phase II of drug metabolism, glucuronidation involves the addition of a hydrophilic compound to make the drug more soluble in water and therefore easier to excrete in the urine. Glucuronidation and sulfation occur with a large number of drugs, and may represent a rate-limiting step for at least some of them, including cyproheptadine (Fischer et al. 1980), oxazepam (Vessman et al. 1973), codeine (Yue et al. 1989), morphine (Yeh 1975), and haloperidol (Someya et al. 1992). Ethnic differences are limited to a report that Chinese are less efficient than Caucasians in the glucuronidation of codeine (Yue et al. 1991). This finding is of special importance because studies in the literature have reported that Asians tend to require lower dosages of codeine yet experience more side effects (Lin et al. 1989). Gender variation in glucuronidation is limited to a report that men had significantly lower glucuronidation metabolic ratios than women (Yue et al. 1989) and the observation that paracetamol and clofibric acid glucuronidation was increased in women taking oral contraceptives (Miners et al. 1983; M. C. Mitchell et al. 1983).

Although these observations suggest that the enzymes responsible for glucuronidation may be polymorphic as well as being important in determining gender and ethnic differences in metabolism, the need for further research is evident.

Plasma Protein Binding

Another genetically determined factor in the pharmacokinetics of drugs is protein binding. Although various proteins as well as cells in the blood provide binding sites for psychotropics and other drugs, and thus function as carriers for these pharmacoactive agents, two categories of plasma proteins—α_1-acid glycoproteins (AAGs) (Baumann and Eap 1988; Kremer et al. 1988) and albumins (Kragh-Hansen 1981)—are generally regarded as the most important. Variations in the concentrations of these drug-binding proteins in the plasma can significantly influence the effect of the drug by changing the free fraction and thus the concentration of unbound (free) drug in the plasma (DeLeve and Piafsky 1981; R. H. Levy and Moreland 1984; Routledge 1986). Because only the free (unbound) fraction of the drugs is usually pharmacologically active and capable of crossing the blood-brain barrier, changes in the concentrations of drug-binding proteins may have profound clinical significance (Baumann and Eap 1991; Crabtree et al. 1991). AAG is a protein in blood that binds many basic compounds with high affinity and that also demonstrates isoenzyme variation. Drugs such as imipramine, chlorpromazine, fluphenazine, loxapine, thioridazine, thiothixene, carbamazepine, and triazolam have been shown to have higher affinity for this glycoprotein than for albumin (Borga et al. 1977; Kornguth et al. 1981; Kroboth et al. 1984; Piafsky et al. 1978). Of particular interest is the increased binding of nortriptyline, amitriptyline, and methadone to a particular S variant of the AAG (Eap et al. 1990; Tinguely et al. 1985).

Interethnic variation has been demonstrated in absolute levels of AAG (Zhou et al. 1990) as well as in distribution of its two variants, S (slow) and F (fast) (Eap and Baumann 1989; Montiel et al. 1990). The S variant of AAG is more efficient in binding with drugs. Population studies reveal that Asians have an S-variant frequency in the range of 15%–27%, whereas African Americans, and Caucasians in the United States and Europe, demonstrate a range of 34%–67%. Inuit People ("Eskimos") as well as Canadian and South American Indians have a frequency of 43%–45%, which is higher than that observed in Asians, while Indians from Mexico are reported to have a frequency of 54%. Information on gender variation in protein binding is sparse. One limited study by Wilkinson and Kurata (1974) suggested that in some circumstances the protein binding of drugs is decreased in women. During pregnancy, the binding of many drugs—including phenytoin and diazepam—is decreased (Adams and Wacher 1968; M. Dean et al. 1980; Ganrot 1972), with the greatest decrease noted during the third trimester (Perucca and Crema 1982). This decreased binding may in part be due to the decreased levels of albumin reported during pregnancy (Yoshikawa et al. 1984).

The concentrations of AAG are reported to vary with the menstrual period (Parish and Spivey 1991). Studies of the effect of oral contraceptives on AAG concentration reveal mixed results. One study of healthy women on oral contraceptives revealed no effect (Blain et al. 1985), whereas three other studies noted lower concentrations of AAG in oral contraceptive users (Routledge et al. 1981; Song et al. 1970; Walle et al. 1993).

It is presently unclear whether or not these qualitative and quantitative differences in AAG could lead to clinical effects. Theoretically, a woman from an ethnic group with a low frequency of the S variant, when pregnant or taking oral contraceptives, could be at risk of developing elevated levels of unbound drugs and resultant increases in side effects and toxicity. Thus far, very few cross-ethnic or cross-gender studies of plasma protein binding have been conducted. The need for more systematic research is apparent.

Acetylation

In addition to the cytochrome P450 system, acetylation is a major route of metabolism for a large number of pharmacoactive agents, including some frequently prescribed psychotropics (Lin et al. 1991; Mendoza et al. 1991) (see Table 7–4). Inherited in an autosomal recessive fashion (Lunde et al. 1977), the liver enzyme N-acetyltransferase also displays bimodal distribution of metabolic phenotypes—poor and extensive metabolizers (PMs and EMs). This phenomenon is important for several reasons: 1) when treated with drugs requiring acetylation, PMs are more likely than EMs to demonstrate improved responsiveness to phen-

Table 7–4.   Drugs subject to acetylation

Acebutolol	Hydralazine
p-aminobenzoic acid	Isoniazid
Aminoglutethimide	Nitrazepam
p-aminosalicylic acid	Phenelzine
Amrinone	Prizidilol
Caffeine	Procainamide
Clonazepam	Sulfadiazine
Dapsone	Sulfamerazine
Dipyrone	Sulfamethazine
Endralazine	Sulfapyridine

elzine, hydralazine, and isoniazid; 2) when treated with drugs requiring acetylation, PMs are at higher risk of developing drug-induced systemic lupus erythematosus, hypersensitivity reactions, polyneuropathy, drowsiness, and nausea from phenelzine (Rieder et al. 1991); and 3) poor metabolizing is a significant risk factor for the development of a number of malignant conditions (Weber 1987). At present, acetylation status and its relevance to health and diseases represents an active area of research (Weber 1987).

Ethnicity is an important factor in determining acetylation status. The frequency of PMs in most Western populations ranges from 38% to greater than 50% (Grant et al. 1990; Weber and Hein 1985), while poor metabolizing rates for Japanese, Chinese, Koreans, and Inuit are in the range of 5%—15% (Dufour et al. 1964; Grant et al. 1983). Recent studies have indicated that the Cuna and Ngawbe Guaymi Amerindians have similarly low rates of PMs for acetylation (Inaba and Arias 1987).

Gender also appears to affect the rate of acetylation, although its effects have rarely been the focus of research. Iselius and Evans (1983) reported that women had higher isoniazid plasma levels than men when treated with equivalent doses of the medication, and several recent studies have indicated that women responded better to phenelzine than did men (Davidson and Pelton 1986; Raskin 1974). The extent and mechanism of such a proposed gender influence on acetylation remain to be further explored.

Alcohol Metabolism

Although not directly involved in the biotransformation of psycho-tropics, the enzymes responsible for the metabolism of alcohol—namely, alcohol dehydrogenase (ADH) and aldehyde dehydrogenase (ALDH)—represent classic examples of how ethnicity influences the metabolism of xenobiotics. In addition, recent studies have demon-strated that gender also plays a significant role in the metabolism of alcohol. Not only is research in this area important for understanding ethnic and gender differences in alcohol-related conditions, but it also points to possible future research directions, including identification of the gene(s) that may be responsible for the development of alcoholism and study of the metabolism of endogenous neurotransmitters, some of which are biotransformed by these two enzyme systems (Agarwal and Goedde 1990; Agarwal et al. 1982).

Ethnicity and Alcohol Metabolism

Racial differences in alcohol sensitivity among Asians and Caucasians have long been recognized. Wolff (1972, 1973) observed that more than 80% of Asians and about 50% of American Indians were alcohol sensi-tive ("alcohol flushers"), whereas less than 10% of Caucasians exhibited alcohol flushing. Blood acetaldehyde level, but not alcohol level, is sub-stantially higher in alcohol-sensitive individuals than in nonsensitive ones (Mizoi et al. 1979). The alcohol sensitivity seen in Asians has now been proven to be due to the genetic differences of alcohol-metabolizing enzymes. Since ALDH plays a major role in determining this phenom-enon, we review it first. To a lesser extent, ADH activities also contribute to ethnic differences in alcohol responses, and we discuss these at the end of this section.

Several ALDH isozymes have been identified (Yoshida et al. 1991). Cytosolic liver $ALDH_1$ and mitochondrial liver $ALDH_2$, which exhibit high activity for the oxidation of acetaldehyde, are considered to play a major role in acetaldehyde detoxification in the liver. $ALDH_1$ is activated only when acetaldehyde concentration reaches significantly high levels, and thus is not as efficient as ALDH$_2$ in the elimination of this potentially toxic substance.

Approximately 50% of Asians lack ALDH$_2$ activity in their livers. The deficiency is due to the genomic mutation in the *ALDH$_2$* locus (L. C. Hsu et al. 1985; Yoshida et al. 1984). The frequency of the variant *ALDH$_2$^{2}* gene is about 30% in Japanese and null (or very low) in Caucasians (Shibuya and Yoshida 1988). Both heterozygous *ALDH$_2$^{1}/ ALDH$_2$^{2}* and homozygous atypical *ALDH$_2$^{2}/ALDH$_2$^{2}* individuals lack ALDH$_2$ activity in their livers (i.e., the variant *ALDH$_2$^{2}* gene is dominant in the expression of enzyme activity) (Table 7–3).

The most remarkable genomic difference between alcohol flushers and nonflushers, and between alcoholic patients and nonalcoholic control subjects, is in the frequency of the wild-type (usual) *ALDH$_2$^{1}* and the atypical Asian-type *ALDH$_2$^{2}* genes. Virtually all Japanese alcohol flushers are either heterozygous *ALDH$_2$^{1}/ALDH$_2$^{2}* or homozygous atypical *ALDH$_2$^{2}/ALDH$_2$^{2}* at the *ALDH$_2$* locus, and conversely, most patients with alcoholic liver diseases are homozygous usual *ALDH$_1$^{1}/ ALDH$_1$^{1}*. Yoshida et al. (1989) concluded that Japanese with genotypes *ALDH$_2$^{1}/ALDH$_2$^{2}* or *ALDH$_2$^{2}/ALDH$_2$^{2}* are alcohol sensitive, cannot drink large amounts of alcohol, and do not have a strong alcohol-seeking tendency. Consequently, these individuals are at low risk of developing alcoholic liver diseases. Harada (1990) and Thomasson et al. (1991) examined the genotypes of the *ALDH$_2$* locus of Japanese and Chinese alcoholic individuals and confirmed this conclusion.

In addition to ethnic variations in the genotypes of ALDH$_2$, there also are clear ethnic differences in ADH activities. The frequency of the wild-type (usual) *ADH$_2$^{1}* gene exceeds 90% in Caucasians but is only about 30% in Asians, whereas the atypical *ADH$_2$^{2}* gene is more common (70%) in Asians. Another atypical gene, *ADH$_2$^{3}*, is fairly common in blacks. Two common genes, the wild-type *ADH$_3$^{1}* gene and the variant *ADH$_3$^{2}* gene, are commonly found in Caucasians, while the frequency of the variant gene is low in Asians. Some of these variants, especially the Asian-type *ADH$_2$^{2}* gene, are more efficient in converting alcohol into acetaldehyde and thus contribute to the accumulation of this substance. This trait is particularly problematic if it is combined with a deficiency in ALDH activity (genotypes *ALDH$_2$^{1}/ALDH$_2$^{2}* or *ALDH$_2$^{2}/ ALDH$_2$^{2}*).

Gender and Alcohol Metabolism

A number of animal studies have suggested that alcohol metabolism differs between males and females (C. J. P. Eriksson 1973; K. Eriksson and Malmstrom 1967; J. R. Wilson et al. 1984) and that hormonal influences are involved in modulating these differences (A. C. Collins et al. 1975; Rachamin et al. 1980). Although similar research in humans has produced inconsistent results (Cole-Harding and Wilson 1987), genetics is felt to play an important role. It is known that women are more susceptible to alcoholic liver injury than are men. Frezza et al. (1990) reported that a significantly larger amount of ethanol was metabolized in the stomachs of men, and that ADH activity of stomach mucous membranes is substantially higher in men than in women. Yasunami et al. (1991) recently cloned and characterized the *ADH6* gene and found that the enzyme produced by the gene exhibits class II ADH characteristics, is expressed in the stomach, and has a hormone-responsive element. The resultant increased amount of alcohol available for absorption (due to the decreased ADH activity) and the decreased volume of distribution in women could potentially explain the higher peak blood alcohol level (BAL) observed in this gender group (Cyr and Moulton 1993). This increased BAL may in part explain why women, especially Native American and African American women, show an increased susceptibility to alcoholic liver disease even with a shorter duration of heavy drinking (Halliday and Bush 1987).

Conclusion

Pharmacogenetics is a relatively new and rapidly expanding field. Although much remains unclarified, the available literature does indicate that definitive differences exist among ethnic groups in a number of important drug-metabolizing enzyme systems as well as in the plasma proteins involved in drug binding.

Even less is known about the influence of gender on pharmacogenetics. However, certain trends are beginning to emerge. First, hormonal regulation appears to play an important role in modulating the function of the cytochrome P450 and the alcohol-metabolizing enzyme systems, as well as in determining the concentration of AAG. Second, at least in animals, there exist critical periods in neurodevelopment during which exposure to hormones determines later expression.

In addition to the separate effects of many drugs, the potential for interactive effects exists. Clinically, this potential is important because it alerts us to the possibility that women from certain ethnic groups may be at increased risk of developing side effects and toxicity due to genetically determined differences in drug metabolism that are related to both ethnicity and gender. Progress in this area will not only allow us to provide dosage guidelines that are rationally and empirically based, but will also further our understanding of the basic mechanisms regulating drug activity and metabolism. To ensure continuing progress in this regard, it is important that future pharmacological researchers pay special attention to the ethnicity, gender, and hormonal status of their research subjects.

Section II

The Life Cycle and Psychopharmacology of Women

Nonpregnant Reproductive-Age Women

Part I: The Menstrual Cycle and Psychopharmacology

Margaret F. Jensvold, M.D.

Women who present for help with psychiatric symptoms related to the menstrual cycle often "fall through the cracks" in current medical care, with psychiatrists tending to know little about the menstrual cycle and gynecologists tending to have little training in or time needed to deal with emotions and behavior. In addition, the menstrual cycle has traditionally been used as justification for excluding women from drug studies rather than being seen as a legitimate subject of scientific study. Because the menstrual cycle has been relatively understudied as an influential factor in pharmacology, answers to many pertinent questions posed by patients are not yet available. However, enough is known to make it clear that the menstrual cycle affects the expression of some women's psychiatric symptoms and influences the need for or response to psychotropic medication, or both.

This chapter and Chapter 9 provide a conceptual framework for understanding and summarize what is known about the influence of the menstrual cycle and exogenous sex steroid hormones on psychotropic drugs in reproductive-age women. This chapter focuses on the normal menstrual cycle and its effects on psychopathology and on psychopharmacological agents. Chapter 9 describes exogenous sex steroid hormonal agents, including psychological side effects and their management, use of reproductive hormonal agents to treat psychiatric conditions, and interactions between contraceptive agents and psychotropic drugs.

The Normal Menstrual Cycle

Reproductive age lasts from puberty (menarche occurs at about age 12) to the menopause, which occurs on average at about age 51 years. The "second transition"—that from reproductive age to menopause—has been described as occurring over approximately a 10-year period, starting after about age 35, with the earliest changes being subtle and imperceptible. *Perimenopause* has not been uniformly defined. The American College of Obstetricians and Gynecologists (ACOG) defines perimenopause as a 5-year period occurring around menopause, whereas the World Health Organization criteria view it as a 10-year period (Grimes 1993).

Menstrual cycles typically range from about 25 to 30 days in length. The follicular phase, during which there is growth of the oocyte in the follicle, lasts 12–16 days, and the luteal phase, named for the corpus luteum, the sac that remains in the ovary after the follicle ruptures at ovulation and the oocyte is released, lasts 10–16 days (Marshall and Odell 1989). Luteal-phase length tends to be constant within the individual (Baird 1989), with follicular-phase length being variable. Menstrual cycle length tends to decrease slightly as the woman becomes older, by an average of 1–2 days, due to shortening of the follicular phase with age (Treloar et al. 1967). As premenstrual syndrome (PMS) researchers well know, some intercycle variability in cycle characteristics or associated symptoms (e.g., cycle length, breast tenderness) is typical.

Markedly irregular menstrual cycles may occur for 12–18 months after menarche, suggesting that it may take some time for the new hormonal interrelationships to be established (Marshall and Odell 1989). Anovulatory cycles are considered normal at puberty and in the late perimenopausal phase.

Between puberty and the perimenopause, occasional, infrequent anovulatory cycles may occur without being disruptive to the general pattern of menses; these are not considered abnormal. Abnormalities of ovulation and/or uterine bleeding may likewise occur, presenting as primary or secondary amenorrhea, oligomenorrhea, menorrhagia, or menometrorrhagia.

The Brain–Reproductive System Relationship

When considering the menstrual cycle, many people tend to think only of the ovaries and uterus. The brain, however, is equally important if not more so. The brain can be thought of as orchestrating the responses of the ovary and uterus. The hypothalamic-pituitary-ovarian axis is an integrally interconnected feedback loop, with suprahypothalamic input and hormones produced in the periphery feeding back upon the brain. The uterus is the end organ whose cyclical shedding provides an external marker that yet another cycle is beginning.[1] The uterus also releases prostaglandins and other hormones.

Figures 8–1, 8–2, and 8–3 depict key events of the menstrual cycle. The hypothalamus releases gonadotropin-releasing hormone (GnRH) into the pituitary portal system. GnRH stimulates the pituitary to release the gonadotropins, luteinizing hormone (LH), and follicle-stimulating hormone (FSH). The gonadotropins act upon the ovaries, stimulating them to produce estrogen and progesterone, which feed back upon the brain in addition to affecting other organs.

---

[1] *Shedding* and *sloughing* are among the traditional terms used to describe the menstrual cycle. E. Martin (1992) provides a critique of traditional language and suggests alternatives, such as "a drop in [hormone levels] creates the environment for reducing excess layers of endometrial tissue" (p. 52).

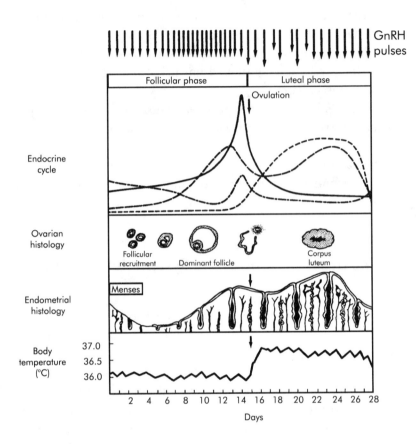

Figure 8–1. Schematic representation of alterations in gonadotropin-releasing hormone (GnRH) secretion and the relationship to gonadotropin and sex steroid hormone, ovarian, endometrial, and basal body temperature changes during the normal menstrual cycle. The arrows represent pulses of GnRH release. The length of an arrow indicates the amount of GnRH secreted, and the distance between arrows represents pulse intervals. E_2 = estradiol; FSH = follicle-stimulating hormone; LH = luteinizing hormone; P = progesterone. *Source.* Reprinted with permission from Carr B, Wilson J: Disorders of the ovary and female reproductive tract, in *Harrison's Principles of Internal Medicine.* Edited by Brunwald E, Isselbacher K, Petersdorf R, et al: New York, McGraw-Hill, 1989, p. 1823; and from Marshall J, Odell W: The menstrual cycle—hormonal regulation, mechanisms of anovulation, and responses of the reproductive tract to steroid hormones, in *Endocrinology.* Edited by DeGroot L, Besser G, Marshall J, et al. Philadelphia, PA, WB Saunders, 1989, p. 1945.

Pulsatile release of hormones is now recognized to be ubiquitous in human physiology. Pulsatile release of GnRH by the hypothalamus is key to the functioning of the reproductive system (Figure 8–1). Changes in GnRH pulsatility drive the dramatic physiological changes occurring at menarche and menopause (Figure 8–3). Changes in GnRH/LH pulse frequency also distinguish ovulation and the follicular and luteal phases of the menstrual cycle (Figure 8–1).

GnRH pulses in the pituitary portal system are not yet directly measurable in humans. However, the frequency and/or amplitude of LH pulses measured in the periphery are thought to accurately reflect pulsatile release of GnRH by the hypothalamus (Marshall and Odell 1989). LH pulses during the early follicular phase have a constant amplitude and a frequency of 1–2 hours. LH pulses during the luteal phase have a more variable amplitude and a frequency of 2–6 hours (Reame et al. 1984). Hypothalamic neurons that produce GnRH have an intrinsic ability to release GnRH in a pulsatile manner. The inherent pattern can be modified, however, by gonadal steroids and other factors (Kalra and Kalra 1983).

The endogenous time clock driving the system is not fully understood in humans. What is known is that "the essential features of the [time clock] system include a modulatory mechanism consisting of opioid peptide and catecholamine-secreting neurons interposed between the suprahypothalamic 'neural clock' and the GnRH secretory neurons. These mechanisms regulate the function of the GnRH neurons, 'the pattern generator' " (Kalra and Kalra 1983, p. 341). Hypothalamic cells in tissue culture retain the ability to release GnRH in a regular pulsatile fashion, suggesting that the hypothalamic cells constitute the endogenous pulse generator. How the hypothalamic cells come to change their functioning dramatically at puberty and at menopause is not well understood but is thought to be in great part genetically determined.

Considerable animal research documents that the extrahypothalamic central nervous system (CNS) may exert influence on reproductive functioning. Suprahypothalamic input to the hypothalamus includes endorphins, norepinephrine, epinephrine, and dopamine. As a generalization, catecholamines, epinephrine, and norepinephrine tend to *increase* GnRH release, whereas β-endorphins *decrease* GnRH

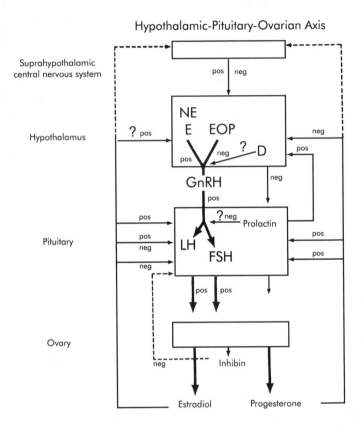

Hypothalamic-Pituitary-Ovarian Axis

Figure 8–2. Schematic representation of the hormones and feedback control mechanisms in the hypothalamic-pituitary-ovarian axis. *Solid lines* indicate established and *dotted lines* putative regulatory pathways. *Pos* indicates stimulatory and *neg* inhibitory regulation. D = dopamine; E = epinephrine; EOP = endogenous opioid peptides; FSH = follicle-stimulating hormone; GnRH = gonadotropin-releasing hormone; LH = luteinizing hormone; NE = norepinephrine.

Source. Reprinted with permission from Marshall J: Regulation of gonadotropin secretion, in *Endocrinology.* Edited by DeGroot L, Besser G, Marshall J, et al. Philadelphia, PA, WB Saunders, 1989, p. 1904.

release by their action on the hypothalamus (Marshall 1989). In fact, the situation is more complicated. For example, norepinephrine's effects ap-

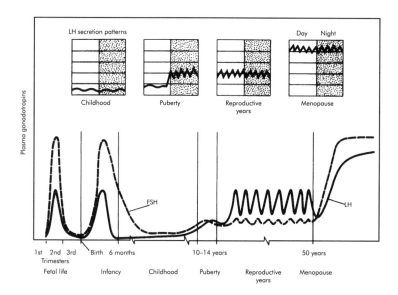

Figure 8–3. Pattern of gonadotropin secretion during different stages of life in women. FSH = follicle-stimulating hormone; LH = luteinizing hormone. The secretory patterns of LH during the waking hours (*clear area*) and at night (*stippled area*) for each stage are indicated in the upper insets.
Source. Reprinted with permission from Carr B, Wilson J: Disorders of the ovary and female reproductive tract, in *Harrison's Principles of Internal Medicine.* Edited by Brunwald E, Isselbacher K, Petersdorf R, et al: New York, McGraw-Hill, 1989, p. 1819, after Faiman et al. 1976.

pear to be dependent on the presence of ovarian steroids, especially estradiol. In steroid-primed rats, epinephrine is more potent than norepinephrine in stimulating GnRH and LH release, but in ovariectomized animals, epinephrine has no effect on LH secretion. This evidence suggests that epinephrine may play a role in the ovulatory surge (Kalra and Gallo 1983). Dopamine's effect on LH secretion is less clear (Marshall 1989).

Serotonin receptor levels have been shown to undergo regular changes during the estrous cycle in the basal forebrain and hippocampus of the rat. There was no effect of the estrous cycle on serotonin receptors in the cortex and caudate (Biegon et al. 1980).

In humans, blood serotonin levels fell during the mid- and late-luteal phases of women with premenstrual mood changes, but not in asymptomatic regularly cycling women (Rapkin et al. 1987).

Belmaker and colleagues (1974) found that human platelet monoamine oxidase (MAO), a major enzyme catabolizing brain biogenic amines, peaked during the ovulatory interval and reached a nadir 5–11 days later. Mood reported retrospectively showed no correlation with the platelet MAO levels (Belmaker et al. 1974). Poirier et al. (1985) found conflicting results, reporting a *decrease* in platelet MAO activity in the ovulatory phase.

Plasma free tryptophan was found to change during women's menstrual cycles (Wirz-Justice et al. 1975), and plasma free tryptophan levels correlated with plasma concentrations of estrogens. However, kinetic parameters of serotonin uptake in platelets did not vary with menstrual cycle stage in women (Wirz-Justice and Chappuis-Arndt 1976).

In the past decade, researchers have discovered "neurohormones"—endogenous hormones in the brain. For example, progesterone and progesterone-related compounds and metabolites produced by neurons in the brain act upon CNS gamma-aminobutyric acid (GABA) receptors (Majewska 1992; Majewska et al. 1986). This discovery has significant ramifications for drug development.

Research suggests a possible mechanism for intraindividual cycle variability. Pheromones, chemical signals that exert their influence via olfactory input to CNS pathways, may play a role. "Positive" pheromones, which phase-advance the estrus cycle, and "negative" pheromones, which phase-delay the cycle, have been documented to exist in mammals (McClintock 1987). Computer models of the competing effects of phase advance– and phase delay–type pheromones predict irregularities in the menstrual cycles of humans, with cycle-to-cycle variability being necessary to maintain overall stability of the system (Schank and McClintock 1992).

A variety of *ultradian* rhythms (< 24 hours; period length may be seconds, minutes, or hours) and *infradian* rhythms (> 24 hours in period length) interact. Terms for monthly rhythms include *catamenial* (of or related to menses) and *circatrigintan* (about 30 days). "Rhythms in the gonadotropic axis cover a wide range of frequencies, from ultrafast oscillations of plasma LH levels occurring at intervals of a few minutes, to episodic release in the circhoral [hourly] range, to diurnal [daily] rhythmicity, and finally to monthly and seasonal cycles. These various rhythms interact to provide a coordinated temporal program governing the development of the reproductive axis and its operation at every stage of maturation" (Van Cauter and Aschoff 1989, p. 2670). Considerable research demonstrates that gonadal steroids play a role in the regulation of circadian rhythms in animals; in humans the interrelationships are, for the most part, still being elucidated (Liebenluft 1993).

Physiological Changes
Over the Menstrual Cycle

The gonadotropins LH and FSH appear to act fairly specifically upon the ovaries, fallopian tubes, and uterus. In contrast, the sex steroid hormones, estrogen and progesterone, act upon many organs, perhaps most organs of the body (Marshall and Odell 1989; Southam and Gonzaga 1965).

Many systemic factors vary in a circadian manner (e.g., thyroid-stimulating hormone, cortisol, body temperature), often with the person unaware of the changes. Similarly, many systemic factors have been shown to fluctuate over the course of the menstrual cycle (Southam and Gonzaga 1965), often with the woman unaware of the changes.

A partial list of systemic factors that have been shown to vary during the menstrual cycle includes pulse, blood pressure, respiration, weight, mucus cytology, gastrointestinal transit time (Southam and Gonzaga 1965), urinary excretion (Christy and Shaver 1974), arteriolar responsiveness to hormones and catecholamines (Altura 1975), heme catabolism (Mercke and Lundh 1976), and oxytocin (M. D. Mitchell et al. 1981; see also Chapter 2).

Psychopathological Changes
and the Menstrual Cycle

With many physiological factors varying during the menstrual cycle, it is not surprising that many medical conditions vary over the course of the menstrual cycle in at least a subgroup of reproductive-age women who have the conditions. Examples are acute porphyria (Herrick et al. 1990), irritable bowel syndrome (Whitehead et al. 1990), systemic lupus erythematosus (Morley et al. 1982), cyclic premenstrual unconjugated hyperbilirubinemia (Yamaguchi et al. 1975), genital herpes, and migraine headaches. In about 60% of reproductive-age women who have migraine headaches, migraines occur in relation to the menstrual cycle. Menstrual migraines appear to be associated with the rapid drop in estrogen premenstrually (Sheftell et al. 1992; Silberstein and Merriam 1993). Why migraines recur in relation to the menstrual cycle in some regularly menstruating migrainous women and independently of the menstrual cycle in others is not known.

Some psychiatric conditions vary over the course of the menstrual cycle in subgroups of women with the conditions (Jensvold 1993a). A number of cases of periodic psychosis or catamenial psychosis—recurrent episodes of psychosis occurring premenstrually or during menses—have been reported (F. Berlin et al. 1982; Brockington et al. 1988; Hatotani et al. 1983). In some, the condition has responded to medroxyprogesterone (Depo-Provera) after failing to respond to other treatments (F. Berlin et al. 1982; Leetz et al. 1988).

In one study (Jensvold and Putnam 1990), both women with prospectively confirmed premenstrual mood symptoms and control women without menstrual cycle–related symptoms had high prevalences of histories of abuse. Patients had somewhat more severe histories of abuse—including significantly more severe abuse and severe physical abuse—than control subjects but comparable sexual abuse. Patients also had a significantly higher lifetime prevalence of posttraumatic stress disorder (PTSD), a longer course of PTSD when it did occur, and more current PTSD. Some patients' symptoms were expressed in relation to the menstrual cycle, constituting menstrual cycle–related PTSD or menstrual cycle–related dissociative disorders.

The initial onset of obsessive-compulsive disorder (OCD) in women has a bimodal peak, with one peak occurring around the time of menarche and the other occurring in the women's 20s, around the peak time of childbearing. Some women experience initial onset of OCD during the postpartum period, and some report premenstrual worsening of OCD symptoms (M. F. Jensvold, unpublished data, April 1989) or trichotillomania (M. F. Jensvold, unpublished data, March 1990).

Premenstrual Dysphoric Disorder

Most women are asymptomatic or minimally or mildly symptomatic with respect to their menstrual cycles. The term *molimina* refers to common, mild symptoms occurring premenstrually that herald the approach of menses but that are not particularly bothersome and are considered normal—including, for example, fatigue and mild breast discomfort. Surveys indicate that at least 75% of women claim to experience one or more symptoms related to their menstrual cycles, although only a small proportion consider the symptoms to be severe or say they would seek treatment for them (C. Wood et al. 1979). Psychological symptoms are often considered to be the most bothersome (Scambler and Scambler 1986).

The concept of "PMS" has an extensive literature that has been discussed at length elsewhere (e.g., Gise 1988; Jensvold 1993a; Severino and Moline 1989). Although space does not allow a full discussion of PMS and the controversy surrounding it, a brief review of the history of the term may be helpful.

When Robert Frank coined the term *premenstrual tension* (PMT) in 1931, he assigned a narrow definition, referring to a severe disorder of primarily psychological symptoms occurring only premenstrually, with relief with onset of menses. Frank specified that PMT is different from systemic illnesses that vary with the menstrual cycle, such as catamenial asthma and catamenial epilepsy, and different from molimina, the mild symptoms occurring premenstrually that are not abnormal (R. Frank 1931).

Over the course of the next few decades, more and more symptoms were added to the definition, culminating in Katharina Dalton's broad definition of PMS as including any symptom varying in any regular manner over the course of the menstrual cycle (Dalton 1977). Even asthma and seizures occurring in regular relation to the menstrual cycle were considered to be symptoms of PMS. This "wastebasket" definition of PMS had popular appeal but contributed to a lack of clarity in conceptualizing menstrual cycle symptomatology that still affects popular and professional thought today.

The *Diagnostic and Statistical Manual, Third Edition, Revised* (DSM-III-R; American Psychiatric Association 1987), in its appendix of conditions requiring further study, recognized a condition with primarily psychological symptoms, occurring only premenstrually with relief with onset of menses, and meeting a severity criterion. The name *late luteal phase dysphoric disorder* (LLPDD) was assigned, and the condition was listed as being a "disorder not otherwise specified"—meaning that it was not identified as being a subtype of any other disorder or class of disorders.

In DSM-IV (American Psychiatric Association 1994), the name of the condition was changed from LLPDD to *premenstrual dysphoric disorder* (PMDD), and the condition was listed in the body of the text as being a subtype of "depressive disorder not otherwise specified"—that is, a subtype of depression. In addition to being listed in the text, PMDD remains in the DSM's appendix of conditions requiring further study (American Psychiatric Association 1993).

The DSM notwithstanding, the research and clinical question still remains whether it is most accurate to consider severe cases of what is colloquially called "PMS" to be a type of affective disorder or whether there exists a unique premenstrual disorder of primarily psychological symptoms, separate from any other category of psychological disorders.

What is clear is that in studies of lifetime psychiatric histories, women meeting criteria for PMS/PMDD have a greater lifetime history of depression compared with women without PMS/PMDD (S. Diamond et al. 1976; Endicott et al. 1981; Halbreich and Endicott 1985b; Kashiwagi et al. 1976; McMillan and Pihl 1987). Complaints of premenstrual depression have been found to have predictive value regarding future depression (Schuckit et al. 1975). Individual women presenting with menstrual cycle–related depressive symptoms may experience major depression, dysthymia with premenstrual worsening, depressive symptoms occurring premenstrually only, and euthymia at different times, demonstrating a dynamic course to their affective symptoms (Jensvold et al. 1992). A number of tricyclic antidepressants (TCAs), MAO inhibitors (MAOIs), and selective serotonin reuptake inhibitors (SSRIs) have each been reported to successfully treat menstrual cycle–related depressive symptoms (Jensvold et al. 1992), with clomipramine (E. Eriksson et al. 1994) and fluoxetine (Freeman and Rickels 1994; Stone et al. 1990) having been documented in controlled trials to successfully treat premenstrual psychological and physical symptoms. In the study by E. Eriksson and colleagues (1994), clomipramine (a serotonergic drug) was significantly more effective in alleviating premenstrual symptoms than either maprotiline (a noradrenergic drug) or placebo; maprotiline and placebo were comparable.

The proposal has been made that a designation of "menstrual cycle pattern" be added to the DSM to denote psychiatric conditions that vary with the menstrual cycle (Jensvold et al. 1992). This would be similar to the DSM's designation of "seasonal pattern" for seasonal affective disorder. Thus, a patient whose panic disorder worsened premenstrually could be diagnosed as having "panic disorder, menstrual cycle pattern."

Psychopharmacology and the Menstrual Cycle

With physiological factors and pathophysiological entities varying over the course of the menstrual cycle, it would be expected that the menstrual cycle would influence psychopharmacological agents. The need for and the metabolism, benefits, and side effects of some drugs vary with menstrual cycle phase in reproductive-age women or in subgroups of these women.

Menstrual Cycle Effects on Psychopharmacological Agents

Findings of studies of psychoactive drugs investigated in relation to the menstrual cycle are detailed in the appendix to this chapter. Additional considerations are discussed below.

Alcohol.   As seen in the appendix, evidence is conflicting regarding menstrual cycle phase effects on alcohol consumption, metabolism, and self-estimates of alcohol blood levels. Sutker et al.'s (1987a, 1987b) studies, which found lower blood alcohol levels (BALs) and increased alcohol clearance in the midluteal phase compared with the early follicular and ovulatory phases with test doses of alcohol, were among the better-controlled studies of effects of menstrual cycle phase on alcohol metabolism. Brick et al. (1986) reported that menstrual cycle phase altered alcohol absorption rate and peak BAL in studies in which dosing of subjects was done by total body weight rather than by water weight. When doses were calculated by body water weight, differences in BAL between men and women were not found (Brick et al. 1986).

Anticonvulsants.   A considerable range exists (10%–70%) in the proportions of epileptic women whose symptoms have been found to increase in the premenstrual or menstrual phase. A study of 7,000 seizures occurring over 1,200 menstrual cycles found a premenstrual association in two-thirds of patients (Rosciszewska et al. 1986).

Serum anticonvulsant levels decreased much more markedly during menses in women with catamenial epilepsy (Kumar et al. 1988; Rosciszewska et al. 1986; Shavit et al. 1984) than in women with noncatamenial epilepsy (Shavit et al. 1984) or in control women (Kumar et al. 1988).

Antidepressant medications.   In an open-trial study (Jensvold et al. 1992) of antidepressant treatment in women whose depressive symptoms varied during the menstrual cycle, three-fourths received adequate relief of their symptoms with constant dosing, whereas one-fourth required variable dosing (low dose early in the cycle, higher dose later) for optimal results. Another study (E. Eriksson et al. 1994) found that three dosing regimens of clomipramine—constant/continuous dosing, intermittent dosing (× 14 days premenstrually only), and variable dosing (very low maintenance dose in first half of cycle, higher dose × 14 days premenstrually)—each adequately treated patients' PMS symptoms; variable dosing was concluded to have some advantages over either constant/continuous dosing or intermittent dosing.

Whether additional benefit to patients from variable dosing compared with constant dosing derives from pharmacokinetic or pharmacodynamic factors is not definitively known. There are several reports of antidepressant medication blood levels being lower premenstrually with constant dosing or constant when medication doses were raised premenstrually. In one case each, serum trazodone and desipramine levels were lower premenstrually than postmenstrually on constant dosing (Kimmel et al. 1992); in one case, variable dosing of nortriptyline over the menstrual cycle kept blood levels relatively constant (within the therapeutic window) (Jensvold et al. 1992). These few reports suggest that pharmacokinetic changes may occur with at least some antidepressant medications during the menstrual cycles of at least some women.

In contrast, in a larger, controlled study of 40 women with PMS taking fluoxetine or placebo, the fluoxetine levels of 27 subjects were measured twice during the menstrual cycle (D. E. Stewart et al. 1994). No significant differences were found in fluoxetine or norfluoxetine levels in the midfollicular phase compared with late luteal phase with constant fluoxetine dosing. The absence of significant net pharmacokinetic changes in fluoxetine over the time frame of the menstrual cycle is not surprising; fluoxetine's long half-life alone may be responsible for lack of significant differences between blood levels in the follicular and luteal phases. In light of the apparent absence of significant pharmacokinetic differences in fluoxetine over the menstrual cycle, the fact that some patients report marked symptomatic improvements with variable fluoxetine dosing compared with constant dosing (Jensvold et al. 1992) suggests a role for pharmacodynamic changes (e.g., differences in receptor populations or sensitivities) over the course of the menstrual cycle for fluoxetine for some patients. Blood levels of antidepressant medications across the menstrual cycle in asymptomatic women have not, to our knowledge, been studied.

A variety of studies in animals and humans demonstrate a number of mechanisms by which antidepressant medications may have varied pharmacodynamic effects or varied metabolism during the course of the menstrual cycle. Animal research suggests that CNS receptor responses to some antidepressant medications are dependent, in part, on the sex steroid hormonal state of the animal (D. Kendall et al. 1982; M. A. Wilson et al. 1989). Estradiol and progesterone affected the concentration and affinity of imipramine binding sites in the hypothalamus but not the cortex of female rats (M. A. Wilson et al. 1989).

In 10 young women without a personal or family history of mental illness, measures of binding (B_{max}) and dissociation (K_D) of imipramine to high-affinity imipramine binding sites on platelets were not significantly modified by the menstrual cycle (Poirier et al. 1986).

In a study of 5 women, binding to α_2-adrenoceptors and imipramine receptors in intact lymphocytes was unchanged during the menstrual cycle, whereas the number of β_2-adrenoceptor sites on intact lymphocytes varied cyclically (Stowell et al. 1988).

In a study of women with premenstrual mood changes and control subjects, serotonin uptake and imipramine receptor binding in platelets were measured in the nonsymptomatic early luteal phase and the symptomatic late luteal phase. Larger interindividual variability was found in the late luteal phase. In contrast, in the early luteal phase, imipramine receptor binding was lower in patients compared with control subjects. This finding suggested the possibility of a "pre-existent vulnerability to the development of premenstrual dysphoric changes that might be related to impaired gonadal hormone modulation of the serotonergic system" (Rojansky et al. 1991, p. 169). Abnormalities occurring in the early luteal phase may have predisposed to late luteal serotonergic instability and symptoms.

Changes were found to occur in MAO, the catecholamine-catabolizing enzyme, over the menstrual cycle (Belmaker et al. 1974).

Buspirone.   Buspirone is an azaspirodecanedione antianxiety agent. The prolactin response to buspirone varied with menstrual cycle phase in healthy females (Dinan et al. 1990). The mechanism of the prolactin response to buspirone may be related to buspirone's activity as a serotonin-1A (5-HT$_{1A}$) agonist or may be partially or completely due to buspirone's dopaminergic activity (Dinan et al. 1990). Why the prolactin response to buspirone varied with menstrual cycle phase is not known.

Mood stabilizers.   Two well-documented cases indicated that serum lithium levels vary in relation to the menstrual cycle in some women with catamenial bipolar symptoms (Conrad and Hamilton 1986; Kukopulos et al. 1985). The changes in serum lithium levels with menstrual cycle phase in these women may be more related to changes in pathophysiology than to normal physiological changes over the menstrual cycle; in six asymptomatic women, lithium levels remained constant over the menstrual cycle (Chamberlain et al. 1990), whereas in bipolar patients followed longitudinally, serum lithium levels were increased during depression and decreased during mania (Hakim and Pichot 1972; Kukopulos and Reginaldi 1978). How bipolar illness becomes entrained to the menstrual cycle in some patients (Conrad and Hamilton 1986; Kukopulos et al. 1985) but not in others (Wehr et al. 1988) is not known.

Propranolol.   Propranolol had increased apparent clearance at the time of onset of menses in one woman with catamenial migraine (Gengo et al. 1984). It has been speculated that variability in one or more of propranolol's partial metabolic pathways may contribute to the change in clearance over the menstrual cycle. Walle et al. (1989, 1992, 1993) found sex differences in two of three metabolic pathways for propranolol. Propranolol clearance was greater in men compared with women for metabolism via the P450-mediated oxidative side chain (137% greater in men) and for glucuronidation (52%). No sex differences were found for P450-mediated ring oxidation of propranolol. Female subjects were tested in the second week of the menstrual cycle.

Summary.   It is not known why the symptoms of some women who have various conditions—including unipolar depression, bipolar disorder, migraine headaches, and seizure disorders—vary in relation to the menstrual cycle and the symptoms of other reproductive-age women with the same conditions do not. We hypothesize that pharmacogenetic differences may distinguish subsets of women, with subgroups of women having inherited different proportions of metabolizing enzymes, or isozymes, which may in turn differentially interact with different inherited (or acquired) predispositions to pathophysiological conditions. Metabolic pathways may be differentially affected by the fluctuating sex steroid hormones during the menstrual cycle. Central neurotransmitters or CNS receptor numbers or sensitivity may vary between subgroups of women for a variety of reasons, accounting for differences in need for or responsiveness to medications in subgroups of women. We hypothesize that the brain's endogenous time clock, which influences the periphery via the hypothalamic-pituitary-gonadal axis and is known to have suprahypothalamic effects, may via its suprahypothalamic CNS effects contribute to menstrual cycle–related symptoms, at times independently of the influence of sex steroid hormones from the periphery.

An estrogen/progesterone challenge test has been proposed as a possible means of distinguishing subgroups of women whose symptoms may be more likely to be affected by the menstrual cycle or other sex-related factors (J. A. Hamilton, personal communication, May 1991).

Psychotropic Drug Effects on the Menstrual Cycle

In a study of 930 menstrual cycles in 240 women whose cycles were regular before taking fluoxetine, a dose-related effect of fluoxetine on menstrual cycle length was found (Fairman et al. 1995). A difference of 4.0 days or more from the average menstrual cycle length for the entire group was defined as cycle disruption. Cycle disruption occurred in 28% of cycles of women on placebo, in 25% of cycles of women taking fluoxetine 20 mg daily (P = nonsignificant), and in 45% of cycles of women taking fluoxetine 60 mg daily (P = .058). Cycle disruption was found to be dose dependent but not time dependent. Shortening or lengthening of cycles tended to occur in the same direction within subjects (Fairman et al. 1995). Patients were not bothered by the changes in cycle length, and benefits of fluoxetine treatment outweighed any consideration of changes in cycle length (M. Steiner, personal communication, February 1995).

Many psychotropic drugs are capable of producing hyperprolactinemia, which may in turn interfere with the menstrual cycle. Psychotropic drugs that can cause hyperprolactinemia include neuroleptics, antidepressant medications (e.g., amoxapine, imipramine, amitriptyline), opiates, and verapamil (Vance and Thorner 1989). Drugs that interfere with dopamine synthesis or with dopamine inhibition of prolactin secretion cause reversible prolactinemia (Vance and Thorner 1989). Dopamine interferes with prolactin secretion and thus is sometimes called *prolactin-inhibiting factor* (PIF). Gallactorrhea occurs in 30%–80% of women with prolactinemia (Franks et al. 1977; Thorner and Besser 1978). Irregular menses also occurs in some cases.

If galactorrhea and/or irregular menses occur in a patient taking psychotropic medication, the prolactin level should be measured. A mildly elevated prolactin level generally does not require an expensive diagnostic workup, discontinuance of the medication, or treatment. If visual-field loss occurs (a possible sign of pituitary hypertrophy) or the patient becomes amenorrheic (defined as absence of menses for 6 months or longer), computed tomography (CT) or magnetic resonance imaging (MRI) of the sella turcica of the pituitary should be obtained to rule out pituitary adenoma. Adenomas may be treated with dopamine-agonist medication (bromocriptine) or surgery. Mild increases in serum prolactin without visual-field loss or amenorrhea in a patient taking psycho-tropic medication generally can be assumed to be due to medication and to be reversible.

The drugs and classes of psychotropic drugs for which irregular menses has been reported as a medication side effect are discussed in Chapter 16.

Some patients whose menses were irregular prior to taking antide-pressant medication have reported anecdotally that their menstrual cy-cles became more regular when an antidepressant medication effectively treated their menstrual cycle–related mood changes (Jensvold 1995). It is well documented that stress can result in irregular menstrual cycles or hypothalamic amenorrhea (Yen 1991). We hypothesize that antide-pressant medication may have indirect salutary effects on the hy-pothalamic-pituitary-ovarian axis, such as indirect effects on the menstrual cycle via interactions of the hypothalamic-pituitary-adrenal axis and the stress system (adrenal axis and locus coeruleus–norepi-nephrine sympathetic system) (Jensvold 1995).

Two cases have been reported of fluoxetine-stimulated ovulation in women with clomiphene-resistant anovulation (Strain 1994).

Practical Approaches to Dosing of Psychotropic Medication for Treatment of Menstrual Cycle–Related Symptoms

Little has been published to assist physicians in taking the menstrual cycle into account in prescribing psychotropic medication (Conrad and Hamilton 1986; Jensvold et al. 1992). The following recommendations are made for management of cases in which psychiatric symptoms and/ or psychotropic drug effects are found to vary in relation to the men-strual cycle. It can be expected that future research findings will refine case management recommendations.

Constant versus variable dosing.   Patients with menstrual cycle–related psychological symptoms who are being treated with antidepres-sant medication may be initially started on a constant daily dose of medication. This regimen should be tried for at least two or three menstrual cycles, with the goal of optimizing the dosage and ascertaining whether sufficient benefit is obtained with constant dosing. Patients should be advised that the response to psychotropic medication during the first menstrual cycle is often not fully representative, as the medication may not have had sufficient time to achieve maximal benefit. In many cases, constant dosing will adequately treat symptoms with acceptable side effects; for such cases, constant dosing is preferred. The ease of taking the same dose every day is a notable advantage and increases the likelihood of compliance.

If breakthrough depressive or other symptoms or unacceptable side effects occur in relation to the patient's menstrual cycle on constant dosing, the dose may be increased (for breakthrough symptoms) or decreased (for excessive side effects) or variable dosing may be considered. Any decision to try variable or intermittent dosing should be made in collaboration with the patient, since patient involvement will be necessary in planning for and carrying out a variable- or intermittent-dosing regimen.

Continuous versus intermittent dosing.   Patients whose symptoms occur only premenstrually may ask whether they can take antidepressant medication during only part of the menstrual cycle and still obtain benefit.

E. Eriksson et al. (1994) found in a controlled trial that PMS patients receiving low-dose clomipramine for 14 days premenstrually experienced substantial reduction in PMS symptoms, with improvement beginning within several days of starting low-dose clomipramine. E. Eriksson and co-workers concluded that PMS patients benefit from both constant dosing of clomipramine (daily throughout the menstrual cycle) and intermittent dosing (14 days premenstrually only), but that many benefited most from a variable-dosing regimen with very low maintenance-dose clomipramine in the first half of the cycle and a higher dose in the latter half. The latter regimen prevented recurrence of initial side effects that occurred when medication was restarted during every luteal phase. In our experience, some patients who have undergone trials of taking antidepressant medication for 10–14 days premenstrually only for treatment of depressive symptoms occurring for 3–7 days premenstrually have reported lack of benefit; when the dose was subsequently extended to daily dosing throughout the menstrual cycle, the premenstrual symptoms were alleviated (M. F. Jensvold, unpublished data, June 1992).

In theory, given the usual lag period of up to several weeks for antidepressants to work, one might expect that antidepressant medication would need to be taken regularly throughout the menstrual cycle in order to be effective. On the other hand, some of the newer medications (e.g., the SSRIs) work within days for some patients. Furthermore, when antidepressants are used with the aim of taking advantage of beneficial side effects (e.g., when low doses of sedating TCAs are taken at bedtime to assist with sleep), benefits may occur almost immediately. The controlled TCA (clomipramine) trial of E. Eriksson and colleagues (1994) found rapid onset of benefit for PMS symptoms.

Furthermore, in theory, it is unclear *when* in the menstrual cycle medication should be taken if it is to be taken during only part of the cycle. It is possible that events occurring during the follicular phase, around ovulation, or during the early luteal phase may influence later symptoms (e.g., Rojansky et al. 1991), so that medication exposure would need to occur earlier in the menstrual cycle for the patient to derive benefit premenstrually.

Serial blood levels.   For medications for which drug levels are not routinely obtained (e.g., most antidepressant medications, benzodiazepines), serial blood levels would be of interest but may not be necessary before embarking on an empirical trial of varying the medication dosage. For medications for which the toxic-to-therapeutic ratio is high (e.g., SSRIs), serial blood levels are less necessary before varying the dosage compared with those with low ratios. Medications for which serial blood levels on constant dosage should be considered are medications 1) for which blood levels are routinely obtained (e.g., lithium, carbamazepine), 2) for which a therapeutic window (e.g., nortriptyline) or therapeutic level (e.g., imipramine) is well defined, and 3) that have a low toxic-to-therapeutic ratio (e.g., lithium). Ideal would be four weekly serum levels obtained over the course of one menstrual cycle during constant dosing. Also of interest would be two levels during the times of greatest contrast in hormone levels (e.g., early follicular and midluteal, or midfollicular and late luteal) or greatest contrast in symptoms (e.g., postmenstrual week and premenstrual week). (See also Chapter 19.)

Start increased dose prior to onset of symptoms (i.e., prophylactically) versus at onset of premenstrual symptoms .   For cases in which large intercycle variability of catamenial symptoms exists (especially when a substantial proportion of cycles are asymptomatic), waiting until onset or worsening of symptoms occurs before starting or changing the dose may be preferable in order to avoid taking unneeded medication or increasing the dose unnecessarily. However, a small amount of evidence suggests that increasing the antidepressant dose several days before onset or worsening of catamenial symptoms may be more efficacious than waiting until symptoms occur to increase the dose. Several patients have reported that waiting until onset of premenstrual worsening of symptoms occurs to increase the antidepressant dose does not effectively treat symptoms, whereas increasing the dose prophylactically several days prior to expected onset of symptoms works well (M. F. Jensvold, unpublished data, June 1992). A definitive answer awaits further research and may vary between medications and conditions.

Methods of varying dosage.   A clinical method of varying antidepressant medication dosage for menstrual cycle–related symptoms that has been shown empirically to be effective (Jensvold et al. 1992) is as follows: Plan to increase the medication dosage starting 3–7 days before the expected onset or worsening of catamenial symptoms. For example, if the woman's average cycle length is 28 days, and symptoms regularly occur for 7 days premenstrually while she is taking constant medication, plan to increase the medication dosage beginning 10–14 days premenstrually, continuing until onset of menses, at which time dosage is returned to the lower dose (Jensvold et al. 1992).

Scheduled versus as-needed (prn) medication.   An alternative to varying the dosage is to add a supplemental medication—either in a scheduled or a prn manner—for a few days during symptomatic phases of the menstrual cycle. For example, if a constant dosage of an antidepressant medication for treating premenstrual symptoms is found to be helpful for depressive symptoms but irritability for a few days premenstrually continues to be bothersome, adding a low dose of alprazolam on a prn basis during those symptomatic premenstrual days and keeping the antidepressant dosage constant works well for some patients (Jensvold et al. 1992).

Controlled trials differ in their assessment of whether benzodiazepines can be taken premenstrually only and result in benefit for PMDD symptoms. Harrison et al. (1990), in a double-blind, placebo-controlled trial, found that alprazolam taken for 6–14 days premenstrually only, beginning when symptoms started, helped PMDD symptoms. P. J. Schmidt et al. (1993) found that alprazolam taken either continuously or premenstrually only showed no significant difference compared with placebo for PMDD symptoms.

Nonmedication treatment approaches.   Worth mentioning is that all menstrual cycle–related psychological symptoms should not automatically be treated with medication. Charting symptoms, thereby learning better the patterns of one's own symptoms, may assist the patient with mastery. Lifestyle changes, including exercise and dietary changes, cognitive work, stress management techniques, assertiveness training, and support groups, may all be helpful. Furthermore, changes over the course of the menstrual cycle should not be assumed to necessarily be bad. Learning to value, honor, and take advantage of one's different experiences over the menstrual cycle may be a key part of the psychotherapeutic work. In cases in which nonmedication interventions have been tried without success, or in which symptoms are severe, or in which the patient clearly has a condition that is known to be treatable with medication, it is appropriate for medication to be considered.

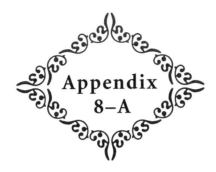

Appendix 8–A

Effects of Menstrual Cycle on Psychoactive Drugs

Alcohol

◆ **Hay et al. 1984**
  ✦ *Subjects and methods.* In 20 female social drinkers (9 not taking oral contraceptives [OCs], 11 taking OCs), ethanol tolerance was measured by using a body-sway procedure.
  ✦ *Findings.* No difference was found in peak blood alcohol level (BAL) as a function of menstrual cycle (MC) phase or in those taking OCs compared with those who were not. High–ethanol-tolerant women were significantly less accurate than low–ethanol-tolerant women at estimating BALs during the midcycle phase.

◆ **B. M. Jones and M. K. Jones 1976**
  ✦ *Subjects and methods.* Alcohol was administered to 20 women at two of three times during the MC. Ten men were tested at 2-week intervals.
  ✦ *Findings.* Females had significantly higher peak BAL than males at equivalent doses. Women in the premenstrual phase had higher peak blood alcohol concentration (BAC) and faster absorption than did women tested in other phases. Performance differences were not found across the MC.

Alcohol (continued)

◆ Sutker et al. 1987a

✦ *Subjects and methods.* Ethanol was administered to 16 women in three MC phases, as above.

✦ *Findings.* The decreased ethanol elimination times, reduced BAC–time curve areas under the curve (AUC), and faster disappearance rates during the midluteal phase compared with the midfollicular and ovulatory phases were associated with decreased levels of progesterone, elevated progesterone-to-estrogen ratio, and decreased follicle-stimulating hormone (FSH). No difference was found in absorption time or peak BAC by MC phase.

◆ Sutker et al. 1987b

✦ *Subjects and methods.* Ethanol was administered three times (early follicular, days 2–7; ovulatory, day 14; and midluteal, days 20–25) in 16 women, and at comparable time intervals in 14 men.

✦ *Findings.* In women, there were significantly shorter elimination times and faster disappearance rates during the midluteal phase of the MC compared with the early follicular and ovulatory phases. Increased anxiety and depression occurred with ethanol in the follicular phase. Men showed no differences between sessions.

◆ Charette et al. 1990

✦ *Subjects and methods.* The ethanol intake and physical and affective symptoms of 82 normally menstruating, nonalcoholic young women—52 at low risk and 30 at high risk of developing alcoholism, based on family history—were monitored over two MCs without subjects' knowledge that MC was being monitored.

✦ *Findings.* Ethanol consumption was not related to MC. Symptoms of physical distress increased premenstrually and during menses; affective symptoms did not change with the MC.

Anticonvulsant Drugs

◆ Bäckström 1976

✦ *Subjects and methods.* Estrogen and progesterone levels were measured on alternate days in 7 epileptic women over 9 MCs.

✦ *Findings.* Six cycles were ovulatory, three anovulatory. In the ovulatory cycles, there was a correlation between seizure frequency and estrogen/progesterone ratio. In anovulatory cycles, there was a correlation between estrogen levels and seizure frequency.

◆ **Bäckström and Jorpes 1979**
   ✦ *Subjects and methods.* In 7 epileptic women, drug levels (phenytoin, phenobarbital, and carbamazepine) and hormone levels (estradiol and progesterone) were each measured every other day for at least one MC.
   ✦ *Findings.* Only small variations occurred in drug levels during the investigation period. No correlation was seen between serum drug levels and serum hormone concentrations. (The relationship of seizure frequency to the MC was not reported.)

◆ **Shavit et al. 1984**
   ✦ *Subjects and methods.* Phenytoin levels were measured in 17 women whose grand mal seizures were more frequent perimenstrually and 7 women with seizures unrelated to menses. Levels were measured twice, on first or second day of menses and 2 weeks later.
   ✦ *Findings.* In women whose seizures were more frequent perimenstrually, serum phenytoin levels were lower during menses. In women whose seizures were unrelated to menses, the drop in phenytoin was much smaller. The decrease in phenytoin levels during menses in women with catamenial epilepsy was due to increased clearance.

◆ **Rosciszewska et al. 1986**
   ✦ *Subjects and methods.* Excretion of estrogen and progesterone metabolites was measured in 37 women whose seizure frequency increased perimenstrually and 27 women whose seizure frequency did not change with MC phase. Serum phenytoin and phenobarbitone levels were measured eight times during the MC in 50 of the women. Hormone levels were compared with those of healthy control subjects.
   ✦ *Findings.* Variation in serum levels of phenytoin was greater for women with catamenial epilepsy; a significant decrease in phenytoin levels occurred in these women between days 27 and 28 and corresponded with increased seizure frequency. There was no correlation between estrogen and seizure frequency. Seizure incidence inversely correlated with progesterone levels.

Anticonvulsant Drugs (continued)

◆ Kumar et al. 1988

✦ *Subjects and methods.* Serum phenytoin levels were measured twice, during ovulatory and menstrual phases of MC, in 8 women with catamenial epilepsy and 8 age-matched control subjects. Pharmacokinetic studies were conducted in 5 patients with catamenial epilepsy.

✦ *Findings.* Phenytoin levels significantly decreased during the menstrual phase in women with catamenial epilepsy; levels were not significantly decreased in control subjects. Clearance of phenytoin was increased during menses compared with the ovulatory phase, although not statistically significantly. Although the fall in phenytoin was within the therapeutic range, it was considered responsible for catamenial epilepsy.

Antidepressant Medications

◆ Stone et al. 1990

✦ *Subjects and methods.* Fifteen women with prospectively diagnosed premenstrual syndrome were treated with a constant dose of fluoxetine ($n = 9$) or placebo ($n = 5$).

✦ *Findings.* Eight of 9 women treated with fluoxetine responded to treatment; 1 of 6 taking placebo responded. In addition, mood symptoms, neurovegetative signs, concentration, and physical symptoms (including bloating and breast tenderness) improved on fluoxetine.

◆ Jensvold et al. 1992

✦ *Subjects and methods.* In an open treatment trial, 37 women with depressive symptoms that varied in relation to the MC were treated with constant dosage of antidepressant medication ($n = 27$) or constant dosage for several months, followed by variable dosing ($n = 10$).

✦ *Findings.* The MC-related symptoms of 26 patients responded well to constant daily dosage with tricyclic antidepressants (TCAs), monoamine oxidase inhibitors (MAOIs), or fluoxetine. In 10 cases, constant dosing was not adequate due to breakthrough depressive symptoms occurring premenstrually or to drug side effects occurring in the follicular phase. In the latter 10 cases, variable dosing, with increased antidepressant dosage beginning 3–7 days prior to expected worsening of symptoms, worked well, better than constant dosing. Only one patient (with a dual diagnosis of catamenial depression and obsessive-compulsive disorder) was a nonresponder to antidepressant medication. Serial blood levels in one patient: on nortriptyline (NOR) 50 mg qd constant dosage, NOR level = 43 ng/mL (therapeutic = 50–150 ng/mL); on NOR 100 mg qd constant dosage, NOR level = 169 ng/mL; with variable dosing, on day 7 (2 days after decreasing dosage from 75 to 50 mg qd), NOR level = 105 ng/mL; on day 14 (9th day of 50 ng/mL), NOR level = 52 ng/mL; on day 28 (8th day of 100 mg qd), NOR level = 97 ng/mL.

◆ **Kimmel et al. 1992**
  ✦ *Subjects and methods.* Two women with premenstrual depressive symptoms were treated with constant antidepressant doses; antidepressant drug levels were measured twice in the MC.
  ✦ *Findings.* Antidepressant drug levels were lower premenstrually than during the follicular phase. Desipramine plasma levels: follicular, 156 ng/mL; premenses, 73 ng/mL. Trazodone plasma levels: follicular, 550 ng/mL; premenses, 280 ng/mL.

◆ **D. E. Stewart et al. 1994**
  ✦ *Subjects and methods.* Forty women with prospectively confirmed late luteal phase dysphoric disorder (LLPDD) were treated with 20 mg or 60 mg of fluoxetine or placebo in a double-blind trial. Fluoxetine and fluoxetine metabolite (norfluoxetine) levels were measured in the follicular and late luteal phases (days 10 and 26) in 27 women.
  ✦ *Findings.* There were no significant differences between midfollicular and late luteal drug levels.

◆ **E. Eriksson et al. 1994 (first study)**
  ✦ *Subjects and methods.* Of 29 women with LLPDD, 15 were treated with clomipramine (CMI, constant continuous doses, 25–75 mg/day, throughout MC) and 14 were treated with placebo. The study was double blind and included three treatment cycles.
  ✦ *Findings.* A marked reduction in symptoms occurred in the CMI group only.

◆ **E. Eriksson et al. 1994 (second study)**
  ✦ *Subjects and methods.* Subjects were given intermittent dosing of CMI (× 14 days premenstrually only). The study was double blind, placebo controlled, and included three treatment cycles.
  ✦ *Findings.* A marked reduction in symptoms occurred in the CMI group only. There were no treatment nonresponders in the CMI group. Subjects tended to respond quickly (within 3–4 days) and to low doses.

Buspirone

◆ **Dinan et al. 1990**
  ✦ *Subjects and methods.* Prolactin response to buspirone was measured in 6 healthy females and 8 healthy males.
  ✦ *Findings.* In males, the prolactin response was consistently reproducible. In females, the prolactin response varied with MC phase, with maximum prolactin responses occurring premenstrually.

Lithium

◆ **Kukopulos et al. 1985**
  ✦ One well-documented case was reported of a woman with a catamenial manic-depressive illness who was taking constant dose of lithium. On lithium, the patient experienced hypomanic symptoms for a few days, followed by depression for a few days that resolved with onset of menses. The lithium levels were highest when depression was greatest (1.1 mmol/L), lowest during hypomania (0.3 mmol/L), and relatively stable at 0.5 mmol/L, when the patient was euthymic.

◆ **Conrad and Hamilton 1986**
  ✦ One well-documented case was reported of an adolescent female with bipolar disorder who, on constant lithium dosage, experienced recurrence of symptoms premenstrually; serum lithium levels also dropped at that time. When lithium dosage was increased premenstrually, premenstrual recurrence of symptoms was prevented and serum lithium levels remained constant.

◆ **Chamberlain et al. 1990**
  ✦ *Subjects and methods.* Six healthy women not taking OCs and 7 women taking OCs took single 300-mg doses of lithium during the midfollicular, midluteal, and premenstrual phases of the MC.
  ✦ *Findings.* There were no significant differences in serum lithium levels between MC phases or between groups.

Propranolol

◆ Gengo et al. 1984
   ✦ One case was reported of a woman who had migraine recurrences despite taking propranolol. Weekly propranolol levels revealed that the serum propranolol level decreased markedly at the time of onset of menses, at about the same time that her headaches worsened. Serial measurements following oral 40-mg doses of propranolol on day 1 and day 16 of the MC revealed a significant (46%) decrease in the area under the serum concentration–time curve from day 16 to day 1, reflecting increased apparent clearance on day 1 compared with day 16.

Nonpregnant Reproductive-Age Women

Part II: Exogenous Sex Steroid Hormones and Psychopharmacology

Margaret F. Jensvold, M.D.

Oral and non-oral (e.g., injectable, implant) hormonal contraceptives are commonly used by women today. Although exogenous sex steroid hormonal agents may cause or contribute to psychological symptoms, such agents may in other circumstances be used alone or in combination with psychotropic agents to alleviate certain psychological symptoms. Complicating matters clinically are potential drug interactions between hormonal agents and psychotropic drugs. In this chapter I review the exogenous sex steroid hormonal agents available for use in reproductive-age women, the prevalence and management of psychological side effects, the use of sex steroid hormonal agents in treating psychiatric symptoms, and the potential interactions of these agents with psychotropic drugs.

Sex Steroid Hormonal Contraception

Oral Contraception

Prevalence of use.   By 1987, oral contraceptives (OCs) had been used by more than 150 million women worldwide, including more than 50 million women in the United States (American College of Obstetricians and Gynecologists 1987). The 1988 Ortho Survey found that 13.8 million women in the United States and 60 million women worldwide were currently using oral contraceptive agents (Hatcher et al. 1990). Table 9–1 shows the proportion of reproductive-age women using contraception and the types used.

Table 9–1.   U.S. reproductive-age women and contraceptive use

In 1988 in the United States:	
Number of women aged 15 to 44 years:	57.9 million
Not using contraception:	39.7%
Reasons for not using contraception:	
Pregnant, postpartum, or seeking pregnancy	8.6%
Noncontraceptively sterile	6.1%
Never had intercourse	11.5%
Had no intercourse in previous 3 months	6.9%
Had intercourse in previous 3 months	6.7%
Using contraception:	60.3%
Contraceptive methods used:	
Sterilization	48.7%
Female	31.4%
Male	17.3%
Oral contraceptives	20.4%
Condom	14.3%
Diaphragm	6.2%
Periodic abstinence	2.8%
Intrauterine device	2.0%
Withdrawal	2.3%
Foam	1.4%
Other (douche, sponge, jelly, or cream alone)	1.9%
Total:	100%

Source.   Adapted from Mosher 1990.

History.   Oral contraceptive medication was approved by the U.S. Food and Drug Administration (FDA) in 1960. In the 1970s, hormone dosages decreased to as little as one-fifth the dosage used in OCs during the 1960s. As dosages have decreased, so have the incidences of side effects and adverse effects. The lower-dose OCs have been found to be relatively safe and relatively free of side effects. The recommendation before 1990 that women over 35 years of age not take oral contraceptive medication has been rescinded. The FDA conducted a review of data and, in 1990, recommended a change in labeling to include the statement that "the benefits of oral contraceptive use by healthy, nonsmoking women over 40 years of age may outweigh the possible risks" (Grimes 1993, p. 10). In 1988, before the change in labeling, only 5% of women aged 35–39 years and 3% of women aged 40–44 years used oral contraceptive medications (Mosher 1990). Today OCs may be used by women until menopause.

Types.   Three main types of hormonal contraceptives are available: combined oral contraceptives (COCs), progesterone-only oral contraceptives (POCs), and progesterone-only contraceptives that are administered by non-oral routes and are generally long acting.

Fifty-two different *combined oral contraceptives* are available in the United States, according to the *Physician's Desk Reference* (1993). The COC formulations differ with regard to 1) monophasic, biphasic, or triphasic formulations, 2) estrogen and progestin dosages, 3) inclusion of a week of placebo pills for use during the pill-free interval (PFI), and 4) brand.

Monophasic pills provide fixed doses of estrogen and progestin throughout the cycle. In biphasic pills, the estrogen dose remains constant throughout the cycle, while the progestin dose is higher in the second half of the cycle. In triphasic OCs, the estrogen dose may stay the same, or may increase and then decrease. The progestin dose varies, either progressively increasing or first increasing and then decreasing. All of these COCs include a PFI.

Two estrogens, ethinyl estradiol and mestranol, are currently used in OCs. Estradiol accounts for 99.5% of the estrogen component in the OCs marketed in the United States. Commercially available progestins are derivatives of 19-nortestosterone or 17-α-hydroxyprogesterone.

Seven progestins currently used in OCs marketed in the United States are norethindrone, norethindrone acetate, ethynodiol diacetate, norgestrel, levonorgestrel, norethynodrel, and norgestimate. Norgestimate, a progestin with less androgenic effect than the earlier progestins, was approved for use in the United States recently. Two other newer progestins related to norgestimate, desogestrel and gestodene, are used outside the United States (Hatcher et al. 1990).

"High dose" combined OCs refer to those containing 80 or 100 μg of estrogen; 30-, 35-, and 50-μg estrogen combined pills are the standard lower-dose pills. The lowest-dose combined pills contain less than 30 μg of estrogen. Most sources recommend that patients start on a 30- to 50-μg pill, adjusting the dose up or down from there as necessary (Hatcher et al. 1990). A tenfold interindividual variability in blood levels of estrogen and progestin may account for the "breakthrough bleeding" or "breakthrough pregnancy" experienced by some women. This interindividual variability may also account for those women with low blood levels who have more than the usual number of side effects compared with women with even higher blood levels of these OC and ovarian hormones (Guillebaud 1989).

A *progesterone-only oral contraceptive* (POC) is available that contains low-dose ("mini dose") progesterone and no estrogen. The POC accounts for 7% of the OC market in the United Kingdom, 4% in Australia, and less than 0.5% in the United States (Fotherby 1989).

In recent years, a variety of *long-acting hormonal contraceptives* have become available on the market, with a number of others currently in testing phases. Table 9–2 lists the long-acting hormonal contraceptive agents available in the United States and summarizes their frequency of administration and reversibility (I. Fraser 1989; Hatcher et al. 1990). Routes of administration include injectable, oral, vaginal ring, biodegradable implant, and nonbiodegradable implant. More than 25 long-acting hormonal contraceptives, each of which contains only progesterone, are being marketed around the world or are in various stages of drug development (I. Fraser 1989). The options for duration of action are 1 month, 2–3 months, 6 months, 1–2 years, and 5 years or longer. The long-acting agents most commonly used in the United States currently are levonorgestrel implant (Norplant subdermal implant) and medroxyprogesterone acetate (Depo-Provera).

Table 9–2. Delivery systems for progestin-only contraceptives and combined oral contraceptives

	Oral Combined OC	Progestin-only OC	Injectable (NET-EN)	DMPA	Implant (Norplant)	Vaginal ring (LNG ring [WHO])
Administration frequency	Daily	Daily	Bimonthly	Trimonthly	5 years	Trimonthly
Progestin dose	Low	Ultra-low	High	High	Ultra-low	Ultra-low
Blood levels	Rapid fluctuation	Rapid fluctuation	Initial peak then decline	Initial peak then decline	Constant	Constant
First pass through liver	Yes	Yes	No	No	No	No
Ovulation suppression	+++	+	++	+++	++	+
Reversibility: Immediate termination possible?	Yes	Yes	No	No	Yes	Yes

Note. DMPA = depo-medroxyprogesterone acetate; LNG = levonorgestrel; NET-EN = norethisterone enanthate; OC = oral contraceptive; WHO = World Health Organization. + = least ovulation suppression; +++ = most ovulation suppression.
Source. Adapted from Hatcher et al. (1990).

Mechanisms of action.   Hormonal contraceptives vary in their mechanisms of action. COCs rely on suppression of ovulation but many other hormone contraceptives do not. COCs and high-dose "depot" progestins act at the hypothalamic level to suppress ovulation. Gonadotropin-releasing hormone (GnRH) superagonists and antagonists act at the pituitary level to suppress luteinizing hormone (LH) and follicle-stimulating hormone (FSH) and therefore ovulation. "Low dose" progestin contraceptives (minipills and implants) act locally at the level of the cervix, uterus, and fallopian tubes (Loriaux 1993).

Psychological Side Effects of Sex Steroid Hormonal Contraceptives

Types, Prevalences, and Mechanisms

Studies examining depression among women taking OCs have found incidences ranging from less than 5% to 30% (Editor, BMJ 1970; Editor, Drug Facts and Comparisons 1993). Current OCs have a lower incidence of depression as a side effect compared with the higher-dose OCs; however, mood effects do occur in some patients on the lower-dose medications (Hamilton and Jensvold 1991).

Depression associated with OCs can be severe, with some cases of suicidal behavior having occurred with OCs. Psychotic behavior has also been reported (American Hospital Formulary Service 1993; Editor, BMJ 1970). Little research has been conducted regarding the psychological side effects of contraceptive agents in populations of women with histories of unipolar depression, bipolar disorder, or other psychiatric conditions. Nevertheless, it has clearly been observed that depression with OCs can be worse in persons with a history of depression (American Hospital Formulary Service 1993; Editor, BMJ 1970).

Little comparative research has been conducted on the psychological side effects of different OC preparations. Summarizing the literature, Hatcher et al. (1990) concluded that "to our knowledge, published double-blind crossover studies have not been reported comparing either the serious complications or the many less serious side effects of the sub–50-μg pills (such as nausea, spotting, 1-year discontinuation rates, premenstrual anxiety, or depression). Only with these data can the clinician or the patient make a fully informed choice from among the 30- and 35-μg pills. However, . . . several differences may be used to make a choice" (p. 257). When unacceptable side effects occur with any particular OC, the relative androgenicity and progestogen potency of various OCs are two factors typically considered in choosing the next OC. Readers are referred elsewhere for detailed discussions of how to choose among the available COCs, depending on which side effects the patient is experiencing (Guillebaud 1989; Hatcher et al. 1990).

The most frequent side effects of the estrogen component of OCs are nausea, breast tenderness, and fluid retention (usually not more than 3–4 pounds). Gestagens are structurally related to testosterone and may produce androgenic side effects. The most common progestin side effects are weight gain (due to anabolic effects of the progestin), acne, a symptom women may experience as nervousness, and amenorrhea (failure of withdrawal bleeding) (Mishell 1989).

Authors differ as to which hormone—estrogen or progesterone—they consider to be responsible for various psychological side effects of OCs. Depression, fatigue, nervousness, dizziness, somnolence, and sedation are attributed to the progestin in COCs by some authors (American Hospital Formulary Service 1993; Dickey 1974, 1984; Hatcher et al. 1990). According to other authors, depression with OCs is due to low estrogen in some cases and to high estrogen or high progesterone in other cases (Hatcher et al. 1990).

Differences among authors may be due to the fact that the information may be mainly anecdotal, or such side effects may be due to combined effects of hormones, or different patients may respond differently to different hormones or dosages (Guillebaud 1989).

Mechanisms that have been proposed for OC-related depression have involved estrogen. Estrogens in OCs may convert tryptophan metabolism from its minor pathway in the brain to its major pathway in the liver, thus decreasing brain serotonin, the end product of tryptophan metabolism, and resulting in depression in some women and in sleepiness and mood changes in others (Mishell 1989; Rose and Adams 1972). This effect is reversible, disappearing when OCs are stopped. It is thought to result in clinically important depression in a small proportion of women (Mishell 1989). Additionally, disturbances in tryptophan metabolism due to OC use may result in pyridoxine deficiency, which has been proposed as a factor in depression (Editor, Drug Facts and Comparisons 1993); this possibility has prompted some authors to recommend 25–50 μg of pyridoxine as a treatment for OC-related depression (Editor, Drug Facts and Comparisons 1993; Guillebaud 1989).

OCs may affect receptors, which in turn may influence depression or response to antidepressant medication. For example, a triphasic OC was found to induce an upregulatory effect, increasing maximal imipramine-binding capacity on platelet membranes, by the second cycle of pill use (Weizman et al. 1988).

The POC has fewer side effects overall than the COCs, but it is also somewhat less efficacious with regard to contraception. Its use is usually reserved for women who do not tolerate estrogen.

The progesterone-only minipill frequently causes menstrual side effects (breakthrough bleeding) but is associated with relatively few nonmenstrual side effects overall (Fotherby 1989). Although it can cause depression, the POC results in less depression, fewer premenstrual symptoms, and less decrease in libido compared with the combination OCs (American Hospital Formulary Service 1993; Hatcher et al. 1990).

With the long-acting, non-oral progesterone contraceptives, various side effects, including mood change and decreased libido, have been reported to occur, generally with frequencies of 5%–15% (Schwallie and Assenzo 1972; Scutchfield et al. 1971)—that is, with prevalences comparable to those found with OCs. In an adolescent population taking depomedroxyprogesterone acetate (DMPA), the prevalence of depression was 35%; of fatigue, 42%; and of headache, 38% (Cromer et al. 1993).

Drugs used in treating infertility, including clomiphene citrate, human menopausal gonadotropin, danazol, and GnRH analogs, are also associated with psychological side effects. Readers are referred elsewhere for a discussion of these (Daniluk and Fluker 1995).

Strategies for Management of Psychological Side Effects of Hormonal Contraceptive Agents

The FDA recommends selecting the oral contraceptive formulation with the least estrogen and progesterone compatible with a low failure rate and meeting the individual's needs (Mishell 1989). It is usually recommended that OCs be initiated with a formulation containing 30–35 µg of ethinyl estradiol and the lowest dose of a particular gestagen (Meade et al. 1980; Mishell 1989). The OC can than be "titrated" up or down, changing to a lower-dose preparation or switching to a POC if side effects are not tolerated, or switching to a higher-dose preparation if breakthrough bleeding or "breakthrough pregnancy" occur. Several authors have issued detailed guidelines for deciding when a change in estrogen versus a change in progestogen is merited, depending on which side effects are problematic (Guillebaud 1989; Hatcher et al. 1990; Editor, Drug Facts and Comparisons 1993).

History of depression should be obtained before starting an OC. Some authors consider a history of depression to be a relative contraindication to OC use (Mishell 1989). A depressed patient who is taking OCs should be asked about onset of depression relative to initiation of OCs, depression experienced on other OCs and before taking OCs, and time in the pill cycle when depression is worst, as well as other standard questions such as severity of depression, suicidality, and other possible contributory factors (Hatcher et al. 1990).

If depression of a serious degree occurs for the first time or recurs on an OC, the OC should be stopped (American Hospital Formulary Service 1993; Editor, Drug Facts and Comparisons 1993). Stopping the OC may be necessary to determine whether the symptom is drug related (Editor, Drug Facts and Comparisons 1993). Later, trying a different-formulation OC containing a lower progestogen dose; changing to the newer, less androgenic progestogen, norgestimate; and/or eliminating estrogen altogether (Guillebaud 1989) can be tried. There is disagreement about whether to stop OCs or to treat OC-induced depression with antidepressants. Some authors recommend against treating OC-related depression with antidepressant medication (Guillebaud 1989). However, in our experience, antidepressant medication has been successful in treating OC-related depression (Hamilton and Jensvold 1991; M. F. Jensvold, unpublished data, January 1993).

Evidence that OCs alter tryptophan metabolism, resulting in a deficiency in brain serotonin (Mishell 1989; Rose and Adams 1972), suggests that selective serotonin reuptake inhibitors (SSRIs) might be particularly effective in treating OC-related depression. However, no comparative study of SSRIs versus other classes of antidepressants for treatment of OC-related depression has been conducted. Pyridoxine (vitamin B$_6$) 25–50 µg per day has been recommended for treating pyridoxine deficiency, which has been cited as a possible factor in OC-related depression (Editor, Drug Facts and Comparisons 1993; Guillebaud 1989), although controlled trials of pyridoxine for treatment of OC-related depression are not, to our knowledge, available.

Some cases of OC-related depression may be due in part to decreased estrogen in the ovulation-suppressed patient. In such cases, increasing the estrogen dose in the OC formulation may be helpful (Hatcher et al. 1990).

If symptoms occur selectively during the PFI of the OC cycle, the physician may recommend "tricycling." Tricycling refers to having a PFI every 3 or 4 months (three to four times per year) rather than every 4 weeks. Tricycling is achieved by taking three or four cycles of monophasic pills consecutively, followed by a PFI. Biphasic or triphasic pills, in which the progesterone dose varies, cannot be used to achieve this effect (Guillebaud 1989). In women with intact uteri, periodic shedding of the uterine lining is necessary in order to avoid an increased risk of endometrial cancer. Shedding at, minimally, 3- to 4-month intervals is thought to be adequate to avoid an increased risk of endometrial cancer.

For some conditions, such as catamenial epilepsy (Guillebaud 1989), phasic pills (i.e., biphasic, triphasic) are relatively contraindicated. The object is to keep hormone levels as constant as possible, since fluctuations may precipitate symptoms.

Some evidence suggests that OCs can induce a rapid-cycling mood state (Hamilton and Jensvold 1991). Stopping the OC and/or treating the condition with mood-stabilizing medication is recommended.

If a patient's psychiatric symptoms occur in relation to an OC pill cycle, stopping the OC may be necessary in order to determine whether the OC is ameliorating the patient's psychiatric symptoms, exacerbating the patient's psychiatric condition, or has no effect. A decision can then be made whether to resume pill use with the same or a different contraceptive agent or whether to discontinue OC use entirely.

Evidence is mixed as to whether hormone replacement therapy (HRT) alleviates the mild psychological symptoms commonly seen in perimenopausal women. Some studies have found some benefit to these symptoms with HRT, others a worsening of symptoms, and yet others no effect. Consensus has been reached, however, that when depressive symptoms in perimenopausal women meet criteria for a depressive disorder, HRT cannot be counted upon to adequately treat these symptoms, and antidepressant medication should be considered (Jensvold, in press).

Two methods have been recommended for determining when to switch a perimenopausal woman from OCs to HRT (Grimes 1993). One method is to discontinue the OC for 3 months beginning in January to see if menses returns. If menses returns, the woman may be asked her preference regarding remaining off the OC or resuming it. If she chooses to resume OC use, a trial off OCs should be planned again a year or two later. Alternatively, in the late reproductive-age woman taking OCs, measure the FSH level on the last pill-free day of a cycle. If the FSH level is elevated, the patient is most likely menopausal. A nonelevated FSH level may mean either that the patient is not yet menopausal or that it simply takes longer for the FSH to desuppress. The exact timing of making the switch from OCs to HRT is not important (Grimes 1993).

Regarding non-oral hormonal contraceptives, long-acting hormonal agents that are removable and reversible should be selected over nonreversible agents for patients with a history of depression. Patients with a history of affective disorders should be monitored closely when they start on any steroid hormonal contraceptive agent.

Use of Reproductive Agents for
Treating Psychiatric Conditions

Reproductive agents are at times used to treat psychological symptoms or psychiatric conditions.

Treatment of "premenstrual syndrome" (PMS) with oral contraceptive medications has had mixed results. In one case report, OCs alleviated premenstrual depression and a subsequent major depressive episode (Roy-Byrne et al. 1984). In a controlled trial, women taking monophasic or triphasic OCs reported no less premenstrual symptomatology than women not taking OCs, although women taking monophasic OCs had less breast tenderness than women in the other two groups (A. Walker and Bancroft 1990). Among women with prospectively confirmed late luteal phase dysphoric disorder (LLPDD) who participated in a research clinic (i.e., women who were significantly bothered by primarily psychological symptoms occurring only premenstrually, many of whom had previously tried without success a variety of treatments for PMS) most of the patients who had previously taken oral contraceptive medication reported that OCs had worsened their PMS (M. F. Jensvold, unpublished data, June 1989). Women presenting to a general gynecology clinic for treatment of PMS might report different results than those presenting to a specialized PMS research clinic due to a selection bias in the latter for women whose previous treatments had failed. Alternatively, the specialized research clinic might attract women with more severe symptoms and a greater component of depression susceptible to worsening with OCs.

Severe premenstrual symptoms have been alleviated by ovariectomy (Casson et al. 1990), as well as by the reversible "chemical menopause" induced by potent GnRH agonists (Bancroft et al. 1987; Hammarback and Bäckström 1988). In one study of 20 women taking a potent GnRH agonist to treat premenstrual symptoms, 2 patients' premenstrual symptoms worsened, 1 patient's premenstrual depression persisted, and 1 patient experienced her first hypomanic episode (Bancroft et al. 1987). The less tightly symptoms are linked to the menstrual cycle, the less likely they are to benefit from GnRH treatment.

We have had experience with a patient whose severe monthly pelvic pain due to ovarian cysts, severe premenstrual depression with suicidal ideation, and numerous brief premenstrual hospitalizations were alleviated with low-dose GnRH agonist plus antidepressant medication after failing to respond to OCs alone, antidepressant medication alone, and OC plus antidepressant medication.

In a double-blind study, high-dose estrogen helped to relieve depression among severely depressed women who had failed to respond to conventional antidepressant treatments (Klaiber et al. 1979).

In a series of studies including both open treatment trials and the largest double-blind, placebo-controlled, randomized studies of PMS treatment to date, 1) oral micronized progesterone and progesterone suppository treatment were not effective in treating PMS, 2) alprazolam was more effective than placebo, 3) GnRH analogs effectively reduced PMS symptoms but not the depressive symptoms of women with co-morbid depression, and 4) serotonergic antidepressants significantly reduced symptoms of both PMS and premenstrual exacerbation of major depression (Freeman et al. 1995).

Numerous controlled trials have found progesterone to be no more effective than placebo in alleviating premenstrual symptoms. Further-more, a hormonal manipulation study used the progesterone antagonist mifepristone (RU486) to truncate the hormonal events of the late luteal phase in a blind fashion. Psychological symptoms continued to cycle in some LLPDD patients despite unlinking from the usual hormonal events of the cycle (P. J. Schmidt et al. 1991). This study documents that at least some women's menstrual cycle–related psychological symptoms occur independently of progesterone levels. Additionally, plasma levels of progesterone and anxiolytic progesterone metabolites, allopreg-nanolone and pregnanolone (Freeman et al. 1993), during the late luteal phase in women with PMS and control women showed no significant group differences and no correlations between mood or behavioral symptoms and plasma levels (P. J. Schmidt et al. 1994). This finding suggests that PMS symptoms occur independently of peripheral proges-terone and progesterone metabolites, although the possibility of CNS mechanisms of progesterone effects is not addressed.

Despite profuse research findings to the contrary, many patients and their doctors continue to report impressions that progesterone—par-ticularly natural progesterone as opposed to synthetic progesterone—is helpful in alleviating premenstrual symptoms. One of the most com-mon arguments of progesterone proponents is that U.S. research fails to find significant beneficial effects with progesterone because of the rela-tively low doses of progesterone used in the United States (on the order of 100–400 mg daily) compared with Europe (800 mg and higher). Free-man and Rickels (1994) addressed this question in a study using high-dose progesterone (1,700 mg/day average) for treatment of women with PMS. Large interindividual variability was found in blood levels for the same dose. No correlations were found between dose, blood levels, and symptom relief, and progesterone was not found to significantly relieve symptoms.

Metabolic Effects of Hormonal Contraceptives

OCs have a wide variety of metabolic effects (American Hospital Formulary Service 1993; Hatcher et al. 1990; Kalkhoff 1982; Mishell 1989). Some of the metabolic effects of estrogen (ethinyl estradiol) in OCs include decreased tryptophan metabolism (possibly associated with mood changes and sleep disturbance), decreased sodium excretion (resulting in fluid retention), decreases in albumin and amino acids (without apparent clinical effect), and effects on the breast (resulting in breast tenderness) and endometrial tissue (possible resulting in hyperplasia).

Some of the metabolic effects of gestagens (19-nortestosterone derivatives) involve changes in carbohydrate metabolism (increasing plasma insulin, decreasing glucose tolerance, increasing the number of insulin receptors), changes in serum lipoproteins (decreasing high-density lipoprotein [HDL], increasing low-density lipoprotein [LDL], and changing the relative amounts of HDL2 and HDL3), and production of androgenic effects (which may increase acne or contribute to a feeling of nervousness). With combined OCs, patients may experience slight increases in glucose tolerance, total HDL may be unchanged, and liver function tests may be altered.

Dosages may significantly affect the incidence of side effects of hormonal contraceptives. A well-documented example is the finding that total deaths from arterial causes, ischemic heart disease, and stroke significantly decreased with estrogen doses of 30 mg compared with 50-mg doses (Mishell 1989). This reduced mortality may be due to the fact that the higher the estrogen dose in OCs, the more serum globulins increase, including angiotensin (which influences blood pressure) and globulins (which may be involved with coagulation and hypercoagulability) (Meade et al. 1980). The incidence of total arterial disease with OCs varies with gestagen dose when estrogen is unchanged (Kay 1982), suggesting that lower-dose progesterone is also preferable.

OC formulations containing gestagens without estrogen (i.e., POCs) have a lower incidence of metabolic effects overall compared with COCs (Mishell 1989).

Contraceptive–Psychotropic Drug Interactions

Interactions between OCs and other drugs have been reviewed elsewhere (American Hospital Formulary Service 1993; Back and Orme 1990; Editor, Drug Facts and Comparisons 1993; Grimes 1992; Guillebaud 1989; Hamilton 1991; Hamilton and Parry 1983; Hatcher et al. 1990; Rizack and Hillman 1991). In this section I discuss interactions between hormonal contraceptive agents and psychotropic drugs.

In general, OCs *stimulate* the metabolism of *conjugatively* metabolized drugs and drugs metabolized by *glucuronidation* and *impair* clearance of some *oxidatively* metabolized drugs. Psychotropic drugs that stimulate hepatic enzyme induction may therefore increase metabolism of estrogen and progesterone and risk contraceptive failure.

While some interactions are well demonstrated, others are only suspected. In some cases, information may be contradictory. Whereas some of the interactions may be clinically relevant, in other cases there is not clinical relevance or the clinical relevance is not clear. Table 9–3 summarizes OC interactions with psychotropic drugs. Additional considerations are discussed below.

Oral Contraceptives

Alcohol.   At least one study showed decreased alcohol metabolism with OCs, which may result in an increased alcohol effect (M. K. Jones and B. M. Jones 1984), although another study failed to confirm this (Hobbes et al. 1985). Patients should be forewarned.

Analgesics.   Acetaminophen may result in less pain relief in OC users (Goldzieher 1989) due to increased metabolism (Abernethy et al. 1982b; Miners et al. 1983; M. C. Mitchell et al. 1983; Rogers et al. 1987). The same may be true for aspirin as well, although the evidence is contradictory (Goldzieher 1989). Monitor analgesia and increase dosages if necessary (Goldzieher 1989). Ethinyl estradiol was found to decrease metabolism of acetaminophen, which may result in toxicity, although the clinical significance is not clear (M. C. Mitchell et al. 1983; Rogers et al. 1987).

Table 9–3.   Oral contraceptive–psychotropic drug interactions

Interacting drug	Documentation	Management
Drugs that may reduce oral contraceptive efficacy		
Anticonvulsants and sedatives		
(carbamazepine, phenytoin, phenobarbital, ethotoin, mephenytoin, primidone, ethosuximide)	Strongly suspected; clinical trial data lacking	With spotting, increase OC dose. Consider switch to valproate or clonazepam.
Drugs whose activity may be modified by oral contraceptive use		
Analgesics		
Acetaminophen	Adequate	Larger doses of analgesic may be required.
Aspirin	Contradictory	Larger doses of analgesic may be required.
Meperidine	Suspected	Decrease dose of analgesic.
Antidepressants		
Imipramine	Suspected	Decrease dosage by about one-third.
Other antidepressants	No data	
Minor tranquilizers		
Diazepam	Suspected	Decrease dose.
Other benzodiazepines	Suspected	Observe for increased effect.
Corticosteroids		
	Adequate	Watch for potentiation of effects; decrease dose accordingly.
Xanthines		
(caffeine, theophylline)	Adequate	Decreased dose may achieve same effect.

Source.   Modified from Goldzieher (1989) and Grimes (1992).

Antidepressants, tricyclic.   In women taking low-dose OCs, there was decreased metabolism of imipramine administered in a single oral dose or by iv bolus (Abernethy et al. 1984). The findings were consistent with impaired oxidative metabolism of imipramine with OCs. The clinical significance of this effect has not yet been shown, nor has the effect been replicated. We recommend adjusting imipramine dosage downward based on the side effects experienced and/or the monitoring of imipramine blood levels.

Anticonvulsant drugs/mood stabilizers.   Some anticonvulsant drugs, including carbamazepine (which is also a mood stabilizer), phenobarbital, and phenytoin, are hepatic enzyme inducers. By inducing liver enzymes, these drugs may increase metabolism of oral contraceptive agents, leading to potentially insufficient sex steroid levels and preventing ovulation suppression (Mattson et al. 1986). The cellular mechanism appears to be that these anticonvulsant drugs induce the $P450_{NF}$ isozyme (P450IIIA subfamily), which results in cytochrome P450 induction of ethinyl estradiol 2-hydroxylation, the major pathway of metabolism of ethinyl estradiol (Back and Orme 1990; Guengerich 1988). The degree of increased metabolism of sex steroid hormones by these anticonvulsant drugs is highly variable and unpredictable for individuals (Mattson et al. 1986). The increased risk of contraceptive failure in women taking these drugs may be managed by 1) starting with 50-μg ethinyl estradiol (rather than 30 or 35 μg) and increasing to a higher dose if breakthrough bleeding occurs (Mattson et al. 1986) or 2) switching to valproate (which is also a mood stabilizer) or clonazepam (which also has some antimanic effect and is a benzodiazepine with antianxiety and antipanic effects). Valproate and clonazepam have no effect on enzyme induction and can be taken with low-dose OCs.

Antipsychotic agents (dopamine blockers).   OCs may potentiate the prolactin response to antipsychotics (Hamilton and Parry 1983).

Benzodiazepines.   OCs may increase clearance of benzodiazepines that undergo glucuronidation (lorazepam, oxazepam, temazepam) (Abernethy et al. 1983; Patwardhan et al. 1981, 1983; Roberts et al. 1979; Stoehr et al. 1984), possibly requiring increased dosages of these benzodiazepines. OCs may decrease clearance of benzodiazepines that are metabolized by oxidation (alprazolam, triazolam, diazepam, chlordiazepoxide) (Abernethy et al. 1982a; Editor, Drug Facts and Comparisons 1993; Patwardhan et al. 1983), possibly resulting in toxicity, although the clinical significance of this effect has not been established (Stoehr et al. 1984). Clearance of a benzodiazepine undergoing nitroreduction (nitrazepam) is also reduced (Back and Orme 1990). Other benzodiazepines for which OC–drug interactions have not yet been documented but are suspected are clorazepate, flurazepam, halazepam, and prazepam; these undergo oxidative metabolism, therefore possibly resulting in decreased clearance and increased toxicity when combined with OCs (American Hospital Formulary Service 1993). Psychomotor impairment due to single doses of diazepam may vary during the OC cycle, being greatest during the PFI, although tolerance may develop with multiple doses (Ellinwood et al. 1984; Kroboth et al. 1985). Regarding clonazepam, see the "Anticonvulsant drugs/mood stabilizers" subsection.

β-adrenergic blockers.   Metoprolol and possibly propranolol may have increased effect with OCs due to decreased metabolism (Jack et al. 1982; D. Kendall et al. 1982; M. J. Kendall et al. 1984).

Corticosteroids.   OCs may result in decreased clearance and prolonged elimination half-life of prednisolone (Back and Orme 1990), resulting in increased effects. Lower dosages may be clinically effective (Back and Orme 1990; Goldzieher 1989).

Mood stabilizers.   See "Anticonvulsant drugs/mood stabilizers."

Thyroid.   OCs may increase thyroid-binding globulin (TBG) and decrease free thyroxine (Hansten 1976). Thyroid dose may need to be increased in women taking OCs or estrogens (Hansten 1976).

Xanthines.   Clearance of theophylline, caffeine, and aminophylline may be decreased by 30%–40% in OC users. Starting doses should be decreased by about one-third (Goldzieher 1989). Caffeine toxicity due to decreased metabolism with OCs is possible. This effect may be clinically significant, particularly with high doses of caffeine or prolonged use (Quigley and Yen 1980; Rietveld et al. 1984).

Contraceptive Implants

The available data relate to interactions of levonorgestrel implant (Norplant subdermal implant) with other drugs.

Anticonvulsants.   Carbamazepine and phenytoin may increase metabolism of levonorgestrel, endangering contraceptive efficacy (Editor, Drug Facts and Comparisons 1993; Haukkamaa 1986; Odlind and Olsson 1986). Use of a different contraceptive agent is recommended.

Estrogens

Antidepressants, tricyclic.   Taking conjugated estrogens and TCAs together may result in akathisia (Krishnan et al. 1984). The effects of the interaction may be related to the dose of estrogen (Editor, Drug Facts and Comparisons 1993; Hamilton and Parry 1983).

Antipsychotic agents.   Estrogens may potentiate chlorpromazine (Martin 1978). Phenothiazine plasma levels may vary with estrogen levels (Hansten 1976). Estrogen facilitates development of parkinsonian symptoms in patients taking neuroleptics (Bedard et al. 1977). Estrogens can precipitate neuroleptic-induced extrapyramidal symptoms (Gratton 1960).

Phenytoin.   Estrogen may decrease the metabolism of phenytoin (J. Griffin and D'Arcy 1975), risking phenytoin toxicity.

Tobacco, smoking.   Possible increased metabolism of estrogen may result in decreased efficacy of estrogen (Jensen et al. 1985). Avoid concurrent use.

Conclusion

It is important for psychiatrists, gynecologists, and other health care providers working with reproductive-age women to have knowledge of the relationships between the brain and the reproductive system, and between psychopharmacology and reproductive pharmacology. Although much research remains to be done, a number of pertinent findings are known to be clinically important in at least some women of reproductive age.

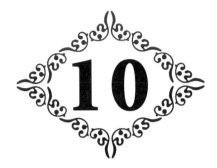

Psychopharmacological Treatment During Pregnancy and Lactation

Katherine L. Wisner, M.D.,
and James M. Perel, Ph.D.

In this chapter we provide a comprehensive review of the issues involved in the treatment of
pregnant women with psychotropic agents. Competent clinical decision
making involves weighing the benefits of treatment against the risks. For
each class of somatic treatment (antidepressants, antipsychotics, lithium, anticonvulsants, benzodiazepines, electroconvulsive therapy),
morphological and behavioral teratological risks are reviewed. Included
is a discussion of pharmacokinetics during pregnancy and pharmacological effects in the newborn. We also present available data about

The authors wish to thank Robert M. Wettstein, M.D., for his suggestions about earlier
drafts.

pharmacotherapy during lactation, because new episodes of psychiatric illness are common in the postpartum period (Kendell et al. 1987; Sholomskas et al. 1993). Of particular importance is a consideration of the *benefits* of pharmacotherapy during gestation, a topic infrequently addressed in reviews. We conclude the chapter with a clinical example that demonstrates the complexity of risk-benefit analysis for somatic treatment during pregnancy.

Risks of Psychopharmacological Treatment During Childbearing

The risks of treating pregnant women with psychotropics can be categorized into two areas: 1) physiological changes of pregnancy and maternal side effects, and 2) fetal teratogenicity and newborn side effects.

The placenta does not prevent psychotropic agents from reaching the fetus. When a woman takes repeated doses of a drug to sustain plasma-level concentrations, as is the case for most psychotropic agents, the drug distribution will be approximately equal in the mother and fetus. Pregnancy is a progressively changing physiological state. Processes that affect drug disposition and dose requirements are 1) increase in volume of distribution (Eadie et al. 1977), 2) decrease in protein-binding capacity, 3) enhancement of hepatic metabolism, and 4) progesterone-induced decrease in gastrointestinal motility. Estrogen, which increases dramatically across gestation, also has central nervous system antidopaminergic effects and inhibits drug metabolism (B. Field et al. 1979; Raymond et al. 1978).

Somatic symptoms that are common during pregnancy must be evaluated before beginning medication to allow differentiation from side effects. For example, gastrointestinal emptying is decreased by 30%–35% during pregnancy (Cupit and Rotmensch 1985), which predisposes to constipation. Adding medication with anticholinergic side effects can create more discomfort.

Teratogenicity is the major concern related to psychotropic use during gestation. A frequent question is whether a particular drug is safe during pregnancy. There is never a guarantee that a pharmacological agent is without teratogenic effects, because low levels of teratogenicity are difficult to distinguish from the spontaneous occurrence of anomalies. An answerable question is whether the risk of a negative outcome is higher in women who use medication at a defined time during gestation than in unexposed pregnant women. The answer clearly depends on which negative outcomes have been observed and reported.

The incidence of major birth defects in the United States is about 2%–4%, and the cause of 65%–70% of these defects is unknown. Only 3% are attributable to environmental causes, including drug exposures (American Medical Association 1983). Therefore, it is unwise to reassure a woman that her infant will be normally developed independent of exposure to a pharmacological agent.

A drug's capacity to act as a teratogen depends upon multiple factors. In his classic chapter, J. G. Wilson (1977) outlined the principles of teratogenicity. His major points were as follows: 1) susceptibility to teratogenesis varies with the developmental stage at exposure; organogenesis (weeks 2 through 8 postconception) is a particularly vulnerable time for the production of anatomical lesions; 2) abnormal development may manifest as death, malformation, growth retardation, functional deficits, carcinogenicity, or altered reproductive capacity; 3) manifestations of deviant development increase in degree as dosage increases from the no-effect to the lethal level; and 4) the presence or absence of maternal toxicity is not a reliable indicator of fetal toxicity.

The term *behavioral teratology* is used to describe deleterious changes in the behavior of offspring exposed to teratogens during fetal development. These effects are due to teratogen-induced neurobiological changes. The behavioral correlates of these changes become evident during postbirth development. Teratological effects include delayed maturation, impaired rates of learning and problem solving, abnormal activity, and pathological arousal states. Behavioral teratogenicity is a manifestation of abnormal development demonstrable at doses of the agent at or below which morphological malformations are induced. Although maximal susceptibility to behavioral teratogenesis corresponds to the first-trimester period of closure of the neural tube, the effects of behavioral teratogens are not limited to this time. Behavioral teratology differs from behavioral toxicity in the neonate, which is due to direct effects of drugs used near term.

Most behavioral teratological data is derived from animal studies, since it is unethical to expose humans to teratogenic agents. Therefore, very little data exist about developmental outcomes in infants exposed to prescribed psychotropics during pregnancy. It is also difficult to isolate effects of the medication from other factors that affect behavior. For example, the quality of the rearing environment has been shown to either attenuate or enhance the long-term biochemical and behavioral consequences of prenatal exposure in rats.

Antidepressant Medication

Choice of Agents

Wisner and Perel (1988) argued that nortriptyline is a favorable antidepressant choice during pregnancy because 1) it has been successfully used for decades, 2) it has lower relative anticholinergic potency compared with other tricyclic antidepressants (TCAs), 3) there is a well-studied relationship between its plasma concentration and therapeutic effect, and 4) its higher potency as an antidepressant reduces other organ exposure because of lower dosage requirements. However, if a woman has responded well to another TCA without major side effects, preferential consideration should be given to the use of the drug known to be effective.

Metabolism During Pregnancy

Wisner, Perel, and Wheeler (1993) found that tricyclic dosages required to contain depressive symptoms increased during the second half of pregnancy. Rapid dose escalation occurred during the third trimester. The final dose achieved during gestation was an average increase of 1.6 times the nonpregnant dose. Serum-level data supported the hypothesis that increased oral dosages were required to achieve constant drug levels across pregnancy.

Morphological Teratogenicity

TCAs.   The Collaborative Perinatal Project was a large, prospective study of children exposed to drugs during gestation (Heinonen et al.

1977). In 42 mother-child pairs exposed to amitriptyline, imipramine, or nortriptyline, 2 malformations were noted. Although this rate was not excessive, the sample size did not allow firm conclusions about malformations. Several clinicians have published case series of women who received imipramine or amitriptyline during pregnancy (Crombie et al. 1972; Kuenssberg and Knox 1972; Scanlon 1969). All concluded that antidepressant exposure did *not* result in an increased risk of malformation. The total number of women in the combined series was 117. There were 3 malformed infants, which yields a rate of anomaly similar to that in the general population. Crombie et al. (1972) studied 81 women who received imipramine (150 mg/day) during gestation and found that none of the exposed infants were malformed. Although these anecdotal series provide valuable information, they are not methodologically rigorous.

Fluoxetine.   Pastuzak et al. (1993) prospectively compared pregnancy outcomes after first-trimester exposure to fluoxetine ($N = 128$) with two matched control groups: one exposed to nonteratogens ($N = 128$) and the other to TCAs ($N = 74$). The mean daily dose of fluoxetine was 25.8 + 13.1 mg/day. Rates of major malformations were comparable within the three groups and did not exceed the expected rate in the general population. The rate of miscarriages tended to be higher (although not significantly so) in both the fluoxetine and the TCA groups compared with women in the nonteratogen-exposed group. If this finding is replicated in other studies, the effect of the psychiatric illness must be separated from that of medication exposure.

Outcomes from 485 prospectively assessed outcomes were recently compiled by Lilly Research Laboratories. The following rates obtained from fluoxetine-exposed infants were similar to those of the general U.S. population: live births, 84.3%; stillbirths, 0.7%; miscarriages, 13.9%; and major malformations 2.8%. Among the live births, 94.6% were full term and 5.4% were premature.

Monoamine oxidase inhibitors.   The Collaborative Perinatal Project monitored 21 mother-child pairs exposed to monoamine oxidase inhibitors (MAOIs), and 3 malformations were observed. Although an elevated risk of malformations was suggested, the sample size was small.

MAOIs should be considered for use during pregnancy only if other options have been exhausted.

Effects in the Newborn

A neonatal behavioral syndrome has been reported in the offspring of women treated with TCAs until delivery. Symptoms included cyanosis, tachypnea, tachycardia, irritability, tremor, feeding difficulties, urinary retention, and profuse sweating. These symptoms may represent either direct effects of the TCA (Schimmell et al. 1991) or withdrawal secondary to cholinergic overdrive (Dilsaver et al. 1983). In women treated during late pregnancy with clomipramine, neonatal withdrawal seizures were described in two infants (Cowe et al. 1982). Wisner and Perel (1988) have recommended gradually tapering or decreasing the dose 1–2 weeks before birth to reduce the risk of withdrawal symptoms.

Breast Feeding

Currently available data do not warrant any absolute recommendation about TCAs and breast feeding. Published studies of tricyclics have demonstrated that the drug concentration in milk is approximately the same as that in maternal plasma. However, the infant's steady-state plasma drug concentration provides a direct and more comprehensive determination of exposure (Atkinson et al. 1988). Therefore, we include only studies of TCAs in which infant serum levels have been obtained in this discussion.

Doxepin.   There is only one report of an adverse outcome in a nursing infant whose mother took tricyclics. Sedation and respiratory depression occurred in an 8-week-old infant whose mother took 75 mg/day of doxepin during lactation (Matheson et al. 1985). The infant's serum doxepin level was just above detectability (3 ng/mL). Two measurements of the infant's serum concentration of the metabolite N-desmethyl-doxepin were 58 and 66 ng/mL (similar to maternal levels). The metabolism of N-desmethyldoxepin includes hydroxylation and conjugation with glucuronic acid, functions which are limited in the newborn. Kemp and colleagues (1985) reported serum levels in a clinically asymptomatic 10-week-old infant whose mother had received 150 mg/day of doxepin. After 43 days of maternal dosing, the infant's doxepin level was not detectable (to 5 ng/mL); the N-desmethyldoxepin level was low (15 ng/mL).

Desipramine.   Stancer and Reed (1986) measured desipramine and its metabolite in the milk and plasma of a nursing mother and in the serum of her 10-week-old infant. Samples were collected 7 and 14 days after the mother reached a dose of 300 mg/day. Neither desipramine nor its metabolite could be detected in the infant's serum when collected 9 hours after maternal dose, even though the measurements were made shortly after peak plasma (and milk) values recorded in the mother. No clinical signs of toxicity were observed.

Clomipramine.   Schimmell et al. (1991) reported serum levels in an infant whose mother was treated with clomipramine (150 mg/day) during pregnancy and breast feeding, which began on day 7 postpartum. The infant remained asymptomatic, and his plasma level (which was 267 ng/mL at birth) decreased over time even though nursing continued. The infant's plasma level was at the lowest detectable level (9.8 ng/mL) at 35 days postpartum.

Amitriptyline.   The total TCA concentration in a nursing mother who had taken 150 mg daily for 3 weeks was 236 ng/mL. No detectable amount of drug was found in her 2-month-old infant's serum (S. H. Erickson et al. 1979). Bader and Newman (1980) described a mother with a serum level of 142 ng/mL of total TCAs while taking 100 mg of amitriptyline. Her infant's serum level was also not detectable. Brixen-Rasmussen and colleagues (1982) studied a mother who took 75–100 mg/day of amitriptyline. At $3\frac{1}{2}$ months postpartum, her total tricyclic level was 121. The infant's serum tricyclic level was below detectability, and there were no signs of drug effects.

Nortriptyline.   Wisner and Perel (1991) studied a series of depressed nursing mothers who were treated with nortriptyline. All of their infants were healthy products of full-term gestations, with the exception of one infant born at 36 weeks. Nortriptyline was not detectable (to 4–5 ng/mL) in infant sera, whereas maternal concentrations ranged from 47 to 164 ng/mL. A metabolite (10-hydroxynortriptyline, 10-OH-NT) was detected at low levels in two infants, the youngest babies (3 and 8 weeks), at the time of sampling. However, five additional cases accumulated since publication have not revealed any 10-OH-NT in these infants, who were all between 2 and 10 weeks of age. There was no evidence of accumulation of nortriptyline or its metabolite in four infants who nursed for 50 days or more. There were no adverse effects, and parents and pediatricians agreed that the children were developing normally. Nonetheless, the possibility that chronic exposure to minute doses of TCAs could affect infant neurodevelopment remains a concern.

Fluoxetine.   Lester and colleagues (1993) studied a 6-week-old breast-feeding infant whose mother was taking 20 mg/day of fluoxetine during the postpartum period. The mother instituted formula feeding and reported a dramatic decrease in her infant's crying 4 days later. The mother continued to pump milk, and returned to breast feeding when the study was completed 3 weeks later. The infant's colic returned within 24 hours. Concentrations in the infant serum were 340 ng/mL of fluoxetine and 208 ng/mL of its metabolite norfluoxetine. The diary records showed increased crying, less sleep, vomiting, and watery stools when the infant received fluoxetine through breast milk.

Sertraline.   Altshuler et al. (1995) studied a nursling whose mother took 100 mg/day of sertraline and 125 mg/day of nortriptyline throughout pregnancy and the postpartum period. The woman delivered a healthy baby at term. Mother and infant serum levels were obtained at weeks 3 and 7 postpartum. At 3 weeks, the maternal sertraline level 12 hours postdose was 48 ng/mL. The infant's serum level was below the limit of detectability (< 0.5 ng/mL). At 7 weeks, the maternal level was 47 ng/mL and the infant again had no detectable level. Nortriptyline levels were measured at 3 weeks only. The maternal level was 120 ng/mL and the infant level was nondetectable (< 10 ng/mL). Routine pediatric evaluations of the child in the first 5 months were within normal limits.

Prevention of Recurrent Postpartum Depression

In an open trial, Wisner and Wheeler (1994) examined 23 pregnant women, each of whom had experienced at least one previous episode of postpartum nonbipolar depression. Significantly more of the women who elected monitoring alone (62.5%) experienced recurrence of postpartum major depression, compared with 6.7% of the women who elected monitoring plus medication. Prophylactic treatment was found to be helpful in preventing recurrences of postpartum depression.

Antipsychotic Agents

Choice of Agents

Wisner and Perel (1988) have recommended the use of high-potency antipsychotics because these agents cause minimal autonomic effects and less sedation, hypotension, and cardiovascular difficulties than their low-potency counterparts. Despite this, more pregnancy data are available for low-potency agents—in particular, chlorpromazine—that have been available for longer periods of time.

Morphological Teratogenicity

Chlorpromazine.   Kris (1961) studied 52 children whose mothers had been treated with chlorpromazine (50–150 mg/day) throughout pregnancy. After following the children for 2–4 years, she concluded that the exposures did not result in morphological or developmental defects. Sobel (1960) studied 52 women who received chlorpromazine for psychiatric conditions during pregnancy and found the rate of anomalies to be similar to that observed in a control group of untreated women. However, 3 women who received high daily doses of chlorpromazine (500–600 mg/day) gave birth to infants with respiratory distress and cyanosis. There were no similar outcomes in the remaining 49 women treated with lower doses. In the Collaborative Perinatal Project (Slone et al. 1977), 142 mothers were exposed to chlorpromazine during the first trimester. No evidence was found for increased risk of malformations, perinatal mortality, diminished birth weight, or lowered intelligence quotient (IQ) at age 4.

Perphenazine.   Data from the Collaborative Perinatal Project included 63 first-trimester exposures and 166 exposures at some point in pregnancy. There was no association with malformations, perinatal mortality, diminished birth weight, or lowered IQ at age 4.

Haloperidol.   This drug was used in hyperemesis gravidarum in the first trimester in 100 women (van Waes and van de Velde 1969). With low-dose treatment, no effects were noted on birth weight, length of pregnancy, fetal or neonatal mortality, or rate of malformations. Haloperidol therapy for chorea gravidarum (1–2 mg/day) has not been related to newborn abnormalities (J. O. Donaldson 1982; Patterson 1979).

Fluphenazine.   Two case reports of pregnant women with schizophrenia who were treated throughout pregnancy have been published. One had a healthy infant (Cleary 1977), who was treated for minor extrapyramidal effects with diphenhydramine at 4 weeks. G. L. Donaldson and Bury (1982) described an infant born with multiple congenital anomalies. General conclusions cannot be drawn from these data.

Summary.   Evidence from the Collaborative Perinatal Project and from most retrospective studies reveals that antipsychotic agents do not cause a rate of malformation distinguishable from that in the general population. No specific organ malformation has been identified. However, the primary indication studied has been nausea (i.e., by Edlund and Craig 1984), and little research has focused on the use of these drugs by *psychotic* women. Data regarding dosage and specific timing are reported infrequently.

Effects in the Newborn

Jaundice has been observed in infants exposed to phenothiazines immediately before birth (Hammond and Toseland 1970) and during labor

(Scokel and Jones 1962). Functional intestinal obstruction occurred in two newborns who were exposed to chlorpromazine and other anticholinergic drugs during late gestation (Falterman and Richardson 1980).

Abnormal behavior has been observed in infants born to women who took antipsychotics during pregnancy. A biphasic pattern with initial postnatal depressed activity (1–5 days) and subsequent agitation (up to 7 months) was described (Desmond et al. 1967). Depression was characterized by decreased movement and crying, vasomotor instability, and feeding difficulties. Infants in the agitated phase displayed hyperreflexia, tremor, excessive sucking, and vasomotor instability.

Breast Feeding

Little information on antipsychotics and breast feeding is available. Whalley et al. (1981) found that a lactating woman taking haloperidol (30 mg/day) had breast-milk levels approximately two-thirds the levels in maternal serum. Clinical observation of the infant revealed no sedation, normal feeding, and achievement of expected developmental milestones at 6 months and 1 year. No behavioral or motor abnormalities were noted.

Adjunctive Agents

Diphenhydramine.   An interaction between diphenhydramine and temazepam resulted in a stillbirth near term, and a high rate of fetal stillbirths was induced in rabbits treated with this combination (Kargas et al. 1985). Whether diphenhydramine combined with other benzodiazepines also carries this risk is unknown; however, the diphenhydramine-benzodiazepine combination should be avoided. The Collaborative Perinatal Project included 595 mother-child pairs exposed to diphenhydramine. First-trimester exposure was related to multiple congenital anomalies. There were no specific data for benztropine or trihexyphenidyl.

Lithium

Metabolism During Pregnancy

Lithium clearance gradually increases by 30%–50% during the second half of pregnancy. The dose must be increased to maintain the therapeutic level as pregnancy progresses (Schou et al. 1973). To avoid dose pulses, lithium carbonate doses should be divided into three to five equal doses throughout the day. With the rapid fall in lithium clearance at delivery, toxic maternal concentrations can occur if the dose is not rapidly decreased.

Weinstein (1980) warned that signs of lithium toxicity may be attributed to somatic symptoms of pregnancy. Typical corrective measures may worsen the toxic state (e.g., sodium restriction for the fluid retention of mild lithium toxicity). Weinstein recommended monitoring lithium levels at least once a month in the first half of pregnancy and once weekly later in gestation.

Morphological Teratogenicity

Lithium exposure during pregnancy was previously thought to be highly associated with a cardiac malformation, Ebstein's anomaly, in offspring. That conclusion was based on biased retrospective reports. More recent epidemiological data and case–control studies document that the teratogenic risk from first-trimester exposure to lithium is lower than was previously thought (L. S. Cohen et al. 1994).

The Register of Lithium Babies collected data from infants exposed to lithium during the first trimester of pregnancy. Weinstein (1980) summarized data for 225 cases: 25 (11%) of the cases resulted in congenitally malformed infants. A total of 18, or 8%, of the malformations were Ebstein's anomaly and other major cardiovascular malformations. He reported that Ebstein's anomaly was 150 times more frequent among the malformed infants reported to the Register than among malformed infants in general, and that cardiovascular malformations of any type appeared about six times as often among the abnormal infants in the Register as among malformed infants generally.

Reports to a register will amplify the frequency of pathology, since abnormal outcomes are more frequently reported. These data do not allow conclusions about the incidence of malformations, because the true number of exposed fetuses is unknown. However, if the drug does *not* have adverse effects, the ratios among *types* of cardiovascular pathology should be similar to the corresponding ratios in the population. This was not the case in the Lithium Registry population, among which Ebstein's anomaly was comparably frequent.

Kallen and Tandberg (1983) studied the offspring of women with bipolar disorder. Infants with a serious heart defect were born to 7% of women who took lithium: women who did not take lithium were not at increased risk. These authors' data suggested that an association exists between the use of lithium in early pregnancy and the birth of an infant with a serious heart defect that is not attributable to the bipolar illness state.

However, two recent case-control studies have suggested that the association between lithium and Ebstein's anomaly was weak. Zalzstein et al. (1990) found that children with Ebstein's anomaly and those with neuroblastoma did not differ in rate of lithium exposure during the first trimester. Kallen (1988) studied children with Ebstein's anomaly or tricuspid atresia and healthy control subjects matched for age and parity. No lithium exposures were detected. These authors concluded that the risk of Ebstein's anomaly is much lower than the rate implied by the Registry data.

S. J. Jacobsen et al. (1992) prospectively studied 138 first-trimester lithium–treated women and 148 age-matched control subjects. The mean daily dose of lithium was 927 mg. Rates of major congenital malformations did not differ between the lithium-treated (2.8%) and the control (2.4%) groups. One patient in the lithium group chose to terminate pregnancy after Ebstein's anomaly was detected by a prenatal echocardiogram. There was one fetus with ventricular septal defect in the control group. Jacobsen and colleagues concluded that lithium was not an important human teratogen and advised that "women with major affective disorders who wish to have children may continue lithium therapy, provided that adequate screening tests, including level II ultrasound and fetal echocardiography, are done" (S. J. Jacobsen et al. 1992, p. 533).

Although this was an important prospective study, the data do not fully support Jacobsen and co-workers' conclusion. The directive to obtain careful obstetrical monitoring is inconsistent with the statement that lithium is not an *important* teratogen. The one cardiac malformation observed was Ebstein's anomaly, which has a rate of occurrence in the general population of 1 in 20,000. The authors have again demon-

strated Weinstein's (1980) contention that first-trimester lithium exposure increases the risk of an extremely low risk anomaly (1 in 20,000)
(Behrman and Vaughan 1987) to a level of greater risk. Jacobsen and
colleagues' (1992) study demonstrated 1 occurrence in a series of 138.
Note that the cardiac anomaly in the control group was a ventricular
septal defect, the most common cardiac malformation (although still
only approximately 2 in 1,000; Behrman and Vaughan 1987). *A more
appropriate conclusion is that cardiac malformations, particularly Ebstein's anomaly, occur at a low rate in exposed fetuses.* Although the rate
is lower than that established by previous studies, it is higher than the
spontaneous rate. L. S. Cohen et al. (1994) concluded that the risk of
major congenital anomalies among the children of women treated with
lithium during early pregnancy was between 4% and 12% compared
with the general population rate of 2%–4%.

Effects in the Newborn

There are many case reports of transplacental fetal lithium exposure
with adverse effects for the newborn. Hypotonia, cyanosis, thyroid depression with goiter, bradycardia, transient atrial arrhythmias, and neph-
rogenic diabetes insipidus have been reported (Wisner and Perel 1988).
Birth weight was significantly higher in lithium-exposed infants than in
control infants despite identical gestational ages (3,475 versus 3,383 g)
(S. J. Jacobsen et al. 1992). Of 241 infants reported to the Lithium Registry, Yoder et al. (1984) found that 39% evidenced premature delivery
and 36% had a birth weight greater than the 90th percentile; in addition,
there was an 8.3% rate of perinatal mortality, including stillbirths.

Behavioral Teratogenicity

Schou (1976) studied 67 normally formed children reported to the Lithium Registry and their nonexposed siblings. These children were at least
5 years old. Data were collected through questionnaires sent to the psychiatrists or general practitioners who had originally reported the exposures. Information was requested about the child's development, with
additional details solicited if the child was abnormal. Schou recovered

50 case questionnaires and 57 sibling questionnaires. The difference in the number of developmental abnormalities between the lithium-exposed and control groups was not statistically significant. Although weak methodologically, this study provides some information about the development of children exposed prenatally to lithium. S. J. Jacobsen et al. (1992) also reported that attainment of major developmental milestones (smiling, lifting head, sitting, crawling, standing, talking, and walking) in 22 children prenatally exposed to lithium did not differ from that of control subjects.

Breast Feeding

Because it is an electrolyte, lithium passes easily into milk. Milk levels average 40%–50% of maternal serum, and infant serum and milk levels are approximately equal (Schou and Amdisen 1973; Sykes et al. 1976). Nurslings have developed toxic symptoms such as cyanosis, hypothermia, and hypotonia (Tunnessen and Hertz 1972). Because infants develop significant blood levels when breast-feeding, lithium is contraindicated in nursing women (Ananth 1978; C. M. Berlin 1981; Wisner and Perel 1988).

Anticonvulsants

Anticonvulsants, particularly carbamazepine and valproate, have been used for treatment-resistant and rapid-cycling bipolar disorder (Post 1990). Women receiving these agents present a clinical challenge during gestation, because fetal toxicity has been described for both. Other somatic treatments, such as antipsychotics or electroconvulsive therapy (ECT), should be considered for pregnant patients with cyclical mood disorder before selecting anticonvulsants.

Morphological Teratogenicity

Data have been collected for women who have taken anticonvulsants throughout pregnancy for seizure disorder. Because anticonvulsants are usually continued throughout pregnancy, little is known about the effects of specific gestational timing, such as whether use beyond the first trimester carries risk. In a Japanese multiinstitutional collaborative study (Nakane et al. 1980), the rate of malformation was 11.5% of live births from first-trimester medicated mothers and 2.3% from non-medicated mothers with seizure disorder. Cleft lip and/or palate and malformations of the cardiovascular system were frequently found in the infants of medicated mothers. The incidence of miscarriage or still-birth was significantly higher in the medicated than in the nonmedicated group. As the number of anticonvulsant drugs used (for polytherapy) in the first trimester increased, the incidence of fetal malformation rose sharply. Higher doses of drugs were related to greater risk of malformations.

Carbamazepine.   K. L. Jones et al. (1989) contacted pregnant women in the first trimester, prospectively followed them throughout gestation, and studied their offspring. They found craniofacial defects (11%), fingernail hypoplasia (26%), and developmental delay (20%) in 35 live-born infants of women exposed to carbamazepine alone. They found no significant difference in major malformations, but a higher rate of 13 minor malformations. Rosa (1991) examined infants of women treated with carbamazepine during pregnancy. Pregnant Medicaid recipients receiving anticonvulsants were assessed, and these data, taken with other published cohort studies, supported the conclusion that exposure to carbamazepine in utero carried approximately a 1% risk of spina bifida.

Hillesmaa et al. (1981) evaluated the mean head circumference (standardized for gestational age and sex) of 20 babies born to mothers on carbamazepine alone. Measurements were significantly lower in drug-exposed than in control babies, and no catch-up head growth had occurred by 18 months of age. Growth variables did not correlate with maternal serum drug levels, etiology or duration of maternal epilepsy, or number and distribution of seizures during pregnancy.

A prospective, controlled trial found no effect on global IQ or language development in children exposed to carbamazepine in utero, whereas IQ and language development were lower in children exposed to phenytoin in utero (Scolnik et al. 1994).

Valproate.   Valproate use has been associated with neural-tube defects (Jeavons 1982; Robert and Guibaud 1982) as well as normal outcomes (Hillesmaa et al. 1980). Bjerkedal et al. (1982) believed that valproate caused spina bifida in 1% of exposed fetuses.

Omtzigt et al. (1992a) studied 92 pregnancies in which valproate was used alone or in combination with other anticonvulsants. In six fetuses, spina bifida was diagnosed prenatally by ultrasound and high α-fetoprotein concentrations in the amniotic fluid. Of these six fetuses, five were exposed to valproate monotherapy and one to a combination of valproate and carbamazepine. The women who carried a fetus with spina bifida used significantly higher daily doses of valproate, which resulted in greater serum levels (73 μg/mL) compared with women with unaffected infants (44 μg/mL). Omtzigt et al. (1992b) also found that maternal serum α-fetoprotein levels were unreliable during prenatal screening for neural-tube defects for women taking valproate. They recommended that amniocentesis and fetal ultrasound be offered. Omtzigt and colleagues also performed pharmacokinetic studies for 52 of 92 pregnancies. Their data suggested that clearance of valproate and its metabolites from the fetal compartment lagged behind that of the maternal compartment (a *deep compartment* model). Therefore, chronic valproate use results in fetal accumulation. Dickenson et al. (1979) also found that the fetal deep-compartment model applied to valproic acid, which crossed the placenta to achieve fetal serum concentrations 1.4 times maternal serum levels. The half-life of the drug in the newborn is increased to 45 hours because of reduced glucuronidation. Unlike carbamazepine, valproate does not induce hepatic enzyme systems in utero.

Effects in the Newborn

Nau et al. (1981) remarked that withdrawal symptoms did not seem to occur in infants born to mothers on valproate.

Breast Feeding

Carbamazepine.   Transient hepatic toxicity has been reported in neonates exposed to carbamazepine during pregnancy and breast feeding.

Frey et al. (1990) reported cholestatic hepatitis. Merlob et al. (1992) described hepatic dysfunction characterized by direct hyperbilirubinemia and high concentrations of gamma-glutamyltransferase. Hepatic dysfunction in the latter case resolved even though the mother breast-fed with continued carbamazepine therapy.

Valproate.   The concentration of valproate in breast milk was between 1% and 25% of the concurrent level in the mother's serum in the study by Dickinson et al. (1979), who concluded that its use was acceptable during nursing. Nau et al. (1981) found the concentration of valproate in mother's milk was 3% of corresponding maternal levels.

Benzodiazepines

Metabolism During Pregnancy

Kanto (1982) thoroughly reviewed the pharmacokinetics of benzodiazepines during pregnancy. As with valproate, the fetus and surrounding tissues functionally become a deep compartment. Prolonged administration of these agents in pregnant women should be avoided. If benzodiazepine use is necessary, a clear time-limited indication should be determined (e.g., severe vomiting secondary to anxiety, agitation secondary to mania). Other drugs that require a longer period of treatment before symptom reduction should be introduced with the intent of eventually tapering the benzodiazepine.

Wisner and Perel (1988) selected lorazepam as the drug of choice during gestation because it is associated with a slower rate of placental transfer than is diazepam (Kanto 1982), it lacks active metabolites, and it has high potency with good absorption. However, little outcome data are available specific to lorazepam use during pregnancy. The general principle of avoidance of chronic or high-dose treatment also applies to this agent.

Lipid solubility affects the rate of absorption of the drug into the bloodstream, the extent of distribution in the body, the rates at which brain sites are entered and vacated, and placental penetrability. As lipid solubility increases, benzodiazepines have faster onset of action, such as sedation/dysphoria, in the central nervous system and expose the fetus to higher initial concentrations. Tables 3–4, 3–5, and 3–6 summarize the pharmacokinetics of commonly used benzodiazepines.

Morphological Teratogenicity

Chlordiazepoxide.   Milkovich and van den Berg (1974) suggested that chlordiazepoxide may be teratogenic during the first 42 days of pregnancy, because the rate of severe malformations was three times as great during this period than in later pregnancy. In a case-control study by Bracken and Holford (1981), mothers of congenitally malformed infants were more likely than mothers of normally formed infants to have used a tranquilizer (usually chlordiazepoxide) in the first trimester. In contrast, data from the Collaborative Perinatal Project (Hartz et al. 1975) did not demonstrate a relationship of chlordiazepoxide exposure to congenital anomalies. No evidence was found that prenatal exposure caused mental or motor score differences at 8 months or IQ score differences at 4 years.

Diazepam.   Retrospective studies have associated the ingestion of diazepam with increased risk of cleft lip with or without cleft palate (Safra and Oakley 1980) but have also failed to find any relationship between first-trimester exposure and oral clefts (Rosenberg et al. 1983). In a study of anticonvulsant use during gestation, Nakane et al. (1980) found that the use of diazepam with anticonvulsants resulted in a higher rate of cleft lip and/or palate, and suggested that the maximum daily dose of diazepam should not exceed 6 mg in early pregnancy.

Benzodiazepines, nonspecific.   In a case-control study, Laegreid and colleagues (1990) evaluated whether infants exposed to benzodiazepines were more frequently affected by four problems assessed in the neonatal period: 1) unspecified congenital malformations of the nervous system; 2) dysmorphic features, unspecified; 3) cleft lip/palate; and 4) congenital malformations of the urinary tract. Retained maternal serum samples drawn at gestational week 12 were evaluated for benzodiazepines after the children were born. Eight of 18 maternal case samples and 2 of 60 control samples were positive for benzodiazepines. The association between one or more of the problems evaluated and benzodiazepine-positive maternal serum samples was highly significant. These findings are important because they do not depend on maternal report of benzodiazepine use.

Alprazolam.   St. Clair and Schirmer (1992) prospectively assessed pregnancy outcome associated with first-trimester exposure to alprazolam. Outcome data were available on 411 pregnancies: 13 live births with congenital anomalies, 47 miscarriages, and 88 elective abortions (1 elective abortion involved an infant with multiple anomalies identified by ultrasound). The 4.7% rate of congenital anomalies is similar to the 3% rate in the general population and the 6% rate quoted by the Collaborative Perinatal Project (Heinonen et al. 1977). There was no consistent anomaly produced. The rates of spontaneous abortion and stillbirth were similar to those in the general population.

Clonazepam.   Fisher et al. (1985) described a 36-week, 2,750-gram premature infant whose mother was treated with clonazepam for myoclonic sleep disorder throughout gestation. The infant developed apnea, cyanosis, and hypotonia within a few hours of birth. Maternal serum clonazepam level at delivery was 32 ng/mL; cord blood was 19 ng/mL (therapeutic range 5–70 ng/mL). The infant's serum level was 4.4 ng/mL. Although the mother breast-fed, the infant's serum level decreased to 1 ng/mL at day 14. Follow-up of the infant revealed excessive apnea episodes until 10 weeks of age, but the neurodevelopmental exam was normal at 5 months. The duration of infant effects may have been due to the long elimination half-life of this agent.

Effects in the Newborn

Two syndromes of neonatal toxicity are associated with the benzodiazepines: the floppy infant syndrome and a withdrawal syndrome. The floppy infant syndrome (Gillberg 1977) occurs after prolonged maternal therapy and produces symptoms such as hypotonia, lethargy, sucking difficulties, hypothermia, and cyanosis. Passive addiction of the newborn also occurs. Neonatal withdrawal consists of tremors, irritability, hypertonicity, and vigorous sucking (Athinarayanan et al. 1976; Rementeria and Bhatt 1977) 2–6 hours after birth.

Breast Feeding

Diazepam.   Erkkola and Kanto (1972) found measurable quantities of diazepam and N-desmethyldiazepam in maternal and breast-feeding infant sera during nursing. The maternal-to-fetal ratio changed from postpartum day 4 (2.8:1) to day 6 (8.1:1) as the concentrations in three infants' sera decreased due to progressively more effective elimination.

Lorazepam.   Lorazepam transfer into breast milk was very low (Whitelaw et al. 1981) in a breast-feeding mother who took 2.5-mg lorazepam twice daily for 5 days after delivery. Her newborn did not appear sedated; however, the effects of longer-term treatment are unknown. There is no information on breast-milk content of these agents when the mother has been treated chronically.

Prolonged benzodiazepine use during lactation is not advisable because of the possibility of accumulation. Alternative treatments should be carefully evaluated. If short-term administration is anticipated, breast-milk production could be maintained artificially until the medication is discontinued.

Other Agents

According to the Collaborative Perinatal Project, atropine exposure in the first trimester did not produce elevated relative risk. However, glycopyrrolate is the anticholinergic drug of choice (Weis et al. 1983; M. G. Wise et al. 1984) because of limited passage across membranes and better suppression of exocrine secretion. In the Collaborative Perinatal Project, exposure to certain barbiturates during the first trimester was associated with cardiovascular malformations. There were 41 cases of prenatal exposure—specifically to methohexital—and 2 malformations were observed.

Electroconvulsive Therapy

ECT has been safely administered in both normal and high-risk pregnancies. Emergency use of ECT is indicated when the illness-related condition of the mother presents hazard for the fetus, such as severe agitation, catatonia, dehydration, malnutrition, or violence (Fink 1981). An advantage of ECT compared with chronic administration of medication for a psychiatric disorder is the brief duration of the pharmacological agents used in ECT.

Effects of ECT During Pregnancy

In later pregnancy, lying in the supine position can cause the gravid uterus to compress the major blood vessels, thereby reducing blood pressure and placental perfusion (Ostheimer and Warren 1984). Use of a wedge under one hip will displace the uterus and avoid this problem.

The effects of ECT on the fetus are minimal. During the ECT procedure, Repke and Berger (1984) monitored the fetal heart rate, which remained stable. These authors also used ultrasonography and noted no significant changes in fetal movements during the procedure. A normal infant was subsequently delivered full term and had favorable Apgar scores and normal neurological exam. Varan and colleagues (1985) reported the successful treatment with ECT and chlorpromazine of a 33-year-old woman who was 18–20 weeks pregnant. Fetal heart rate monitoring revealed that a bradycardia (80 beats per minute) occurred during the tonic phase of the ECT treatment, but the heart rate quickly returned to normal. No uterine contractions were observed during or after any of the ECT administrations. The child was delivered vaginally at term and had excellent Apgar scores and no congenital anomalies. Remick and Maurice (1978) suggested guidelines for ECT during gestation, which included the involvement of an obstetrician to study fetal well-being.

Medications During ECT

Succinylcholine, a neuromuscular blocking agent, is used to prevent muscular contraction during the induced seizure. Succinylcholine is rapidly metabolized by plasma pseudocholinesterase activity to 60% of normal during the first trimester (Ostheimer and Warren 1984). The rare woman who possesses impaired pseudocholinesterase activity may be at particular risk for prolonged apnea. Because of the additional risk posed for the vulnerable mother and fetus, Wisner and Perel (1988) recommended that pregnant women be screened for pseudocholinesterase deficiency as part of the pre-ECT medical evaluation. Such screening is particularly important for women with a personal or family history of postoperative anesthetic recovery problems.

When administered in usual clinical doses, succinylcholine does not cross the placenta in demonstrable quantities, and infants are unaffected (Weis et al. 1983). When maternal cholinesterase activity is low, succinylcholine use near term may affect the fetus, with resultant muscle weakness at birth (Owens and Zeitlin 1975).

There were 26 pregnancies with first-trimester exposure to succinylcholine in the Collaborative Perinatal Project, all of which resulted in normal infants. Because the sample size was small, the power to detect an elevated rate of malformations is very low.

Morphological Teratogenicity

The largest sample that has been reported is that of Impastato and associates (1964), who compiled data on 318 patients. Although the study was performed 30 years ago, succinylcholine and oxygen supplementation were used. Thirteen patients (4%) delivered malformed fetuses; four of these patients also received insulin coma treatment, which was the likely cause of the malformations. In 4 patients, the procedure occurred after the sixteenth week of pregnancy, which made it unlikely that ECT was the cause of the abnormalities. From these data, the authors concluded that there was no increased risk of fetal damage beyond that in either the general population or the population of psychiatric patients.

Behavioral Teratogenicity

Forssman (1955) studied 16 children whose mothers had received ECT (1–6 treatments) during the first and second trimesters. All of the children had normal psychomotor development and physical examinations. Impastato and colleagues (1964) followed 71 children born to mothers who received ECT. Children varied in age from 2 weeks to 19 years, but all were considered normally developed "except two who were mentally defective and four who showed neurotic traits" (Impastato et al. 1964). Descriptions such as these are difficult to evaluate.

Benefits of Psychopharmacological Treatment During Childbearing

Control of Physiological Consequences of Stress

In animal models, stress—independent of chemical agents—can cause behavioral teratogenicity. In a review, Istvan (1986) provided evidence that maternal stress was associated with fetal hypoxia, low birth weight, diminished litter size, higher rates of miscarriage, and fetal hypotension in animal models. Barlow et al. (1979) published an interesting study in which groups of pregnant rats on gestational days 12–14 were 1) treated with restraint stress alone, 2) treated with restraint stress plus diazepam (1 mg/kg bid), 3) treated with diazepam alone, and 4) not treated (controls). Offspring of mothers subjected to restraint stress alone were significantly delayed on a number of developmental measures, including growth, ear-opening, cliff avoidance response, auditory startle response, and midair righting reflex. When adult, these offspring also showed significantly impaired learning ability in a swimming maze. However, the rate of development and learning ability in the restraint-plus-diazepam and the diazepam-alone groups was comparable to or slightly advanced of that in untreated controls. Barlow and colleagues concluded that concurrent administration of a low dose of the antianxiety agent diazepam during restraint stress prevented the adverse postnatal effects of maternal restraint stress during pregnancy.

Prevention of Adverse Outcomes

Consider the physiology of a pregnant woman with an agitated depression: major weight loss, agitation with pacing, circadian rhythm disruption with sleep loss and fragmentation, and extreme fatigue. Psychosocial consequences of failing to treat this patient aggressively can include long-term hospitalization, marital discord and divorce, inability to care for other children, and loss of employment. L. J. Miller (1991) defined the possible risks of withholding pharmacology during gestations as 1) malnutrition, secondary to loss of appetite or impaired judgment; 2) attempts at premature self-delivery, perhaps because of delusions; 3) fetal abuse or neonaticide, secondary to command hallucinations, delusions, or denial of pregnancy; 4) refusal or inability to engage in obstetrical care; and 5) precipitous delivery, if the patient is unable to identify labor and seek care.

Few data exist regarding the risks of *not treating* with psychotropics during gestation. L. S. Cohen et al. (1989) published a case of a woman who suffered a panic attack that was followed by placental abruption. Direct consequences of psychiatric illness, such as the risk of suicide and infanticide, need to be considered in the risk-benefit analysis.

Promotion of Positive Mother-Infant Interactions

The risk-benefit analysis must include a consideration of the interactional capabilities of the mother with her family. The relationship between the infant and the primary caregiver is of vital importance in infant emotional development. Ample evidence supports that uncontrolled maternal psychiatric illness has negative effects on the development of infants. Sameroff et al. (1982) found that the chronicity and severity of maternal psychiatric illness were related to suboptimal interactions.

Sameroff et al. (1982) found that, compared with children of nondepressed control mothers, children of depressed mothers were more active, distractible, and less responsive at 4 months of age. T. Field et al. (1990) found that infants of depressed mothers played less than infants of nondepressed mothers. Insecure attachment in young children occurs more often if their mothers are depressed (D'Angelo 1986). Older children are also negatively affected by parental depression (Downey and Coyne 1990). Consequences of parental mental illness, such as income loss, family disruption, and placement out of the home, further impair child development (Rutter and Quinton 1984).

Prevention of Postpartum Psychiatric Episodes

Ideally, recurrence of psychiatric illness in the postpartum period will be prevented by pharmacological intervention *before* the onset of symptoms in newly delivered women. Investigators have suggested that psychoses can be prevented or attenuated with postbirth lithium treatment (D. E. Stewart et al. 1991), and that major depression can be prevented with antidepressant treatment (Wisner and Wheeler 1994).

Applications of Data to Patient Care

The Physician-Patient Relationship

The stance that medication is never appropriate during pregnancy is unrealistic. In some situations (e.g., severe suicidality, violent behavior), the risk of failing to treat is greater than any known (or unknown) risk of pharmacotherapy. The physician's role in treating the pregnant woman is to 1) provide information about the risks and benefits of available treatments, 2) review the efficacy of various treatments for the patient's specific clinical condition, 3) discuss the influence of pregnancy on the treatment choices, 4) assist the patient in exploring the treatment options and defining the most reasonable approach, and 5) include the father of the baby (or significant other) if the woman desires. The woman's sense of caring for herself and her baby is facilitated by appropriate medication monitoring.

Medicolegal Issues

Informed consent.   In nonresearch situations, written informed consent for treatment with psychotropic medication is neither required nor recommended (Wettstein 1988). Verbal informed consent procedures are more likely to have therapeutic value, to assist in the treatment alliance, to give the patient responsibility for her own care, and to provide an opportunity for continual reassessment of the patient's competence to consent to treatment. Written consent forms may improperly substitute for the informed consent process. These forms will not necessarily defend the physician against charges of failure to disclose alternatives to and risks of treatment or failure to obtain consent. However, this practice may be required by law in some states.

Documentation.   Documentation of the woman's competency to consent includes a description of the content of the discussion and the patient's questions. The woman's ability to repeat the information in her own words is documented. If the father of the baby or significant others are involved, their questions or concerns are also noted. Consent to discuss the treatment with the woman's obstetrician is obtained, and the content of this conversation is also noted. The treatment planning and clinical decision making are documented by the process of "thinking aloud on paper" (Wettstein 1989), which provides evidence that the patient's care was approached responsibly. Other prescribed and over-the-counter or illicit drug use (including smoking) and other circumstances that might affect the pregnancy outcome are also documented. Diagnostic tests (and their results) performed by the obstetrician are recorded.

Liability.   Careful documentation is vital to avoiding legal proceedings. The plaintiff must prove that the physician deviated from the *standard of care* (Wettstein 1989). The deviation may be due to the psychiatrist's *error of omission* (failure to treat or to inform) or *error of commission* (failure to treat in accordance with the standard of care). The psychiatrist is not a guarantor of a good result for the patient, and an adverse clinical outcome does not presume malpractice.

If the practitioner is uncomfortable with the risk-benefit analysis, expert consultation is advisable (Wettstein 1989). Academic medical centers usually have telephone access to pregnancy drug-prescribing information. Obstetrical hospitals or departments often can provide information.

Behavioral teratogenicity is a relatively new area and consists largely of animal studies. No published data exist that firmly establish the behavioral teratogenicity of prescribed psychotropics in humans. Therefore, at this time, the risk is a theoretical one, but its reality and magnitude have not been established. In risk-benefit analyses, it is very difficult to weigh this factor, because there are no data. One approach is to discuss this theoretical risk with mothers directly and to admit relative ignorance in the field. In legal proceedings, the physician's conduct is judged with regard to the standard of care *at the time of treatment* rather than that at a later time when clinical advances may have occurred (Wettstein 1989).

Approach to Risk-Benefit Analysis

Clinical Information

What factors are used to weigh risks and benefits of somatic treatment during gestation?

1. What is the disorder (or disorders) being treated? There is little information about the natural history of common psychiatric illnesses during gestation. Panic disorder may generally improve during pregnancy, but this is certainly not the case for all women (Villeponteaux et al. 1992). Bipolar episodes and major depression can present for the first time or recur during gestation.

2. What is the patient's history? For example, if the patient invariably becomes psychotic when medication is tapered, discontinuation during pregnancy carries a higher risk of recurrence than for a patient who has been treated for a single episode. Recurrence during pregnancy carries risk not only for the patient but also for her fetus.

3. To which medications has the patient responded? Are there alternative medications for which more information about use in gestation is available?

4. What is the patient's attitude about continuing this pregnancy? Explore whether the pregnancy was planned and her experience with past pregnancies.

5. What is the patient's perception of her psychosocial stability as she manages the additional stress of pregnancy?

6. Who are the patient's significant others, and how do they perceive her illness and behave during episodes? Will they support and help monitor her?

7. Is the patient comfortable discussing her mental health with her obstetrician? Are there obstetrical evaluations that will assist in the patient's psychiatric care (for example, a normal ultrasound often significantly relieves anxiety in pharmacologically treated women)?

Before recommending pharmacotherapy or ECT, alternative treatments should be considered, such as specific psychotherapies, behavioral treatments, or light therapy. The choice of treatment will largely be dictated by the severity of symptoms. The clinician will need to evaluate the urgency of symptoms; for example, psychosis with self-abuse and severe vegetative symptoms of major mood disorder dictate pharmacotherapy or ECT. If a nonpharmacological approach is attempted, careful symptom monitoring and pharmacological intervention for intensifying symptoms (ideally, previously agreed upon) can follow. Monitoring of symptom response is vital, since pharmacological intervention cannot be justified if the response that defined its benefit does not occur. Monitoring instruments such as the self-report Inventory to Diagnose Depression (Zimmerman et al. 1986) and the clinician-rated Hamilton Rating Scale for Depression (J. Hamilton 1961) are useful for documenting treatment response.

Case Example: Consultation on an Inpatient Unit

We close this chapter with a case example, which is provided to demonstrate the application of the risk-benefit model. Every clinical issue inherent in this type of work cannot be addressed; however, the reader can obtain a sense of the evaluative process.

Consultation Request

Mrs. E is a 25-year-old white married woman referred for evaluation of the risks and benefits of reintroduction of medication (lithium and haloperidol) at gestational week 16.

1. **Current medications:** Prenatal vitamins.
2. **Laboratory evaluations:** All within normal limits. Sleep-deprived EEG is normal. There is no β-HCG [human chorionic gonadotropin] or gynecological exam on record.
3. **Vital signs:** Pulse 80 regular; blood pressure 110/92 on admission.
4. **Psychiatric history:** Diagnosis is atypical psychosis; rule out bipolar disorder. No history of violent behavior. Patient has not been able to function without pharmacological control of illness for at

least 10 years. Previous withdrawal of haloperidol during a pregnancy resulted in decompensation. Although psychotherapy was provided during gestation, her symptoms continually worsened. Full functional capability returned 1 year after the infant's birth. Recovery required reinstitution of haloperidol and addition of lithium. Her psychosis cleared with haloperidol alone. Lithium was added to treat residual irritability and mild mood instability, with significant improvement. The chart states that the patient's outpatient psychiatrist favors pharmacological treatment during this pregnancy.

5. **Past obstetric history:** Gravida 3, para 1, abortion 1 at age 19. Hypertension and mild hyperglycemia during past pregnancy, which resulted in a full-term 8-pound, 11-ounce girl. No neonatal distress.

6. **Psychosocial history:** Mrs. E was admitted because of inability to function as a homemaker and mother secondary to the cognitive disorganization of psychosis. She is a college graduate.

Patient Interview

1. **Mental status:** Significant for cooperative, mildly euphoric woman with circumstantial and tangential communication; expansive mood. She denies auditory, visual, olfactory, tactile, or gustatory hallucinations. She states that she is occasionally aware of another *presence* inside herself that has pleasant thoughts. At times, she wonders if these are the baby's thoughts. Mrs. E denies thought projection/insertion.

   Mrs. E is excited about her planned pregnancy and frequently speaks of her love for children. She states that she will not consider another abortion. She mentions marital problems but has difficulty being specific. She denies physical abuse. She claims to be in the hospital for psychiatric help and because she does not want her daughter to be affected by the marital discord.

   Mrs. E is an intelligent woman. Despite her cognitive disorganization, she is able to attend to the interview and understands the concept of risk versus benefit regarding medication during pregnancy. She can repeat these concepts back to the examiner in her own words.

2. **Medication exposure history:** Last menstrual period (LMP) 11/25. Last haloperidol dose (5 mg) on 12/29. Lithium discontinued about 20 days postconception. Penicillin 2/19 through 3/1. Mrs. E denies other drugs, alcohol, and smoking.
3. **Family history:** Positive for thyroid disorder (maternal grandmother), rheumatoid arthritis (mother), myocardial infarction, arthritis (father), alcoholism with early death (paternal grandmother), toxemia with postpartum demise, and infant death (paternal grandmother).
4. **Current symptoms of pregnancy:** Nausea that is improving, occasional emesis, fatigue. No constipation, back pain, headache, abdominal cramping, vaginal bleeding, or dizziness. Mild dry mouth reported.

Assessment and Recommendations

1. Mrs. E first learned of her pregnancy via a urine test. She states that her obstetrician, Dr. Smith, performed a serum pregnancy test.
   Recommendation: Confirm the positive serum pregnancy test through Dr. Smith's office. Alternatively, at 16 weeks post-LMP, the fetal heartbeat is audible. Confirm the presence of a viable fetus, because a) a nonviable fetus or other pathological condition will obviate concern about medication, b) beginning medication and subsequently finding a nonviable fetus may result in faulty attribution of fetal demise to the medication, and c) delusional pregnancy, although rare, can be very convincing.
2. Mrs. E is competent to understand, evaluate, and make a decision about the risk-benefit analysis required because she can repeat the information in her own words, ask relevant questions that demonstrate her understanding ("Are my baby's body organs formed at this point in pregnancy?"), and justify her decision with this information.
   Recommendation: Involve Mrs. E in the risk-benefit discussion and decision making and document this discussion in the medical record.
3. Table 10–1 presents a suggested basis for the risk-benefit discussion.

Table 10–1.   Suggested basis for risk-benefit analysis for Mrs. E

Risks of not treating with haloperidol

1. Continued marital dysfunction, minimal capacity for work toward resolution.
2. Estrangement from 3-year-old daughter.
3. Inability to perform daily functions of housewife and mother.
4. Long-term hospitalization; financial obligations.
5. Possible progressive deterioration, which is characteristic of this patient's past history and prolonged period of recovery.

Risks of haloperidol therapy

1. At this point in pregnancy, the risk of major physical malformation is that in the general population (3%). A theoretical risk is behavioral teratogenicity.
2. Maternal discomfort secondary to side effects of haloperidol, which is unlikely, since she previously had none.
3. Possible extrapyramidal symptoms in the newborn (usually without long-term effects).

Benefits of haloperidol therapy

1. Improved cognitive functioning with ability to make optimal use of psychotherapy, adjust to and manage the pregnancy and facilitate attachment to the fetus and newborn.
2. Appropriate interactions with the 3-year-old daughter.
3. Improved ability to function at home.
4. Decreased hospitalization time.

Summary

There is no current risk to the fetus due to maternal poor oral intake or violent behavior. The patient weighs 142 pounds and her usual weight is 131 pounds; weight gain—11 pounds during pregnancy.

The risks of medication at this point are outweighed by the significant psychosocial consequences of no pharmacological treatment for Mrs. E and her family. However, Mr. and Mrs. E should assign their own values to the risks and benefits as active participants in the decision making. If the patient elects pharmacotherapy, lithium use should be deferred until the therapeutic effects of haloperidol alone can be determined.

Effects of exposure that have already occurred due to haloperidol are minimal and approximate the risk of malformation in the general population. The exposure to lithium ceased at the time of cardiac differentiation (20 days postconception) and was clearly discontinued before tricuspid/mitral valve formation. However, the exact time window of exposure to lithium in relation to cardiac malformation is unknown.

The risk for Mrs. E's fetus is probably less than for a fetus who experienced lithium exposure during the course of cardiac differentiation. This would put her risk of fetal cardiac malformation at a maximum of 4%–12% (L. S. Cohen et al. 1994). Mrs. E also carries the general population risk of 3% for fetal malformations (of any type), as any pregnant woman would.

Recommendations

1. Obtain consent to discuss Mr. and Mrs. E's decision with Dr. Smith. In the obstetrical setting, haloperidol has been used for hyperemesis and is currently used for chorea gravidarum in low doses (2 mg/day) without reported ill effects on the mother or the fetus.

   Also, obtain further information about the course of Mrs. E's last pregnancy. Since she currently has an elevated diastolic blood pressure, Dr. Smith may suggest other monitoring while Mrs. E is hospitalized. For example, more frequent blood pressure evaluations, urine protein checks if blood pressure is increased, or weight monitoring might be required. Finally, discuss with Dr. Smith the possibility of fetal echocardiography or high-level ultrasound to determine if a cardiac anomaly exists. Because Mrs. E is very likely to have a normal fetus, these tests may be very reassuring. Alternatively, if a problem exists, optimal obstetrical and pediatric management at labor and delivery can be arranged.

2. Advise staff *not* to give false reassurance that the baby is normal. Mrs. E can be correctly told that she has a far greater probability of carrying a normal fetus than an abnormal one.

3. The consultant offers to follow Mrs. E's progress with the treating physician/staff.

Final Comment

Difficult clinical issues are inherent in treating childbearing women. Which is more deleterious, the uncontrolled psychiatric illness or the medication that allows symptom relief? The task becomes one of working to maximize positive outcome for both mother and baby within the limitations of existing data. The task is worthwhile, since passage through this major life event is usually a positive experience for the new mother, her family, and her physician.

Menopause, Early Aging, and Elderly Women

Barbara B. Sherwin, Ph.D.

Menopause, a universal reproductive event, is associated with psychological symptomatology in a considerable proportion of women. Of course, the occurrence of two events in temporal contiguity does not imply a causal relationship, and, indeed, numerous psychosocial and cultural factors are known to influence the manner in which women experience menopause. On the other hand, menopause is fundamentally a biological event that involves fairly drastic alterations in the endocrine milieu. To the extent that sex hormones have known psychotropic properties, it is reasonable to suppose that changes in their production are manifested in specific changes in psychological functioning.

The preparation of this manuscript was supported by a grant from the Medical Research Council of Canada (#MT-11623) awarded to B. B. Sherwin.

Hormonal Changes at Menopause

In premenopausal women, the ovary secretes 95% of the estradiol that enters the circulation (Lipsett 1986). From about the age of 40 years, the ovary becomes less and less efficient and produces decreasing amounts of estradiol. On average, by the age of 51 years, there is insufficient ovarian production of estradiol and progesterone to sustain monthly menstrual cycles, which finally cease altogether. After menopause, the ovary virtually stops producing estradiol. Then, estrone, a much weaker steroid, becomes the predominant estrogen that arises from peripheral conversion from androstenedione (Longcope 1981). Although it used to be thought that the drastic decrease in ovarian estradiol secretion at the time of menopause was due solely to follicle depletion and ovarian senescence, it is now clear that age-related alterations in hypothalamic function also occur (P. M. Wise et al. 1989). Thus, the transition to menopause is a multifactorial process involving both neural and ovarian factors.

Another well-documented—but less well-acknowledged—endocrine change at menopause is concerned with androgen production. In women, both the adrenal and the ovary contain the biosynthetic pathways necessary for androgen synthesis and secretion. In premenopausal women, the ovary produces approximately 25% of plasma testosterone, 60% of androstenedione, and 20% of dehydroepiandrosterone (DHEA), whereas the adrenal produces 25% of circulating testosterone, 40% of androstenedione, 50% of DHEA, and 90% of dehydroepiandrosterone sulfate (DHEAS). The remainder of circulating androgens in the female are thought to arise through peripheral conversion, which likely accounts for the production rate of 50% of testosterone and 25% of DHEA (Longcope 1986). After menopause, the blood production rate of testosterone, the most potent androgen, changes substantially. For example, in a naturally postmenopausal woman, the blood production rate of testosterone is about one-third the amount in reproductive-aged women and is decreased even more profoundly in women who have had bilateral oophorectomy (Longcope 1981; Poortman et al. 1980). Therefore, possible androgen-deficiency symptoms in postmenopausal women need to be considered as well.

Menopause actually marks one phase of a process called the climacteric, which describes the transition from the reproductive to the nonreproductive stage of a woman's life. Menopause indicates the final menstrual period, and perimenopause includes the premenopausal years of declining ovarian function and extends to several years after menopause until virtual cessation of ovarian function. This typically encompasses the period between 48 and 53 years of age, after which all women are said to be postmenopausal. A premenopausal woman who undergoes bilateral oophorectomy (usually in association with hysterectomy), of course, becomes postmenopausal immediately after surgery.

Neurobiological Effects of the Sex Hormones

Autoradiographic studies have demonstrated that neurons containing specific receptors for estrogen are found in several areas of the brain, predominantly in the pituitary, hypothalamus, limbic forebrain (including the amygdala and lateral septum), and cerebral cortex (McEwen 1980). Receptors for testosterone are found mainly in the preoptic area of the hypothalamus, with smaller concentrations in the limbic system and in the cerebral cortex (Chamness et al. 1979). Thus, it is clear that the brain is a target organ for the sex hormones that are capable of acting in areas that subserve emotion and sexuality.

Recent advances in neuroscience have demonstrated that sex steroids cause synaptic and dendritic plasticity. During the estrus phase of the cycle in rats, when circulating estrogen levels are at their lowest, there is a 30% decrease in apical dendritic spine density in CA1 hippocampal pyramidal cells compared with the proestrus phase, which is characterized by high estrogen levels (Woolley et al. 1990). Moreover, the decrease in dendritic spine density after bilateral ovariectomy is obviated by estradiol replacement (Gould et al. 1991). The electron microscopic evidence that new spines are accompanied by new synapses suggests that estrogen deprivation would decrease neurotransmission in an area of the brain critically implicated in memory functions (McEwen 1992).

Estrogen can also influence the concentration of neurotransmitters by a variety of means. For example, estrogen decreases monoamine oxidase (MAO) activity in the amygdala and hypothalamus in a dose-dependent fashion (Luine et al. 1975). If the same mechanism occurs in the human brain, then the result would be higher central levels of serotonin (5-hydroxytryptamine [5-HT]). Indeed, measurement of peripheral levels of MAO under different estrogen concentrations provides supportive evidence for such an estrogenic effect in humans. In healthy reproductive-aged women, there was an inverse relationship between levels of plasma MAO and plasma levels of estradiol at several phases of the menstrual cycle (Briggs and Briggs 1972; Klaiber et al. 1971). There is also some evidence that in depressed, regularly cycling women, exogenous estrogen decreased plasma MAO levels and enhanced mood (Klaiber et al. 1972). Taken together, these studies provide evidence that the estrogenic influence on MAO levels documented in rat brain (Luine et al. 1975) also occurs in the plasma of human females.

A second mechanism that may explain the estrogenic enhancement of mood is that tryptophan, the precursor of 5-HT, is displaced from its binding sites to plasma albumin by estrogens in vitro and in vivo (Aylward 1973), thereby increasing the amount of free tryptophan available to the brain. Indeed, in bilaterally oophorectomized women, a significant negative correlation was found between depression scores and free plasma tryptophan levels, and an improvement in depression scores occurred subsequent to estrogen administration (Aylward 1976). When estrogen or placebo was added to lithium, a significant increase in the level of free plasma tryptophan occurred with estrogen but not with placebo administration (Coppen and Wood 1978). Either or both of these estrogenic actions could conceivably affect mood.

Estrogen also affects another neurotransmitter, acetylcholine, a relative deficit of which is a hallmark of Alzheimer's disease. Specifically, estrogen increases the amount of choline acetyltransferase, the enzyme needed for the synthesis of acetylcholine in the basal forebrain, the frontal cortex, and the CA1 layer of the hippocampus in female rats (Squire 1992). Moreover, decreased choline acetyltransferase activity is associated with impaired memory performance in aged rats (Luine and Hearns 1990), underscoring the importance of this enzyme for the maintenance of memory functions.

Estrogenic Effects on
Neurotransmitter Receptors

Estrogen induces changes in the density of receptors for a number of neurotransmitters. This steroid hormone enhances central norepinephrine availability (Paul et al. 1979) and sensitizes dopamine receptors (Chiodo and Caggiula 1983). Chronic estrogen treatment reduces α-adrenergic receptors in rat cortex (H. R. Wagner et al. 1979), an effect similar to that observed with chronic antidepressant treatment.

Estrogen also alters serotonergic transmission. In ovariectomized rats, there was a biphasic effect of exogenous estradiol on 5-HT receptor density. A significant decrease in serotonergic binding occurred within 1–2 hours after injection, followed by a 30%–40% increase in 5-HT receptor levels in the amygdala, the mediobasal hypothalamus, and the preoptic area by 72 hours postinjection (Biegon and McEwen 1982).

Finally, it has been demonstrated that estrogen affects the density of tritiated imipramine binding sites, which are thought to modulate the presynaptic uptake of 5-HT in the brain and in platelets (Paul et al. 1984). Both tritiated imipramine binding and tritiated 5-HT uptake increased by 20%–30% in the frontal cortex and hypothalamus of ovariectomized rats after 12 days of treatment with estradiol (Rehavi et al. 1987). Moreover, a significant increase in the density of tritiated imipramine binding sites on platelets occurred after estrogen treatment in surgically menopausal women, in association with an improvement in their depression scores (Sherwin and Suranyi-Cadotte 1990).

In summary, the ability of estrogen to increase the concentration of certain neurotransmitter levels, to upregulate receptor densities, and to induce synaptogenesis in specific brain areas provides support for the idea that this steroid hormone may play an important role in the regulation both of affect and of memory. To the extent that estrogen enhances serotonergic mechanisms, the decrease in endogenous estrogen at the time of menopause could explain the occurrence of dysphoria or depression in vulnerable women.

Consideration of the neurobiological and psychotropic properties of progesterone is also important, because progestins are usually administered in association with estrogen after menopause to prevent endometrial hyperplasia. Whereas estrogen increases the electrical excitability of the brain, progesterone decreases it, acting as an anticonvulsant (Bäckström 1977). Progesterone also has sedative and hypnotic effects (Arafat et al. 1988) and, at high doses, induces deep sleep (Merryman et al. 1954). Importantly, whereas estradiol reduces plasma MAO activity, progestins increase it (Klaiber et al. 1971).

Menopausal Symptoms

Physical Symptoms

Hot flushes, the cardinal menopausal symptom, occur in 60%–90% of menopausal women, albeit with a high degree of variability in frequency and intensity. For 65% of postmenopausal women, the vasomotor phenomena of hot flushes and cold sweats persist for at least 1 year, and for 20%, these symptoms continue for more than 5 years (Brenner 1988). Because hot flushes occur more frequently at night, sleep is often disrupted.

Because the integrity of the tissues of the female reproductive tract is dependent on estrogen, degenerative changes in these structures ensue when levels of estrogen decrease after menopause. The vaginal mucosa of untreated women becomes attenuated and pale due to a decrease in vascularity. Atrophic vaginitis may, in turn, lead to a severe diminution in vaginal lubrication and/or dyspareunia (Bergman and Brenner 1987). Both hot flushes and atrophic vaginitis are estrogen-dependent symptoms and are reliably relieved by estrogen-replacement therapy.

Psychological Symptoms

Epidemiological studies of nonpatient populations have generally failed to find that an increase in depression occurs at the time of menopause (McKinlay and Jeffreys 1974; B. Thompson et al. 1973). Other studies, however, have documented an increase in depressive symptomatology around the time of menopause (Bungay et al. 1980; Green and Cooke 1980; Hunter and Whitehead 1989). In Canadian and American survey studies of female midlife, the percentage of perimenopausal women who reported feeling blue or depressed was 23% and 38%, respectively (Avis et al. 1993). Whether or not there is a distinct subtype of depression that occurs during menopause is still in dispute (P. J. Schmidt and Rubinow 1991). What does seem clear, however, is that, among women who seek medical consultation for menopausal symptoms, 79% have physical symptoms and 65% have varying degrees of depression (Anderson et al. 1987). Even acknowledging the influential role of adverse psychosocial factors in the genesis of these midlife depressions and dysphorias, it is likely that the coincident drastic changes in sex hormone production are also causally related to affective disturbances at this time.

Estrogen and Depressive Symptoms

One experimental paradigm that has been used to assess the effects of estrogen on mood involves preoperative testing of women scheduled to undergo total abdominal hysterectomy (TAH) and bilateral salpingo-oophorectomy (BSO) for benign disease. Subjects are tested again postoperatively after treatment with hormones or placebo. In one such study, women who received placebo after surgery had significantly higher scores on the depression scale of the Multiple Affect Adjective Checklist compared with those who had received estrogen or a combined estrogen-androgen preparation (Sherwin et al. 1985). Although depression scores covaried with circulating levels of estradiol in that study, they remained within the limits of the normal, nondepressed range. These findings were confirmed in a study of women who had undergone TAH and BSO approximately 4 years before their recruitment (Sherwin 1988a). Women who had been receiving either a combined estrogen-androgen preparation or estrogen alone since their ovaries had been surgically removed had more positive moods and higher levels of plasma estradiol compared with a control group of healthy untreated oophorectomized women. Moreover, those treated long-term with both estradiol and testosterone felt more composed, elated, and energetic than women who were given estrogen alone. The results of this study, therefore, confirmed that mood covaries with circulating levels of both estradiol and testosterone in healthy, nondepressed women.

Results of studies of naturally menopausal women generally support our findings that estrogen enhances mood in nonpsychiatric populations of postmenopausal women. Ditkoff et al. (1991) administered either 0.625 mg of 1.25-mg conjugate equine estrogen or a placebo to postmenopausal women who were not experiencing hot flushes. Scores on the Beck Depression Inventory decreased significantly in both groups of women treated with estrogen, while no changes in depression scores were evident in the placebo group after 3 months. These findings also serve to underline the likelihood that estrogen exerts a direct effect on mood rather than having an indirect mode of action secondary to its alleviation of estrogen-dependent symptoms such as hot flushes. Finally, a recent epidemiological study of the Rancho Bernardo cohort in California provided suggestive evidence that long-term postmenopausal estrogen-replacement therapy might protect against the development of depression in older women (Palinkas and Barrett-Connor 1992). In this cross-sectional study of 1,190 women over 50 years of age, mean depression scores (measured with the Beck Depression Inventory) worsened significantly in the untreated but not the estrogen-treated women.

Surprisingly, only a few studies have tested possible therapeutic effects of estrogen on major depression in postmenopausal women. In one such study, the mood of 9 of 10 postmenopausal women whose pretreatment scores were less than 16 on the Beck Depression Inventory improved with conjugated equine estrogen 1.25 mg daily, whereas 6 of the 10 women who had pretreatment scores above 20 at baseline actually became more depressed over time with the same treatment (M. A. Schneider et al. 1977). Taken together, these findings suggest that the administration of estrogen in doses conventionally used to treat menopausal symptoms enhances mood in nondepressed women but is therapeutically ineffective, in and of itself, with respect to mood disturbances of a clinical magnitude.

The recommendation to add a progestin to the estrogen-replacement regimen of naturally menopausal women in order to protect the uterus from the stimulatory effects of estrogen has made clear the dysphoric-inducing effects of some synthetic progestins. Women given estrogen and a progestin had more fatigue, tension, irritability, and depression than did women treated with estrogen alone (Holst et al. 1989). A prospective, controlled study of two doses of conjugated equine estrogen with the addition of medroxyprogesterone acetate or placebo demonstrated that the addition of the progestin to the hormone replacement regimen attenuated the beneficial effect of estrogen on mood in a dose-dependent manner: the higher the estrogen-to-progesterone ratio, the less the negative impact on mood (Sherwin 1991).

Hormones and Sexuality

Survey data on the frequency and type of sexual problems experienced postmenopause show that one-third to one-half of all women complain of disturbance in one or more aspects of sexual functioning at this time (Hällström and Samuelsson 1990; Pfeiffer and Davis 1972). Although numerous psychosocial circumstances such as the availability and health of a partner undoubtedly influence a woman's sexual life at this time, hormonal factors may also play an important role. Because the integrity of the tissues of the female reproductive tract is dependent on estrogen, degenerative changes in these structures ensue when levels of estrogen decrease after menopause. Exogenous estrogen increases vaginal blood flow (Semmens and Wagner 1982) and restores the thickness of vaginal tissues in postmenopausal women.

On the other hand, a decrease in libido, or sexual desire, reported by between 10% and 85% of postmenopausal women (Sherwin 1991) has not usually been found to respond to exogenous estrogen alone. By now, a considerable number of well-controlled psychophysiological (Myers and Morokoff 1986) and hormone replacement therapy studies (Burger et al. 1984; Sherwin and Gelfand 1987; Sherwin et al. 1985) have found that the administration of combined estrogen-testosterone preparations to postmenopausal women enhances sexual desire and interest in those who had experienced a decrease in libido after either natural or surgical menopause. Furthermore, the findings from these studies have provided evidence that in women, just as in men, testosterone has its major impact on sexual desire and not on physiological response. It would seem, therefore, that the decrease in the ovarian production of testosterone after menopause can account for some of the changes in sexual functioning experienced by a considerable number of postmenopausal women and that these changes can be successfully reversed by adding physiological doses of testosterone to the hormone replacement regimen.

Estrogen and Cognitive Functioning

Disturbances in memory are prominent among the symptoms subjectively reported by women around the time of menopause. Recent advances in neuroscience have provided explanatory mechanisms for the ways in which decreases in estrogen may be causal in some of these memory changes due to the influence of this sex hormone on neurotransmitters (especially acetylcholine) and on the morphology of brain areas critically important for memory functions (especially the hippocampus). Within the past 5 years, evidence has become available from controlled clinical studies of estrogenic effects on specific cognitive functions in postmenopausal women.

No effects on tests of visual memory were seen in 57-year-old women given either 4 mg estriol or placebo (Vanhulle and Demol 1976) or in those given 0.625 mg or 1.25 mg of conjugated equine estrogen (Ditkoff et al. 1991). The 15-year follow-up of the Rancho Bernardo cohort of over 1,000 women also failed to find an enhancement by estrogen of visual memory but did determine that long-term users of estrogen had significantly higher scores on a test of semantic memory (category fluency) compared with never-users (Barrett-Connor and Kritz-Silverstein 1993).

In our own laboratory, we have been conducting studies of estrogenic influences on various aspects of memory and other cognitive functions for the past decade. All studies have been carried out using intramuscular preparations of estradiol valerate 10 mg, given once a month. In the first prospective study, we tested premenopausal women who needed to undergo total abdominal hysterectomy (TAH) and bilateral salpingo-oophorectomy (BSO). After surgery, they randomly received either estrogen alone, an estrogen-androgen combined preparation, or placebo and were tested again after 3 months of treatment. Women who received either of the active hormonal preparations performed significantly better on a test of immediate verbal memory (paragraph recall) compared with those given placebo (Sherwin 1988b).

A second prospective study of estrogenic effects on memory used a more extensive battery of cognitive tests. Forty-eight-year-old women underwent TAH or BSO for benign disease and then randomly received monthly injections of either estradiol valerate 10 mg or placebo for the first 3 postoperative months. Once again, women treated with estrogen had higher scores on a test of immediate verbal memory (paragraph recall) in comparison with their own preoperative scores, and these score improvements were associated with their higher levels of circulating estradiol during treatment. In contrast, verbal memory scores of placebo-treated women who had undergone TAH and BSO did not change pre- to posttreatment (Sherwin and Phillips 1990). It was also the case that women who received placebo had lower scores by the third postoperative month on a test measuring the ability to learn new material (paired-associates test), whereas scores of estrogen-treated women remained stable after TAH and BSO (Phillips and Sherwin 1992). There were no changes in scores in either group on measures of attention and of visual memory. It is interesting to note that mood remained stable in both groups pre- to postoperatively. Also, women who complained of severe hot flushes were dropped from the study for ethical reasons so that those who remained in the study for its duration were experiencing only trivial frequencies of hot flushes that were not disturbing to them. These observations lend further support to a previous suggestion (Campbell and Whitehead 1977) that the estrogenic enhancement of memory in postmenopausal women does not occur secondary to this hormone's alleviation of other menopausal symptoms, but rather is due to a direct effect of estrogen on brain functioning. Moreover, we have recently shown that healthy 65-year-old women who had been taking estrogen since menopause had higher scores on immediate and delayed verbal memory as compared with age-matched nonusers (Kampen and Sherwin 1994).

In summary, results of these studies of the role of estrogen in cognitive functioning in postmenopausal women support the conclusion that estrogen enhances short-term verbal memory and helps to maintain the ability to learn new material but is without effect on general attention or visuospatial memory. Thus, there is a specificity of estrogen's action on cognitive functions. It should be noted, however, that although estrogen-treated women performed better on tests of short-term verbal memory in these studies, it was not the case that 48-year-old women given placebo after their TAH and BSO were obviously impaired in their daily functioning in the real world after 3 months. Therefore, the long-term clinical implications of these results are yet to be determined. However, the finding of a preliminary open trial that exogenous estrogen given to a small number of women with Alzheimer's disease resulted in an improvement in aspects of their daily functioning in an American study (Fillit et al. 1986) and in an improvement in memory scores in women with Alzheimer's disease in a Japanese study (Honjo et al. 1989) suggests that estrogen deprivation may indeed play an important role in the pathogenesis of memory dysfunctions in aging women.

Summary

It has long been observed that certain women appeared vulnerable to the development of behavioral changes in association with alterations in the endocrine milieu that occurs during reproductive events such as the premenstrual period, postpartum, and menopause. The commonality in these reproductive events associated with the induction of dysphoric mood in some women is that they are all characterized by a considerable decrease in the ovarian production of estradiol. However, it is only within the past two decades that research in basic neuroscience has provided specific and fascinating information on the fairly profound manner in which estradiol, testosterone, and progesterone influence brain morphology and function. We are now able to use this information regarding sex steroids and brain mechanisms to formulate and test increasingly well-honed and specific hypotheses concerning these hormone-behavior relationships in women. Although much work remains to be done, there is now abundant evidence to support several conclusions. First, estrogen enhances mood in a dose-dependent manner. Second, the physiological role of testosterone in women includes its promotion of feelings of well-being and general energy level and the maintenance of sexual desire or libido. There is some evidence that synthetic progestins may dampen both mood and sexual desire, although the effect and its intensity probably depend on the chemical constitution of the specific progestogenic compound under investigation. Finally, although the literature on estrogenic effects on memory in women is still in its infancy, there is a growing body of knowledge that is beginning to suggest that estrogen also enhances specific aspects of memory in women (Sherwin 1994).

The clinical implications of these findings relate, first, to the considerable proportion of women who become symptomatic after the normal, physiological changes in ovarian hormone secretion during the menstrual cycle and during pregnancy and the postpartum period. Of increasing importance is the dramatic increase in female life expectancy over the past half-century, which means that women now live one-third of their lives beyond the cessation of their ovarian function. Our ability to enhance the quality of life for women and to prevent degenerative diseases during the latter one-third of their life spans depends, in part, on our ability to determine the role of the sex hormones on the brain and other organ systems so that we may have the tools to preserve and protect the psychological and physical integrity of aging women.

Section III

Pathophysiological Entities and Psychopharmacological Agents

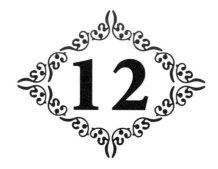

Sex and Treatment of Depressions

When Does It Matter?

Jean A. Hamilton, M.D., Merida Grant,
and Margaret F. Jensvold, M.D.

Clinical depression has been highlighted as a key mental health issue for women (Eichler and Parron 1987; McGrath et al. 1990). There are numerous subtypes of clinical depression, and many occur more commonly in women than in men. The most widely recognized sex—or more precisely, sex-related—difference is in rates of unipolar or major depression (as opposed to bipolar disorder), which is twice as common in women as in men (Hamilton and Halbreich 1993; Nolen-Hoeksema 1990; Weissman and

This work was supported by the Maurice Falk Medical Fund.

Klerman 1977). There is also a 1.5- to 3-fold excess of dysthymic disorder—a chronic, mild form of depression—in women (Weissman et al. 1988).

The higher use of antidepressants by women in comparison with men results, in part, from the excess of depression found among women. Survey data from 1984 show that about two-thirds (67%) of prescriptions written in the United States for certain antidepressants (tricyclics and newer cyclic products) went to women (Baum et al. 1988), a finding that appears to be in keeping with the sex ratio for depressive illness. However, Hohmann (1989) observed that 82% of prescriptions went to women, instead of the expected rate of 67% (representing an excess of 15% over that expected), which suggests biased rates of prescribing.

More than 20 years ago, Raskin (1974) first speculated that sex-related differences may exist in response to antidepressant treatment, stating that "[although] twice as many women as men are treated for depression, the depression literature suggests that it is the men rather than the women who benefit most from antidepressant drugs" (p. 120). Increasing evidence suggests that sex is an important factor in predicting the course of depressive illness and response to treatment (Hamilton and Halbreich 1993). However, the field arguably has been slow to follow up on Raskin's hypothesis. The American Psychiatric Association (1993), for example, first recognized one of the sex-related findings to be discussed here only recently.

In this chapter, therefore, we critically examine the evidence suggesting that sex-related differences exist in response to antidepressant treatment with selected psychotropic medications. We rely heavily on other reviews (Hamilton 1995, in press a; Hamilton and Grant 1993; Hamilton and Jensvold 1991). In particular, we *summarize* quantitative analyses that were presented by Hamilton and Grant at a meeting in 1993.

The first antidepressant used in the United States was imipramine (von Kuhn 1958), and it continues to be considered the "gold standard" for evaluating treatments for nonbipolar depressions (e.g., Elkin et al. 1989). For this reason, imipramine will be used as a model for examining possible sex-related effects on treatment outcome and pharmacokinetics in depression research.

One problem with previous reviews is that they have not been comprehensive. Instead, authors have cited examples of sex differences that happened to come to their attention. There is no way of knowing whether such anecdotal findings are representative. Even if a MEDLINE search were done using keywords such as sex, many studies that potentially show sex differences will be missed, since studies rarely analyze data or report findings by sex. To avoid this bias, we examined all published imipramine treatment outcome studies of depression and all pharmacokinetic studies of steady-state plasma concentrations of imipramine in humans. The comprehensive reviews of imipramine will be supplemented with other information that has come to our attention about other antidepressants.[1]

A second problem of previous reviews of possible sex-related differences in psychopharmacology is that they have been *qualitative*, in that the investigators have provided a narrative summary of studies. However, techniques for *quantitative* analysis are increasingly recommended for summarizing clinical treatment trials (J. C. Bennett 1993; Hamilton 1985). Meta-analysis is a technique used to quantitatively review and summarize research findings across individual studies (F. M. Wolf 1986). Importantly, meta-analysis has been empirically shown to be superior to qualitative reviews (H. M. Cooper and Rosenthal 1980; R. Rosenthal 1991). Effect sizes also provide a way to summarize and display the relative size of findings (J. Cohen 1992; R. Rosenthal and Rubin 1982). Here we summarize (but do not exhaustively present) a *quantitative* review for imipramine by sex.

---

[1] The present review was informed by a MEDLINE search (through October 1993) using the following search terms: sex; contraceptive agents, female/ad; sex hormones/ad,pk,pd; menopause/de,me; estrogen replacement therapy; menstrual cycle; pharmacokinetics. These terms were crossed with: gastric acid; gastric oxidation; gastric emptying; lean body mass; total body water; tissue concentration; biotransformation; cytochrome P450; protein binding; renal blood flow; liver blood flow; brain blood flow; glomerular filtration; and creatinine clearance. In addition to searches for imipramine, selected newer psychotropics were individually cross-searched (serotonin reuptake inhibitors; prazepam; clonazepam; oxazepam; lorazepam; alprazolam; barbiturates; clonidine; propranolol; clomipramine; buspirone; carbamazepine; clonazepam). Despite this approach, our mention of other antidepressants must be considered anecdotal until comprehensive meta-analyses, similar to those mentioned here for imipramine, are completed.

A third problem with previous reviews is that possible sex-related differences in antidepressant efficacy have not been carefully examined for subtypes of depression. Here we examine what is known about the relative efficacy of drug treatments for dysthymic disorder and for double depression (i.e., major depression with superimposed dysthymic disorder). Specifically, we consider the relative efficacy of tricyclic antidepressants (TCAs) and monoamine oxidase inhibitors (MAOIs). And finally, we argue that inadequate attention has been devoted to possible confounding variables in depression treatment trials.

Treatment Outcome in Response to Imipramine

A review by J. B. Morris and Beck, entitled "The Efficacy of Antidepressant Drugs," appeared in 1974. This paper became the basis for subsequent reviews. For example, it provides the basis for Baldessarini's discussion of imipramine efficacy that appeared in 1979. Unfortunately, sex differences were not examined in either of these reviews.

Hamilton (in press a; Hamilton and Grant 1993) recently provided a systematic review of imipramine treatment outcome studies in humans that addressed possible sex differences. A total of 205 papers on clinical imipramine trials from 1957 through 1991 were evaluated. Of these, 180 were suitable for further quantitative review.

The majority of the studies clearly stated that both sexes were included in the research population. In most of them, however, the distribution of subjects by sex was not described, nor were outcome data analyzed by sex. Of the final sample, only 19% ($N = 35$)—or less than one-fifth—were "sex-relevant" (i.e., allowing an examination of possible sex differences in outcome). Characteristics of sex-relevant outcome studies for the treatment of depression with imipramine are detailed elsewhere (Hamilton 1995). Sex-relevant studies sampled a total of 711 women and 342 men, resulting in a 2:1 sex ratio, which corresponds to the rates of illness.

Sex differences were first examined by calculating the excess of good responders in men compared with women (i.e., by subtracting the proportion for women from that for men, with a positive percentage representing a male advantage). In some cases sex was discussed, but precise findings by sex and relevant statistics were not reported.[2] Other studies included pertinent data but did not analyze them by sex.[3] For reasons such as these, data for 61% of sex-relevant studies required reanalysis. The methods of analysis used were, if anything, conservative (e.g., Yates correction was used for small sample sizes).

In 53% of the sex-relevant studies, men were found to show more benefit from imipramine than women. In contrast, women were found to receive more benefit in only 19% of studies, and no sex difference in response was observed in about 28%. Few sex differences (19%) reached statistical significance. This should not be surprising, however, since potentially confounding pharmacological variables (e.g., smoking, menstrual cycle phase, menopausal status, and other contextual factors, as discussed in Hamilton and Yonkers, Chapter 2, this volume) were not typically assessed. Such variables may create "noise" that tends to obscure observation of clear group differences.

The average rates of good responding were 62% for men and 51% for women. *Men responded well an average of 11% more frequently than did women* (Hamilton 1995, in press a). Fisher's combined test was used to calculate an overall chi-square statistic. Meta-analysis confirms that *men respond significantly better than women* when data are combined across studies (Hamilton, in press a; $\chi^2 = 128$, $df = 60$, $P < .001$).

The average effect sizes for these studies were 0.18 (for values derived from chi-square) and 0.20 (for values derived from the correlation coefficient r). According to J. Cohen's (1992) guidelines, *the effects of sex are well beyond "small" in size and might be termed moderate.* But the variance accounted for by sex is only about 6%. Using the approach of R. Rosenthal and Rubin (1982), however, we find that this corresponds to the interpretation that *male sex increases the clinical improvement rate from about 38% to 62%* (Hamilton, in press a). In comparison, drugs

---

[2] See Appendix 12–A; H. C. Abraham et al. 1963; Angst et al. 1974; Gerner et al. 1980; M. Greenblatt et al. 1964; Holt et al. 1960; Isaksson et al. 1968; D. F. Klein and Fink 1962).

[3] Examples include Beckmann and Goodwin 1975; Costa et al. 1980; Donnelly et al. 1979; Gram et al. 1976; Kemali et al. 1972; Perier and Eslami 1971; and Reisby et al. 1977.

that exceed placebo response rates by 20% are considered effective. Thus, the effects of sex on clinical outcome may be clinically meaningful, especially in heterogeneous populations such as those that practitioners actually serve.

Other Antidepressants

Steiner and colleagues (1993) recently reported that the selective serotonin reuptake inhibitor (SSRI) paroxetine may be more beneficial in women than in men. Their study is difficult to interpret, however, because males showed an unusually high placebo response rate. Other data have failed to show a sex difference in response to another SSRI, fluoxetine, versus placebo for treatment of major depression (D. J. Goldstein, personal communication: gender analyses of fluoxetine versus placebo in major depressive disorder [efficacy, reasons for discontinuation, adverse events, statistical methods], Lilly Research Laboratories, Lilly Corporate Center, Indianapolis, IN, November 16, 1993).

Although other antidepressants have not been reviewed exhaustively, there is some evidence suggesting that the male advantage is not limited to imipramine or to TCAs (Gerner et al. 1980). The male advantage for imipramine (and possibly for other antidepressants such as trazodone) may, however, be relatively specific to treatment of *depression*. For example, a *female advantage* has been observed in several antidepressant treatment outcome studies of *pain* (Blumer and Heilbronn 1984; Edelbroek et al. 1986).

Clinical Implications: Sex and Outcome

Although the meta-analytic study of sex and imipramine outcome is comprehensive, it combines studies that used different diagnostic criteria and methods. It is possible that the apparent sex difference in response to imipramine results from the use of relatively heterogeneous populations in early clinical trials (e.g., in terms of DSM-IV [American Psychiatric Association 1994] Axis I depressive diagnoses and Axis II personality disorder diagnoses, as well as patterns of comorbidity). That is, sex differences in imipramine outcome may be an artifact of having more women with atypical, dysthymic, or anxious depressions and more men with endogenous depression (for a review, see Hamilton 1995).[4] This might affect outcome rates because there is some evidence suggesting that subtypes of depression differ in responsivity to various types of antidepressants. For example, MAOIs may be more efficacious than TCAs in women with atypical or anxious depressions (Davidson and Pelton 1986; Quitkin et al. 1988; J. W. Stewart et al. 1989). This issue is discussed further in the section "Sex and Selection of Treatment Agent," below.

More recently, use of "pure" major depression populations has resulted in studies of much more homogeneous groups (with exclusion rates on the order of 50%). These pure studies have generally failed to observe sex-related differences in antidepressant treatment outcome (Croughan et al. 1988; Kocsis et al. 1989; Paykel et al. 1988; Sotsky et al. 1991). Instead of discounting the possibility of sex-related differences in antidepressant treatment outcome, the latter findings firmly support the need for "effectiveness" research on this topic. That is, studies assessing sex as it may relate to outcome in *actual populations seeking treatment* in community or other *real-life practice settings* are needed, as opposed to only those using narrowly selected (and in some ways unrepresentative) subjects in academic or other strictly controlled research settings (Keller and Lavori 1988; Roper et al. 1988).

Pharmacokinetics of Imipramine

A systematic review of imipramine steady-state plasma concentrations was recently presented (Hamilton and Grant 1993). Here we summarize (but do not exhaustively explicate) these findings. Human imipramine pharmacokinetics were identified by MEDLINE search, regardless of whether sex was used as a keyword. Of 106 studies, 12% ($N = 13$) were sex-relevant, meaning that data could be examined by sex.[5]

---

[4] On the other hand, the male advantage is less likely to be entirely an artifact, because Gerner et al. (1980) observed the male advantage even among a more homogeneous group of patients with endogenous depression.

[5] Bjerre et al. 1981; Brosen et al. 1986; Costa et al. 1980; Glassman et al. 1977; Gram et al. 1976, 1977, 1983; Kocsis et al. 1986; Moody et al. 1967; Muscettola et al. 1978; Nagy and Johansson 1977; Reisby et al. 1977; and Sutfin et al. 1988.

In all studies, data were tabulated by sex but either analyses were *not* reported by sex or exact statistics were not given. Thus, secondary re-analyses of these data were undertaken.[6] When possible, plasma concentrations were adjusted for dose (mg/day). Dose-controlled data were available for a smaller number of cases ($N = 9$ for imipramine, $N = 8$ for desmethylimipramine).

Women had 18% higher raw plasma concentrations of imipramine and nearly 12% higher desmethylimipramine levels compared with men. Total plasma levels (imipramine + desmethylimipramine) were about 10% higher in women overall than in men. As shown in Table 12–1, Fisher's combined test (F. M. Wolf 1986) confirmed that *women have significantly higher dose-adjusted (mg/day) plasma concentrations of imipramine and desmethylimipramine than do men* (see Yonkers and Hamilton, Chapter 3, this volume).

Only three studies were available in which imipramine plasma levels could be controlled by dose and weight (mg/kg; Gram et al. 1977; Moody et al. 1967; Sutfin et al. 1988). Although firm conclusions are impossible given such limited data, it appears that dose-by-weight adjustment of plasma concentrations may remove the apparent effect of sex, as the Fisher's combined test failed to reach significance.[7]

Of the three studies that allowed rigorous adjustment of plasma levels, only one was restricted to a premenopausally aged (50 years or younger) sample (Gram et al. 1977). Thus, age or menopausal status may confound dose-by-weight–controlled studies. In the most homogeneous (albeit small) study, dose-by-weight–adjusted imipramine levels averaged 12.1 (standard deviation [SD] = 1.0) for two women compared with 17.1 for three men (SD = 8.3), and dose-by-weight-adjusted desmethylimipramine averaged 21.5 in the women (SD = 10.4) compared with 28.0 in the men (SD = 13.8). Thus, women at or below the median age for menopause had *lower*—not higher—dose-by-weight-adjusted plasma levels.

---

[6] In two studies, data were provided for low and high doses; when these data were analyzed separately, the total number of cases was 15. In all 15 cases, total concentrations were available. Concentrations of imipramine and desmethylimipramine were available, however, in only 12 cases.

[7] We realize that meta-analysis is usually reserved for at least 10 studies.

Table 12–1.   Meta-analysis of imipramine plasma concentrations:
summary statistics

| | Raw data | | Dose-adjusted data (mg/day) | |
	Imipramine	DMI	Imipramine	DMI
Fisher's combined test (χ^2)	39.189[*]	45.651[**]	27.236[*]	31.449[*]
$df\,(N{*}2)$	24	22	16	18
Criterion for significance	33.9	36.4	26.3	28.9

Note.   DMI = desmethylimipramine. [*]$P < .05$; [**]$P < .005$.
Source.   Hamilton and Grant 1993.

In two other studies, both younger and older subjects were studied (Moody et al. 1967; Sutfin et al. 1988). Even when dose and weight were controlled, women had *higher* overall imipramine and desmethylimipramine levels compared with men. Data from these studies were reanalyzed and subjects categorized as premenopausally aged (< 50 years) or postmenopausally aged (> 50 years; see rationale in Hamilton and Yonkers, Chapter 2, this volume). In the study by Moody et al. (1967), women in both age groups had higher dose-by-weight-adjusted imipramine levels compared with men (77% higher among younger and 20% higher among older women). Dose-by-weight-adjusted desmethylimipramine levels were lower in younger women and higher in older women compared with men (17% higher and 32% lower). In Sutfin and colleagues' (1988) study, however, younger women had marginally lower dose-by-weight-adjusted imipramine and desmethylimipramine levels (7% and 39%, respectively). This study included older women but not men.

None of the three studies stated whether subjects smoked, used oral contraceptives (OCs), or received hormone replacement therapy (HRT). Thus, data are inconsistent and may be confounded, making firm conclusions impossible. The apparent sex difference in dose-adjusted plasma concentrations might, for example, be an artifact of higher rates of smoking in men (tending to decrease plasma levels) and of OC use in women (tending to increase levels), thus spreading the male vs. female plasma concentrations apart (Hamilton and Yonkers, Chapter 2, this volume). To the exceedingly limited extent that patterns can be discerned, however, it appears that *women may have **higher** dose-by-weight-adjusted imipramine and desmethylimipramine, **but only in older age groups**.* What is perhaps most striking about these data is how little good information we have about plasma levels of imipramine in humans by sex. Clearly, the paucity of data (including small sample sizes) prohibits firm conclusions at this time.

Other Antidepressants

Preskorn and Mac (1985) found that increasing age and female sex were associated with higher amitriptyline plasma levels. Although suggestive, studies for amitriptyline or other antidepressants have not been reviewed systematically, and thus it is unclear whether these findings are representative.[8]

Effects of synthetic sex steroid hormones and of menstrual and menopausal status are reviewed in the chapter on pharmacokinetics for specific psychotropics (Yonkers and Hamilton, Chapter 3, this volume). Briefly, OCs heighten the sex-related differences on plasma concentrations or clearance, such that higher blood levels occur in women on OCs; and the menstrual cycle will tend to have an opposing effect in a small group of women premenstrually such that lower blood levels may occur.

Clinical Implications: Sex and Pharmacokinetics

While speculative, several sex-related pharmacokinetic findings for antidepressants may be clinically meaningful. By clinically meaningful, we refer to alterations with respect to dosing, monitoring of treatment, and selection of the treatment agent. As examples, recommendations have been made for 1) a lower dose of the TCAs amitriptyline (Preskorn and

---

[8] Van Harten (1993) has reviewed pharmacokinetics for SSRIs. Plasma concentrations of sertraline were found to be higher in young women compared with men, but this finding is not believed to require adjustments in dosage by sex (Warrington 1991).

Mac 1985) and imipramine (Hamilton and Grant 1993), especially for women over 50 years of age; 2) a lower dose of imipramine for women chronically taking OCs (Abernethy et al. 1984; American Psychiatric Association 1993); and 3) a higher dose premenstrually for women with symptomatic breakthroughs and lowered plasma levels during that cycle phase (Conrad and Hamilton 1986; Jensvold et al. 1992; Kimmel et al. 1992). Thus, while not conclusive, some evidence suggests the need to consider sex-related factors both in dosing and in monitoring treatment for depressed female patients. At present, there is enough evidence to support the need for further research; in the meantime, clinicians may want to increase their "index of suspicion" with regard to sex-related factors, especially when depressed women are refractory to usual treatment regimens.

Also, women may respond more slowly to TCAs, necessitating longer treatment trials (E. Frank et al. 1988). There is some evidence that thyroid augmentation is especially beneficial in speeding treatment response in women (Prange et al. 1972). It remains uncertain whether women with an adolescent onset of depression and/or those with persistent premenstrual breakthrough symptoms should more often be offered long-term maintenance therapy.

Some evidence suggests that non-TCAs (SSRIs or MAOIs) should more often be used as first-line treatments for women as compared with men. For example, women are more likely to present with anxious and so-called atypical depressions, whereas men more frequently present with "usual" depressions (classic major depression). Because women may be more sensitive to and troubled by anxiety-like side effects, consideration should be given to adjunctive use of alprazolam or other antianxiety agents early in the course of treatment.

There has been a great deal of concern about undertreatment of depressive disorders (Goethe et al. 1988; Keller and Lavori 1988). Brosen et al. (1986) have emphasized that the daily dosage recommended for imipramine in textbooks, 100–200 mg, " . . . is *often too low* but sometimes too high" (p. 48, emphasis added). We hypothesize that the recommended dosage is more often too low (e.g., in the case of women with premenstrual exacerbations of illness) or too high (e.g., in the case of older women or women on OCs) because of sex-related factors for females than for males.

Sex-related differences in plasma concentrations are most likely to be clinically meaningful, if at all, for antidepressants with a narrow therapeutic index (see Hamilton and Yonkers, Chapter 2, this volume)—for example, nortriptyline. Low plasma concentrations can be related to lack of efficacy and high concentrations to increased side effects or toxicity, potentially leading in either case to dropouts and to lack of benefit from treatment (although the latter would be easily apparent only in *effectiveness* studies, not in pure, controlled trials, which rarely report dropout rates by sex). As one example, a female excess in type, number, or severity of side effects has been reported for TCAs (e.g., Mindham 1973; Raskin 1974; Rickels et al. 1967; L. G. Schmidt et al. 1986; Schulterbrandt et al. 1974; however, for a more complete review, see Hamilton 1995), fluoxetine (D. J. Goldstein, personal communication: gender analyses of fluoxetine versus placebo in major depressive disorder [efficacy, reasons for discontinuation, adverse events, statistical methods], Lilly Research Laboratories, Lilly Corporate Center, Indianapolis, IN, November 16, 1993; Steiner et al. 1993), and an MAOI antidepressant (Hamilton et al. 1984a; Middlefell et al. 1960), as well as for lithium (Connelly et al. 1982; Jamison et al. 1979).

Sex and Selection of Treatment Agent for Subtypes of Depression

M. Grant (unpublished data, November 1993) has taken the lead in considering the role of sex in selection of treatment agents for dysthymic disorder, major depression, and double depression. Unfortunately, despite the excess of dysthymic disorder in women compared with men (Weissman et al. 1988), sex has virtually never been considered in reporting treatment outcome in studies of dysthymic disorder.

When left either untreated or "undertreated," as the case may be, the course of depression may become protracted, waxing and waning without complete syndromal remission for years. The typical course of dysthymia involves the presence of a long-standing chronic depression, with recurrent episodes of major depression resulting in pervasive interpersonal impairment. Keller et al. (1992) report that if recovery is to occur at all, it typically takes place early on, within the first 6 months of treatment—hence the importance of early detection, accurate diagnosis, and effective treatment strategies.[9]

Like MAOIs for treatment of atypical depression, Howland (1991) has speculated that MAOIs are more effective than TCAs for treatment of dysthymia. It is unclear, however, to what extent symptoms of dysthymia overlap with those of atypical depression.[10] In clinical settings, there is a greater prevalence of atypical symptom presentation in depressed women (e.g., Quitkin et al. 1989; J. W. Stewart et al. 1989). Therefore, apparent differences in response to type of medication (MAOIs versus TCAs) in dysthymic disorder may actually represent underlying differences in rates of illness or types of symptoms by sex.

Only three studies have directly compared TCAs and MAOIs in treatment of dysthymic disorder (Quitkin et al. 1989; Rowan et al. 1982; J. W. Stewart et al. 1989). Rates of responding are shown by drug type in Figure 12–1. Contrary to Howland's (1991) hypothesis, these data suggest that TCAs and MAOIs are similar in efficacy.[11] Thus, findings from direct comparisons of MAOIs and TCAs in treating chronic minor forms of depression do not confirm the superiority of MAOIs. Other, more recent, reviews of the literature also report no significant differences in efficacy by drug type (Conte and Karasu 1992). Here, again, the paucity of the data is striking.

A somewhat larger number of studies allow comparison of TCAs or MAOIs versus placebo (see Appendix 12–A). We calculated the magnitude of effects for a TCA versus an MAOI using r. As shown in Fig-

---

[9] These findings seem to suggest the existence of a critical period during which proper treatment is crucial to prevent long-term chronicity, since the longer a person remains depressed, the lower his or her chance of recovery. This period is also crucial because it is a time during which both full recovery and relapse into major depression are equally likely, depending on the level of effectiveness of the treatment received (Keller et al. 1992).

[10] Ironically, the Howland (1991) review was based on a small number of studies with MAOIs, one of which did not report percentages (Vallejo et al. 1987) and another of which did not assess atypical depression.

[11] Fisher's combined test reveals that effectiveness does not differ between TCAs and MAOIs in treatment of dysthymic disorder ($\chi^2 = 5.75$, $df = 6$, which is not significant as the criterion at $P = .05$, one-tailed is 12.59). Again, however, we are aware that meta-analytic techniques are generally reserved for summarizing 10 studies or more.

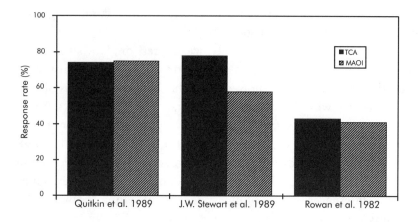

Figure 12–1. Response rates for dysthymia/double depression: tricyclic anti-depressant (TCA) *(solid bars)* versus monoamine oxidase inhibitor (MAOI) *(crosshatched bars).*
Source. M. Grant, unpublished manuscript, November 1993; Hamilton and Grant 1993.

ure 12–2, the effect size for the TCA versus placebo ($n = 6$) was $r = .332$ and for the MAOI versus placebo ($n = 4$), $r = .276$. The difference in these effect sizes was not significant. Overall, TCAs account for 11% of the variance in outcome, and MAOIs, for 8%. The binomial effect size display (R. Rosenthal and Rubin 1982) is shown in Figure 12–3. These findings should be interpreted cautiously, however, due to the small number of studies.[12]

In general, there is little evidence that sex is related to choice of agent in treatment of chronic depression. This hypothesis deserves greater research attention.

---

[12] Quitkin et al. (1989), in a study of intermittent chronic minor depression, compared the efficacy of imipramine and phenelzine. They found that failure to respond to either drug could not be attributed simply to inadequate dosage. For both medications, initial nonresponders were prescribed higher doses to address their lack of response. Plasma levels for imipramine and platelet inhibition for phenelzine were unexpectedly higher for nonresponders than responders. Nonetheless, no subsequent improvement was associated with this increase in drug availability.

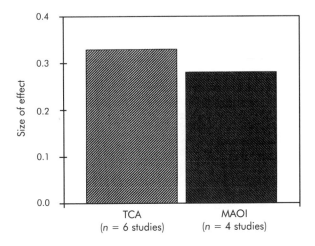

Figure 12–2. Magnitude of drug effects: drug (TCA/MAOI) versus placebo. TCA = tricyclic antidepressant; MAOI = monoamine oxidase inhibitor. *(Note.* No significant differences.)
Source. Hamilton and Grant 1993.

Other Confounding and Contextual Effects

Confounding effects may also include sex- or *gender*-related differences (Deaux 1993; Jackson 1993) for the following patient characteristics at baseline: 1) illness presentation (e.g., diagnostic subtype); 2) other illness characteristics (e.g., chronicity, initial severity or prognosis of the illness or condition being treated); 3) comorbidity (which may relate to severity of illness or to treatment failures); and 4) patterns of concurrent drug use that may influence the course of illness or alter pharmacokinetics (e.g., smoking, caffeine, alcohol, OCs) (Hamilton 1995, in press a, in press b; Hamilton and Halbreich 1993; Hamilton and Jensvold 1991; Hamilton and Yonkers, Chapter 2, this volume).

Pharmacological treatment trials can also be confounded by the following sex- or gender-related differences arising during the course of a study (Hamilton 1995, in press a, in press b; Hamilton and Halbreich 1993; Hamilton and Jensvold 1991): 1) as suggested earlier,

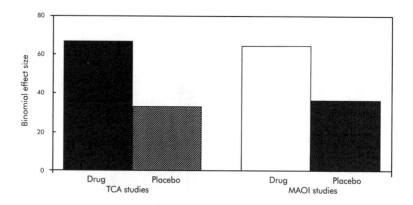

Figure 12–3. Binomial effect size: drug (TCA/MAOI) versus placebo. TCA = tricyclic antidepressant; MAOI = monoamine oxidase inhibitor.
Source. Hamilton and Grant 1993.

prevalence or salience of and tolerance to side effects, because these could lead to differential dropout rates; 2) speed of response; 3) spontaneous rates of relapse or remission; 4) placebo response; and 5) strength of the therapeutic alliance (i.e., patient cooperation with the treatment plan may depend, in part, on the therapeutic relationship; these issue are discussed further in Hamilton, in press a, in press b, and in Hamilton and Jensvold 1991).

With regard to antidepressant trials, Raskin (1974) cited studies that documented sex differences in a variety of such confounding variables. There is some evidence that women may benefit from initial cotreatment with antianxiety agents to prevent or reduce early dropouts due to cardiovascular side effects that mimic anxiety (see Hamilton and Jensvold 1991).

Conclusion

There is increasing recognition that sex is a critical variable to consider in psychotropic drug research (J. C. Bennett 1993; Merkatz et al. 1993a,

1993b). Even though women may not respond to TCAs such as imipramine as well as men, this does not mean that use of TCAs should be avoided in women. Although newer agents are of high interest, the TCAs remain important, especially from the public health perspective, due to their much lower cost. We should pay increased attention to strategies for enhancing treatment efficacy in women (Prange et al. 1972). Given that dose-by-weight correction apparently removes the sex difference in drug plasma levels (at least in younger women), it is unclear whether *raw* plasma concentrations should be interpreted using sex-blind norms, as is common clinical practice. Alternatively, perhaps guidelines for interpreting plasma levels should be normed separately for men and women. These are empirical questions.

The ultimate goal of sex and gender-sensitive research is to optimize pharmacotherapy for women (and men) by maximizing therapeutic benefits and minimizing negative side effects. Evidence increasingly suggests that sex should be considered—both in dosing and monitoring treatment and potentially in selection of treatment agent—in treatment of depression; this may be especially true for the subgroup of women who appear refractory to usual treatments. The magnitude of certain sex-related effects suggests that such efforts will result not merely in "fine tuning," but may for some individuals be much more profound. Such considerations, when firmly grounded, should be incorporated into practice guidelines (Munoz et al. 1994).

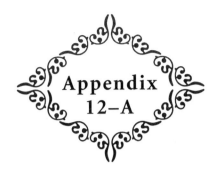

Appendix
12–A

Abbreviated Bibliography: Treatment of Dysthymia and Double Depression

Davidson JRT, Giller EL, Zisook S, et al: An efficacy study of isocarboxazid and placebo in depression, and its relationship to depressive nosology. Arch Gen Psychiatry 45:120–127, 1988

Goldberg HL, Rickels K, Finnerty R: Treatment of neurotic depression with a new antidepressant. J Clin Psychopharmacol 1 (suppl):35S, 1981

Guelfi JD, Pichot P, Dreyfus JF: Efficacy of tianeptine in anxious-depressed patients: results of a controlled multicenter trial vs. amitriptyline. Neuropsychobiology 22:41–48, 1989

Kocsis JH, Frances, AJ, Voss C, et al: Imipramine treatment for chronic depression. Arch Gen Psychiatry 45:253–257, 1988

Quitkin FM, McGrath PJ, Stewart JW, et al:. Phenelzine and imipramine in mood-reactive depressives: further delineation of the syndrome of atypical depression. Arch Gen Psychiatry 46:787–793, 1989

Rosenthal J, Hemlock C, Hellerstein DJ, et al: A preliminary study of serotonergic antidepressants in treatment of dysthymia. Prog Neuropsychopharmacol Biol Psychiatry 16:933–941, 1992

Rowan PR, Paykel ES, Parker RR: Phenelzine and amitriptyline: effects on symptoms of neurotic depression. Br J Psychiatry 140:475–483, 1982

Stewart JW, Quitkin FM, Liebowitz MR, et al: Efficacy of desipramine in depressed outpatients: response according to RDC diagnoses and severity of illness. Arch Gen Psychiatry 40:202–207, 1983

Stewart JW, McGrath PJ, Quitkin FM, et al: Relevance of DSM-III depressive subtype and chronicity of antidepressant efficacy in atypical depression. Arch Gen Psychiatry 46:1080–1087, 1989

Anxiety Disorders in Women and Their Pharmacological Treatment

Kimberly A. Yonkers, M.D.,
and James M. Ellison, M.D., M.P.H.

nxiety disorders are the most prevalent class of psychiatric disorders, affecting as many as 1 in 10 individuals (Bland et al. 1988; Robins et al. 1984). Women develop anxiety disorders at a far greater rate than men (see Table 13–1). Panic with agoraphobia is seen two to three times more commonly, social phobia is found one and one-half times as often, simple phobias three to four times more frequently, generalized anxiety disorder (GAD) about two times more often, and posttraumatic stress

The authors wish to thank Sabrina Popp, M.D., for her assistance and contribution to the posttraumatic stress disorder section and Judith Kando, Pharm.D., for her interest and assistance in researching previous work on gender-related differences in response to pharmacotherapy.

disorder (PTSD) twice as frequently (Bourdon et al. 1988; Robins et al. 1984; Schneier et al. 1992) in women as in men. Symptoms of anxiety motivate women to seek medical and psychiatric care and are a leading cause for women's disproportionate consumption of minor tranquilizers and other psychotropic agents (Balter et al. 1974; Baum et al. 1988). Despite the fact that the majority of anxiety-disorder patients are women, little is known about gender-related features, mechanisms, and treatment issues of anxiety disorders. In this chapter we review what is known regarding anxiety disorders in women and discuss the pharmacotherapy of female patients suffering from anxiety disorders. This discussion has been informed by other work from the authors (Yonkers 1994; Yonkers and Gurguis 1995).

Overview of Anxiety Disorders

Panic Disorder

Panic disorder with or without agoraphobia is frequently seen in medical and psychiatric treatment settings. A panic attack, the hallmark of panic disorder, is a sudden paroxysm of somatic symptoms including shortness of breath, hyperventilation, heart palpitations, chest discomfort, trembling, shaking, and paresthesias. These are accompanied by catastrophic cognitions such as feeling out of control or having a sense that something disastrous will imminently occur. Symptoms crescendo

Table 13–1.   Lifetime rates of DSM-III anxiety disorders in men and women from community surveys

	Men (%)	Women (%)
Panic with agoraphobia	2.9	7.7
Simple phobia	7.2	13.9
Social phobia	2.3	3.2
Posttraumatic stress disorder	6	11.3
Obsessive-compulsive disorder	2.0	3.1

Note.   DSM-III (American Psychiatric Association 1980).
Source.   Adapted from Robins et al. 1984, Breslau et al. 1990, and Bourdon et al. 1988.

over several minutes before gradually dissipating. The initial panic attack may be triggered by a stressful event or may occur without an identifiable precipitant. To meet DSM-IV (American Psychiatric Association 1994) criteria for panic disorder, an individual must have suffered recurrent attacks (with no identifiable precipitants) during a 1-month interval and must experience concern about subsequent attacks, worry about the implications of the attack, or show changes in behavior because of the attack.

Often, panic disorder is accompanied by agoraphobia or another anxiety disorder (Bourdon et al. 1988). Agoraphobia, the fear and avoidance of a place from which escape might be difficult, may develop as a consequence of panic attacks (D. F. Klein and Gorman 1987), although some authors believe that phobia occurs before panic (Marks 1987).

Panic disorder has several unique features in women. In addition to the frequent accompaniment of agoraphobia, other disorders such as simple phobia, GAD, and/or depression are more likely to co-occur in women with panic disorder, whereas alcohol abuse and dependence are frequently noted in men with panic symptoms (see Table 13–2) (Yonkers 1994). Hafner (1981) found that men are more likely to fear harming another person than to express fear of an object or of exposure to a situation. However, several research groups have failed to find any gen-

Table 13–2. Panic disorder and co-occurring psychiatric disorders

| | Lifetime | | |
| | Men | Women | |
Comorbid diagnosis	($n = 160$), %	($n = 367$), %	P
Agoraphobia	72	82	.013
Alcohol abuse	43	23	< .001
Generalized anxiety disorder	19	27	.043
Major depression	52	57	NS
Obsessive-compulsive disorder	17	12	NS
Posttraumatic disorder	6	10	NS
Simple phobia	12	21	.015
Social phobia	20	20	NS

Note. NS = nonsignificant.
Source. Adapted from Yonkers and Gurguis 1995.

der divergences in the profile of DSM-IV panic symptoms (Chambless and Mason 1986; Scheibe and Albus 1992; Yonkers 1994).

Many women with panic attacks complain of premenstrual worsening, although this effect has not been confirmed in several small prospective studies (Cameron et al. 1988; Cook et al. 1990; Stein et al. 1989). On the other hand, preliminary work from a larger study has found evidence for premenstrual worsening of panic (L. Cohen, personal communication, May 1993). Of note, for women with premenstrual syndrome, the late luteal phase is a time of vulnerability to lactate or CO_2-induced panic (Facchinetti et al. 1992; Harrison et al. 1989). Similarly, some women first experience panic shortly after childbirth (Metz et al. 1988).

Biological factors may play a role in the high rate of panic in women, particularly during certain phases of the menstrual cycle or during the postpartum period. Progesterone elevations during the luteal phase of the cycle cause chronic hyperventilation (Fadel et al. 1979), which may lead to panic in vulnerable groups. Recently, D. F. Klein (1993) suggested that the decrease in a woman's chronically compensated hyperventilation during the late luteal phase triggers a suffocation alarm and hence panic attacks. Panic may be further compounded by withdrawal of ovarian hormones, since progesterone and several of its metabolites are bioactive and soporific by virtue of binding at the gamma-aminobutyric acid–A ($GABA_A$) receptor complex (P. C. MacDonald et al. 1991; Majewska et al. 1986). Some evidence suggests an increase in noradrenergic sensitivity during the middle part of the menstrual cycle (Ghose and Turner 1977; S. B. Jones et al. 1983). Heightened noradrenergic sensitivity may increase susceptibility to panic in genetically vulnerable individuals. Withdrawal of substances that act as agonists at the $GABA_A$ receptor would be expected to further increase noradrenergic activity.

Finally, as shown in Table 13–3, the frequent occurrence in women of certain medical disorders—such as mitral valve prolapse and hyperthyroidism—long associated with panic disorder may provide a sufficient trigger for panic. It may be that somatic sensations caused by these medical disorders are catastrophically misinterpreted by the individual (Yonkers 1994). D. M. Clark (1986) has suggested that in a subsequent chain of events, anxiety and somatic sensations increase, catastrophic cognitions worsen, and a panic attack ultimately occurs.

Table 13–3.   Panic disorder and concurrent medical disorders

Medical illness	Men ($n = 160$), %	Women ($n = 367$), %	P
Allergies	36	52	.001
Gastrointestinal ulcer	17	7	.001
Headache	30	45	.001
Low blood pressure	7	23	< .001
Migraine	21	37	< .001

Source.   Adapted from Yonkers 1994.

As noted by Yonkers (1994), a role for developmental and sociological factors in the disproportionate expression of phobias and panic among women has been proposed by several authors. Through the process of sex role socialization, women learn "helplessness, avoidance of mastery experiences, competition and lack of assertiveness" (Fodor 1974, p. 140), which in some women results in fewer tools with which to overcome fear. In support of this hypothesis, another group has found that agoraphobia in women is inversely correlated with scores on masculinity scales (Chambless and Mason 1986).

Although such explanations are only speculative, they suggest fertile areas for investigation. Given the extensive overlap found among the various anxiety disorders, these potential mechanisms of anxiety may also be relevant to other anxiety disorders (White et al. 1992).

Generalized Anxiety Disorder

Changes in the diagnostic criteria for GAD between DSM-III (American Psychiatric Association 1980) and DSM-III-R (American Psychiatric Association 1987) virtually created a new diagnostic category that has been further refined in DSM-IV. As originally conceived, GAD was designed to encompass the anticipatory anxiety often seen with panic and phobic states, the anxious prodrome before full-blown panic disorder, and the residual anxiety after treatment of acute panic attacks. Changes in diagnostic criteria have included an emphasis on worry or apprehension, a lengthened illness episode (6 months), and a greater allowance for comorbidity with other anxiety and nonanxiety disorders. In particular, the longevity requirement of 6 symptomatic months defines a disorder with great chronicity and a low likelihood of complete remission. Little is known about gender differences in the expression of GAD other than that the disorder has higher prevalence in women. In one study, the co-occurrence of GAD with dysthymia was high, and the two disorders remitted concurrently (Shores et al. 1992). The overlap between GAD and dysthymia may also be due to the fact that both disorders occur frequently in women (Robins et al. 1984).

Obsessive-Compulsive Disorder

A discussion of gender differences in obsessive-compulsive disorder (OCD) is also found in Yonkers and Gurguis (1995). As shown in Table 13–4, data from the Epidemiologic Catchment Area (ECA) study (Robins et al. 1984) show that OCD ranks fourth in lifetime prevalence among psychiatric disorders. Diagnostic features of OCD include obsessions, defined as images or thoughts that are ego-dystonic, irrational, or meaningless but recurrent. The individual attempts to suppress them and knows they are not real. The other component of OCD, compulsions, are defined as behaviors that are repetitive, senseless, yet difficult to control; these behaviors are carried out by patients in an attempt to reduce anxiety.

Early clinical studies claimed that OCD occurred more frequently in men (Insel et al. 1983; Rasmussen and Tsuang 1984), although subsequent ECA data found similar prevalence rates for men and women (Robins et al. 1984). It appears, however, that the average age at onset differs by sex. One study found a preponderance of early-onset OCD (i.e., at 5–15 years old) in males and a mostly later onset (i.e., at ages

---

Table 13–4.   Gender-divergent features of obsessive-compulsive disorder (OCD)

- ◆ Women have older age at onset.
- ◆ Depression and anorexia frequently occur in women with OCD.
- ◆ Women suffer from compulsive washing.
- ◆ Checking rituals are frequently reported in men.
- ◆ Course may be worse in men.

26–35) in females; the associated length of illness is also longer in males (Noshirvani et al. 1991). A lifetime history of depression if found significantly more often in women than in men (Noshirvani et al. 1991), although this may be due to the fact that depression occurs more often in women. The later-onset type of OCD, which occurs more often in women, may begin with an episode of depression that improves but leaves residual obsessions and compulsions (Welner et al. 1976).

A prospective study of OCD showed that the only subjects who recover from OCD are women with OCD and depression (White et al. 1992). Some evidence suggests that early onset of OCD is a poor prognostic factor and that males may have a more treatment-resistant variant of the illness (Rasmussen and Tsuang 1984). The fact that males may seek treatment at an earlier age and may receive longer periods of treatment might account for the male preponderance of OCD found in earlier clinical studies. Symptom profiles often differ between men and women with OCD. Compulsive washers are more often women; men are more likely to have checking rituals (Noshirvani et al. 1991). In addition, obsessions about food and weight, as well as diagnoses of anorexia, are more common in women (Kasvikis et al. 1986).

Posttraumatic Stress Disorder

PTSD can be difficult to diagnose and treat; its sufferers are heterogeneous, its symptoms are varied, and it often overlaps symptomatically with comorbid psychiatric disorders. PTSD in women may represent an underlying problem in borderline personality disorder, dissociative identity disorder, and dissociative states. The essence of PTSD is a distinctive symptom cluster developing in the aftermath of a traumatic event that transcends normal human experience. In addition to resulting from combat exposure or natural disasters, PTSD can be induced by a wide range of other stressors. In female patients, PTSD is commonly the unfortunate sequela of rape, incest, or childhood abuse. According to DSM-IV, PTSD symptoms fall into three categories: 1) reexperiencing of a traumatic event, 2) avoidance or general numbing of responsiveness, and 3) increased arousal. Symptoms must have been present for at least 1 month to satisfy diagnostic criteria for PTSD. In contrast with the other anxiety disorders, which tend to have an early onset, PTSD can occur at any age. Two community surveys have provided estimates for the prevalence of PTSD. Helzer and colleagues (1987) found a surprisingly low lifetime rate of 1% for PTSD. Combat veterans had an incidence of 9%, whereas 3% of assault victims developed PTSD. Using a sample drawn from a large Detroit-based health maintenance organization (HMO), Breslau and colleagues (1990) found an overall rate nine times as great as that noted by Helzer and colleagues—11% of women and 6% of men. Among individuals exposed to trauma, nearly 24% developed PTSD. This difference likely reflects variations in the methods used to probe for traumatic events and to identify PTSD patients. In the Breslau report, as in the Helzer study, a higher rate of trauma exposure occurred in men. In Breslau's sample, among those exposed to trauma, 31% of women and only 19% of men developed PTSD. Female sex, neuroticism, and family history of anxiety or depression were risk factors for PTSD in a logistic regression model (Breslau et al. 1990). A differential effect of stress or "psychological distress" in males and females was also found by Kessler and McLeod (1984). Again, despite exposure to a greater number of traumatic events, men were less likely to suffer psychological stress than women. To investigate the mechanism behind this finding, the authors conducted analyses that showed that women are exposed to greater amounts of "network events"—events befalling people intimate with the patient. Such events lead to increased cumulative stress and higher psychological distress. The importance of staying in "connection" with other people is noted by Miller (J. B. Miller 1976; J. B. Miller and Stiver 1993) in her theory of women's psychology. This factor may also explain the relatively larger impact of traumatic "network events" on women; psychological distress often develops as a consequence of losing valuable connections with close friends or family members.

As noted above, PTSD in women may occur as a result of childhood trauma, sexual abuse, or incest. An association between early traumatic events and dissociative experiences, borderline personality disorder, and multiple personality disorder has been observed by several research groups over the past decade (Herman et al. 1989; Putnam et al. 1986; Soloff and Millward 1983). Herman and colleagues (1989) found that 81% of patients with borderline personality disorder had histories of trauma, and rates at least as high occur with multiple personality disorder (Putnam et al. 1986). The strikingly elevated incidence of trauma among patients diagnosed with borderline personality disorder has led some to question whether this condition is a "personality disorder" or a variant of chronic PTSD (Saunders and Arnold 1991). Given the invasive, shameful, and secretive nature of childhood abuse and incest and the fact that such experiences occur during the time when an individual is developing a sense of self, it makes sense to many clinicians that the pathological sequelae would appear as pervasive and enduring as a personality disorder.

Recent neurobiological theories of PTSD have focused on limbic system dysfunction and the actions of neurotransmitters and endogenous opiate peptides (EOPs). The state of chronic arousal that accompanies PTSD suggests an overactivity of the noradrenergic and possibly dopaminergic systems (Charney et al. 1993). The model of *inescapable shock* has been proposed by van der Kolk (1987). In this paradigm, an animal is repeatedly exposed to an inescapable stressor and, as a result of the stress response, is depleted of the neurotransmitters dopamine and serotonin, which leads to noradrenergic and dopaminergic supersensitivity and autonomic hyperarousal. As noted earlier, adrenergic activity may vary across the menstrual cycle, suggesting increased vulnerability to stress at these specific times (although not confirmed by stress testing across the menstrual cycle [Polefrone and Manuck 1987]). A synergistic role may be played by endogenous opiates, which are released as part of the stress response in animal models of "stress-induced analgesia" (Charney et al. 1993). After administration of acute, uncontrollable shock, animals develop endogenous opiate–dependent analgesia to subsequent aversive stimuli. In humans, reexperiencing the trauma or self-mutilation may also lead to an increase in endogenous opiate activity; the soothing opiate response may be the driving force behind these behaviors (van der Kolk 1987). It is also possible that secretion of EOPs leads to certain dissociative phenomena. In some studies, levels of EOPs also vary across the menstrual cycle. Incremental increases occur during the follicular and early luteal phases, with an acute withdrawal just before menses (Giannini et al. 1990). Worsening of PTSD symptoms, particularly dissociative episodes during the luteal phase of the cycle, has been reported (Jensvold and Putnam 1990). Whether fluctuations in levels of EOPs or in adrenergic activity correlate with PTSD symptoms—particularly symptoms of dissociation and arousal (respectively)—is unknown.

These specific characteristics, in terms of possible mechanisms and expression of PTSD symptoms in women, argue for special considerations, such as monitoring symptoms across the menstrual cycle and assessing premenstrual onset or worsening (Hamilton and Jensvold 1992). These features also suggest that certain populations of women, particularly those diagnosed with borderline personality disorder, should be carefully assessed for histories of trauma and that such experiences be addressed in the treatment plan.

Social Phobia

Social phobia, a persistent fear of one or more situations in which the person may be exposed to embarrassing scrutiny by others (American Psychiatric Association 1994), can cause patients to go to great lengths to avoid the feared situation. Avoidance and fear impairs daily functioning.

According to community data, social phobia occurs more often in women than in men, with a prevalence rate of 2.4% (Schneier et al. 1992) Men with social phobia are seen more frequently in clinical settings. Risk factors include female sex, single status, youth, and lower socioeconomic status (Schneier et al. 1992). Patients with social phobia are considered at increased risk for depression, suicide, and alcohol abuse (Liebowitz et al. 1985). One study showed a depression risk of 94% in social phobia patients who did not meet panic disorder criteria (Uhde et al. 1991). Other studies of social phobia have shown rates of concurrent alcohol abuse as high as 39% (Liebowitz et al. 1985). It is speculated that social phobia and panic disorder overlap (Uhde et al. 1991). Social phobia typically begins in early adulthood and may follow a variety of courses. Little is known about specific gender differences in the symptoms or correlates of this disorder.

Therapeutic Issues and Treatment

Pharmacotherapeutic principles important in women include dosage considerations, drug interactions (especially those with exogenous hormones), menstrual cycle effects, and modifications required during pregnancy (Table 13–5).

Table 13–5.   Pharmacological treatment principles in women

◆ Adjust starting medication dose for smaller weight and body size.
◆ Assess for changing drug levels or efficacy across the menstrual cycle.
◆ Monitor potential drug interactions with oral contraceptives.
◆ Counsel patient regarding drug effects in instances of unanticipated or accidental pregnancy.
◆ Consider effects of psychotropic drug on oral contraceptive efficacy.

Benzodiazepines

Benzodiazepine anxiolytic agents are among the first choices for pharmacotherapy of anxiety, including panic disorder with or without agoraphobia. Their antianxiety effect is very rapid, giving this class of medication special appeal. Considerable research on their mechanism of action suggests that benzodiazepines work by binding to a cell-membrane receptor essential to the effects of the neurotransmitter GABA. Benzodiazepines augment the action of GABA, an inhibitory neurotransmitter, by controlling ion flow through the chloride ion channel associated with this receptor, thereby raising the threshold necessary for the neuron to fire. Raising this threshold is also thought to modulate neurotransmission of norepinephrine, serotonin, and perhaps other neurotransmitters.

Schatzberg and Cole (1992) subclassify benzodiazepine anxiolytics on the basis of structure into three groups: 2-keto, 3-hydroxy, and triazolo benzodiazepines. The 2-keto group includes agents oxidized in the liver. Drugs in this category, which include chlordiazepoxide, diazepam, clorazepate, prazepam, and clonazepam, are slowly metabolized and therefore have long half-lives (20–60 hours). In addition, each of these agents has an active metabolite with its own path of metabolism. Members of the 3-hydroxy group, comprised of lorazepam and oxazepam, have shorter half-lives (9–14 hours) and are cleared via conjugative phase II metabolism in the liver. No active metabolites are produced, and the conjugates are renally excreted. In contrast, the triazolo compounds alprazolam and adinazolam are oxidized to active metabolites. Half-lives of the parent compounds are, respectively, 14 hours and 2 hours (Schatzberg and Cole 1992).

Gender differences in the metabolism of benzodiazepines have been suggested by several researchers (see also Hamilton and Parry 1983; K. Wilson 1984; Yonkers et al. 1992a). Clearance of benzodiazepines that undergo metabolism via conjugation (lorazepam and oxazepam) appears to be slower in women than in men (D. J. Greenblatt et al. 1980b). Nitro reduction of the anxiolytic nitrazepam does not differ with respect to gender (Jochemsen et al. 1982), but the clearance of chlordiazepoxide is probably slower in women (Roberts et al. 1979). The evidence regarding diazepam is conflicting, and other oxidatively metabolized compounds (prazepam and clonazepam) show no gender-related differences in metabolism (Abernethy et al. 1982a; Giles et al. 1981; D. J. Greenblatt et al. 1980a; MacLeod et al. 1979).

Concurrent oral contraceptive (OC) use affects serum levels and the side effects of benzodiazepines by influencing benzodiazepine metabolism. OC preparations differ in their content of estrogen, progestin, and gestagen. Current evidence suggests that *estrogen*-dominant OCs inhibit microsomal oxidase, induce conjugative enzymes, and elevate levels of binding protein (Abernethy et al. 1982a; Fazio 1991; Teichmann 1990). The net effect for women receiving both benzodiazepines and estrogen-dominant OCs may be an increase in serum levels of oxidatively metabolized benzodiazepines and a decrease in serum levels of OCs that are conjugated and excreted. Studies of psychomotor and cognitive performance of women using OCs and undergoing benzodiazepine treatment suggest psychodynamic properties independent of pharmacokinetic effects. Kroboth and colleagues (1985) found that women taking lorazepam or temazepam and an OC had significantly greater impairment of psychomotor performance despite plasma levels that were nearly equal to those of women not taking OCs. In some situations, the effects of benzodiazepines may fluctuate between weeks on and off exogenous hormones. Ellinwood and colleagues (1984) demonstrated relative intoxication from diazepam in women OC users who were in the hormone-free week. These authors suggested that during the 3 weeks on hormones, the rise in benzodiazepine levels is slower, whereas during the fourth, hormone-free week, benzodiazepine levels sharply increase, thus causing "intoxication."

These findings suggest a need to closely monitor benzodiazepine side effects in OC users, with the understanding that simple pharmacokinetic explanations might fail to predict all of the adverse reactions observed, especially since our data are based on peripheral plasma levels whereas the effects occur in the central nervous system (CNS). Empirical studies of newly marketed drugs in OC users would be helpful in guiding clinicians, since some effects may be unpredictable (Hamilton 1991).

Benzodiazepine Treatment Considerations

Benzodiazepine anxiolytics are widely beneficial, either as a primary treatment in anxiety disorders such as phobia, GAD, and panic or as adjuncts in the treatment of OCD and PTSD. Many patients, particularly those with PTSD, panic, and OCD, require both an antidepressant and a benzodiazepine.

Several controlled studies have shown that alprazolam is effective in the treatment of panic disorder with or without phobia (Ballenger 1990; Charney and Heninger 1986; Sheehan 1982). Optimal doses average 3 mg/day (Ballenger 1990), although a recent report found lower doses (2 mg/day) to be very effective (Lydiard et al. 1992). Sheehan (1982) noted that some patients require doses up to 6 mg/day for adequate control of panic.

For women with anxiety disorders, starting doses of alprazolam should be between 0.25 mg and 0.5 mg, three times daily. Multiple daily doses are given because the therapeutic effects of a single dose last between 8 and 12 hours. Alprazolam dosage may be increased to a daily total of 6 mg, depending on efficacy and side effects. Although research does not suggest that women require much smaller dosages, clinicians often begin with smaller dosages on the basis of body size. For women on OCs, serum levels are likely to be marginally higher; this, however, does not usually alter physical or cognitive functioning to a significant degree.

Another short-acting, high-potency benzodiazepine, lorazepam, is effective in the treatment of panic disorder. Suggested daily doses are around 3 mg (Ballenger 1990), beginning with doses around 0.5 mg twice daily and titrating upward to the lowest effective amount. Some patients will require three doses per day. Women may metabolize lorazepam more slowly than men, although the drug is cleared with greater rapidity in patients taking OCs. Serum levels do not reflect the degree of psychomotor or cognitive impairment (Kroboth et al. 1985).

Clonazepam, a high-potency, oxidatively metabolized benzodiaze-pine, effectively alleviates panic disorder at average daily doses of 1.5–2.5 mg (Pollack et al. 1982). The longer half-life for this medication allows for once-per-day dosing, although some patients may feel the need for doses twice daily. As with the other benzodiazepines, clonaze-pam is started at a low dose, and attention is given to increased side effects when OCs are also used. Diazepam, too, has been used to treat a variety of anxiety disorders, including panic disorder, although it is more often used for generalized anxiety disorder.

Benzodiazepine Side Effects

Among the side effects associated with benzodiazepines, sedation is the most important. At higher doses, both psychomotor and cognitive im-pairment occur. As previously mentioned, women vary in their suscep-tibility to the sedating properties of benzodiazepines, even at equivalent doses, and particularly when they are also taking OCs. Over the long term, there is a risk of dependency. One report suggests that more women in general are at greater risk for developing dependency by virtue of receiving more medication prescriptions (Trinkoff and Anthony 1990). However, when risk is assessed after controlling for the number of prescriptions written, the gender difference disappears and a history of previous substance abuse emerges as a key risk factor for predicting benzodiazepine abuse or dependence.

A very important aspect of benzodiazepines is their capability to in-duce withdrawal symptoms. Seizures are the most serious withdrawal symptom and may occur in the wake of abrupt discontinuation. Other withdrawal symptoms include sleeplessness, jitteriness, palpitations, clammy hands and feet, nausea, confusion, lightheadedness, and hy-persensitivity to light or sound (Rickels et al. 1982a, 1982b; Schatzberg and Cole 1992). These symptoms resemble those of the initial anxiety disorder, making it difficult to distinguish withdrawal from a return of the disorder that initially required treatment. Withdrawal reactions can be more intense or prolonged when the duration of treatment is lengthy, a common feature of treatment for anxiety disorders. High-potency ben-zodiazepines are more likely to cause withdrawal complications, man-dating gradual dose reduction. One authority recommends tapering alprazolam by 0.25 mg/day per week (C. S. Brown et al. 1991). A similar recommendation can be made for discontinuation of clonazepam.

Benzodiazepine Use During Pregnancy

When psychotropic drug use becomes necessary during pregnancy, careful attention must be given to potential effects on both the mother and the fetus. The physiological changes associated with pregnancy include increases in volume of distribution, cardiac output, and glomerular filtration rate (Mortola 1989). These are somewhat counterbalanced by an increase in absorption secondary to slowed gastric emptying, a decrease in hepatic metabolism, and a decrease in binding protein production (Wald et al. 1981). The net effect is generally less available drug, but there may be no change in plasma level.

Animal data on the teratogenicity of benzodiazepines suggest an association with malformations, particularly cleft palate, decreased fetal weight, and neural-tube defects (Elia et al. 1987). These concerns are supported by several small human case series that have correlated benzodiazepine use during pregnancy with congenital cleft palate (Aarskog 1975); other studies, however, have not confirmed this association (Delaney 1983; Rosenberg et al. 1983). A recent study of 500 patients who reported exposure to alprazolam during pregnancy (St. Clair and Schirmer 1992) and a larger prescription monitoring survey (J. G. Edwards et al. 1991) both failed to find a significantly elevated risk of malformations associated with use of the drug. Still, the evidence is not conclusive, and thus it is prudent to avoid benzodiazepines, particularly during the first trimester, when fetal cells are differentiating.

Further concerns regarding benzodiazepine medication use relate to effects of the drug on the fetal CNS. The CNS continues to develop well beyond parturition, and the effect of psychotropic drugs in causing behavioral teratogenicity is not known. Finally, benzodiazepines may affect parturition. The newborn infant's immature liver, deprived of maternal metabolic assistance, is unable to rapidly dispose of certain drugs. Benzodiazepine levels may persist in the newborn and produce symptoms of withdrawal, including muscle weakness, sedation, or hypotonia (Elia et al. 1987). Near the expected date of delivery, benzodiazepine use should be minimized (see also Wisner and Perel, Chapter 10, this volume).

Benzodiazepine Use in GAD

The medication used in most clinical trials of generalized anxiety is diazepam; doses range between 5 and 40 mg, with an average dose around 15–20 mg (Schatzberg and Cole 1992). Because diazepam is very lipophilic, it is absorbed quickly and crosses the blood-brain barrier rapidly. Patients may require doses two to three times daily because the drug's action is shortened by rapid uptake and storage in adipose tissues. As noted in the previous section, many women require lower dosages, and treatment should be started at 2 mg tid (Schatzberg and Cole 1992). Drug interactions with OCs may increase the effective dose (Abernethy et al. 1982a; Giles et al. 1981; D. J. Greenblatt et al. 1980a; Kroboth et al. 1985; MacLeod et al. 1979), and physicians should monitor their patients for this effect. Because these agents are tranquilizing, patients should be instructed to start the medication when they are not under obligation to drive, use other potentially dangerous machinery, or complete tasks that would put them at risk should they become sedated.

The length of time for which a patient should be treated with a benzodiazepine for generalized anxiety has not been established. Many practitioners have concerns about the addictive potential of these agents and the possibility of dosage escalation over time. On the other hand, GAD is a chronic condition and the risk that symptoms will return if the drug is stopped is probably as high as 50% (Rickels and Schweizer 1990). Rickels and colleagues (Rickels and Schweizer 1990; Rickels et al. 1982a, 1982b) found low rates of dose escalation in a maintenance study of diazepam; they also found elevated rates of relapse after discontinuation and high levels of ongoing symptoms despite continued treatment. For patients terminating long-term diazepam treatment, these authors suggest decreasing the dose of diazepam by 2.5–5.0 mg/day, but not more than one-fourth the daily dose, every 1–2 weeks.

Other benzodiazepine anxiolytics can be used in the treatment of generalized anxiety. Patients require lower doses of the higher potency benzodiazepines; for alprazolam and lorazepam, this is around 1.0–3.0 mg. Long-term users of these agents require an even more careful dose reduction.

Benzodiazepine Use in PTSD

Benzodiazepines are helpful in treatment of many symptoms associated with PTSD. As with other anxiety disorders, the benzodiazepine alprazolam is effective for anxiety symptoms but less helpful for intrusive symptoms (Braun et al. 1990). Sleep disturbances associated with PTSD can be profound, and benzodiazepines are helpful in treating this problem. Generally, higher doses are required to achieve sedation, perhaps because patients with PTSD have a high degree of autonomic arousal. Although the sedating properties of benzodiazepines are beneficial, they may lead to behavioral disinhibition (Cowdry and Gardner 1988) and increases in self-mutilating behavior for patients who suffer from these symptoms. Substance abuse can also confound treatment, and patients should be assessed for this before starting and after commencing treatment.

Antidepressants

Antidepressants are primary treatment agents for panic disorder and OCD. They are also useful for treatment of the depressive symptoms that accompany PTSD or that secondarily arise from any of the anxiety disorders.

In 1964, D. F. Klein reported that imipramine was effective in treating panic attacks. Subsequent studies have concurred, and more recent work suggests that doses as large as those required to treat depression—at least 150 mg/day of imipramine or its equivalent—are necessary for optimal response in many patients (Lydiard 1985). Other tricyclic antidepressants (TCAs) shown useful in the treatment of panic disorder include desipramine, nortriptyline, doxepin, amitriptyline, and clomipramine (Balestrieri et al. 1989; Liebowitz et al. 1988).

The monoamine oxidase inhibitor (MAOI) phenelzine has been used to treat anxiety disorders for more than 30 years (D. F. Klein 1964) and may be more effective than TCAs in alleviating panic disorder (Sheehan et al. 1980). An additional benefit is that it is less likely to induce the "hyperstimulation" symptoms that can accompany TCA treatment and that occur more often in women (Noyes et al. 1989; Pohl et al. 1988). Other MAOIs, including tranylcypromine, have also been shown useful for treating panic disorder (Liebowitz et al. 1988). When taking this class of medication, patients must restrict their intake of foods high in tyramine and avoid medications such as meperidine, which can cause a hyperthermic reaction. Patients should be given a list of foods and medications that are potentially dangerous. Some psychopharmacologists choose to give patients an emergency 10-mg pill of nifedipine to chew and place under the tongue in the event that a hypertensive crisis occurs. If a patient suspects that a reaction has occurred, she should proceed to an emergency room, whether or not she has taken protective medication. The risks of either a hypertensive or a hyperthermic crisis make MAOIs undesirable as first-choice treatment of panic disorder or agoraphobia.

The new selective serotonin reuptake inhibitors (SSRIs) are now being evaluated for the treatment of panic disorder. One group (Schneier et al. 1990) has demonstrated fluoxetine's effectiveness in an open trial. Other SSRIs, sertraline and paroxetine, await definitive evaluation. Anecdotally, however, they seem to be effective.

Antidepressant Treatment Considerations

TCAs, in the treatment of anxiety disorders, should be started at very small doses. With nortriptyline, imipramine, desipramine, or amitriptyline, for example, a beginning dose of 10 mg/day is usually well tolerated. The dosage is then increased as slowly as 10–25 mg/day every few days until clinical improvement is attained.

Patients who experience excessive sedation can be told to take their medication at bedtime. When using TCAs, particularly in women, it is important to watch for the emergence of a "jittery syndrome" or "hyperstimulatory reaction," characterized by agitation and tremulousness and occurring in the early stages of TCA treatment (Noyes et al. 1989; Pohl et al. 1988). Jitteriness may occur more often during treatment of anxiety disorders, particularly when using desmethylated compounds (e.g., nortriptyline, desipramine) (Pohl et al. 1988). The distress caused by this syndrome can be minimized by warning patients in advance and reassuring them that these side effects are treatable. Symptoms of hyperstimulation usually abate within the first few weeks (Noyes et al. 1989). Patients can temporarily take a benzodiazepine to control these TCA side effects. Small doses of propranolol may also help with the jitteriness, although Noyes and colleagues have had greater success with the benzodiazepines for this purpose.

Antidepressant Side Effects

Side effects caused by TCAs are predominantly anticholinergic or antihistaminic. TCAs also have adrenergic-blocking properties, responsible for orthostatic hypotension. In addition to sedation or hyperstimulation, as mentioned above, TCAs may cause dry mouth, constipation, sexual dysfunction, cardiac arrhythmias, orthostatic hypotension, blurred vision, urinary retention, and increased appetite and weight gain. They can also precipitate an emergency in patients with narrow-angle glaucoma. In elderly patients, TCAs can induce or aggravate delirium.

As in the treatment of depression, TCAs require several weeks to develop maximal therapeutic effect. The full response may not be evident until 4 weeks at a therapeutic dose. If a benzodiazepine is required to reduce initial adverse effects, it is often possible to discontinue it once TCA response becomes established.

Similar principles of treatment pertain to pharmacological management of MAOIs. For phenelzine, doses in the range of 15–75 mg/day for 4 weeks are needed to achieve therapeutic effect. Patients may feel relief at lower doses, but full doses are usually required for optimal sustained response. MAOI side effects, in addition to the dietary considerations, include orthostatic hypotension, mild dizziness, dry mouth, headache, constipation, urinary hesitancy, sleep disturbance, sedation, and blurred vision.

SSRIs share some of the activating properties found with TCAs and, particularly in women, fluoxetine may cause an initial increase in anxiety and agitation. Fluoxetine, in liquid form or capsules of 10 mg or 20 mg, can be started at the low initial dosage of 5–10 mg/day. For patients who are sensitive but who require higher doses, the medication can be increased by 5 mg/day every week until a daily dosage of 20 mg is reached. Sertraline, available in 50-mg scored caplets, can be started at 25 mg/day. This dosage can be increased to 50 mg/day the following week and augmented as appropriate on a weekly basis. Similarly, paroxetine can be started at 10 mg ($^1/_2$ of the scored caplet) and increased to 20 or 30 mg/day if needed.

Antidepressant Use During Pregnancy

Case reports of first-trimester TCA exposure suggest a weak association of the drug with fetal malformations, particularly limb deformities (Elia et al. 1987). The largest study surveyed the rate of malformations in more than 1 million newborns whose mothers were prescribed tricyclics, including a group with first-trimester exposure. The absence of a large excess of fetal malformations in this group argues that these agents are *not* potent teratogens (Elia et al. 1987; Rowe 1973). TCA use during pregnancy is not risk free, however. Exposure at specific times, in particular weeks 5–9, may be more dangerous. In addition, these agents frequently cause orthostatic hypotension which, if severe, can compromise blood flow through the utero-placental unit. Side effects that make TCAs less desirable for use in pregnant patients include constipation and sedation, problems that are already common and annoying in many pregnant women, even without medication treatment. On the other hand, these agents have been used for decades, and a much larger body of literature on their relatively safe use in pregnancy is available.

MAOIs can cause a hypertensive crisis with attendant high blood pressure or hyperthermic reactions. These potentially severe adverse reactions make MAOI use undesirable in pregnancy, particularly since women may require anesthesia at delivery.

The new class of antidepressants, the SSRIs, includes fluoxetine, the first compound to be marketed in this class. These drugs do not cause orthostatic hypotension, constipation, or sedation, and this makes them more tolerable in pregnancy. First-trimester fluoxetine use has been compared with standard tricyclics and nonteratogens, and no group differences were found (Pastuszak et al. 1993). This medication has been available for only 6 years and, thus, experience with it is far less than with other antidepressant agents (see also Wisner and Perel, Chapter 10, this volume).

Antidepressant Use in GAD

Historically, benzodiazepine anxiolytics were thought to be effective for GAD, whereas antidepressants were felt to have no role in treatment (D. F. Klein 1964). Currently, however, many clinicians and researchers feel that antidepressants are also effective for treatment of GAD (Liebowitz et al. 1988; Rickels and Schweizer 1990). The majority of studies have examined the efficacy of doxepin, but as pointed out in a review by Liebowitz and colleagues (1988), other TCAs probably have equivalent efficacy. In a manner similar to treating women with panic disorder, one should start low and gradually increase the dose to a therapeutic level.

Antidepressant Use in OCD

Tricyclics. The mainstay of pharmacological treatment for OCD is the TCA clomipramine. Clomipramine has been studied and shown effective in a number of trials (Ananth et al. 1981; Insel et al. 1983; Thorén et al. 1980). Clomipramine blocks serotonin reuptake to a greater degree than do other TCAs, a property that is considered responsible for its superior anti-OCD effects. The drug has a long half-life, 20–40 hours, and has active metabolites (Trimble 1990). Clomipramine levels are slightly higher in young women than in young men because of slower hydroxylation of the parent compound (Gex-Fabry et al. 1990). This effect is not likely to be of great clinical significance.

Gastrointestinal side effects are often diminished by using a twice-daily dosing regimen. Clomipramine should be started at 25 mg bid and gradually increased as high as 250 mg/day, the maximum recommended dose, as tolerated. Improvement may be gradual, and patients may not experience the full therapeutic effects of the medication for several months. Other TCAs have been used to treat OCD, and their efficacy is probably between clomipramine and placebo (Insel and Zohar 1987).

SSRIs. Fluoxetine is also effective in the treatment of OCD. In open trials, it has been used in doses between 20–80 mg, and in one study it was found to be as effective as clomipramine (D. L. Murphy et al. 1990). The investigational SSRI fluvoxamine was superior to placebo in two clinical trials (Perse et al. 1988). Peak responses to treatment may require 6–10 weeks (Insel 1990). Other SSRIs, sertraline and paroxetine, also hold promise for this disorder.

Antidepressant Use in PTSD

For nearly every type of antidepressant medication, uncontrolled case reports have reported reduction of PTSD symptoms. Current prescribing practices for PTSD treatment vary widely. To date, only five double-blind placebo-controlled studies have examined the pharmacotherapy of PTSD, and most of these studied male war veterans. These studies measured responses to phenelzine, imipramine, amitriptyline, desipramine, and alprazolam (Solomon et al. 1992). J. B. Frank and colleagues (1988) found either phenelzine or imipramine superior to placebo, with phenelzine performing slightly better than imipramine. The most responsive symptoms in this study were the intrusive ones, with little effect on avoidance symptoms (J. B. Frank et al. 1988). Amitriptyline is effective in decreasing depression and anxiety symptoms but may have less impact on avoidance (Davidson et al. 1990). Like the benzodiazepines, amitriptyline has the additional benefit of helping patients initiate and maintain sleep. Similarly, desipramine is helpful in depression but less so with other symptoms of PTSD (Davidson 1992).

The SSRIs also appear promising for PTSD treatment and may work by normalizing serotonergic neurotransmission (Davidson 1992). In preliminary open trials, these medications have relieved PTSD avoidant symptoms (Davidson 1992). Medication doses should start low, at about 10 mg of fluoxetine or 25 mg of sertraline. Patients should be monitored for exacerbation of sleep disturbance as dosages increase. Trazodone, cyproheptadine, or amitriptyline (at a low dose) may be added to manage sleep disturbances.

Other Agents

Azapirones

A new class of agents, which act as agonists at the 5-hydroxytryptamine$_{1A}$ receptor, has been successfully used in the treatment of GAD. Published studies indicate that the prototypic drug in this category, buspirone, is as effective as diazepam in treatment of GAD (Rickels et al. 1982a); the related compounds ipsapirone and gepirone are under development. Several properties of these anxiolytics set them apart from benzodiazepines. They do not bind at a site associated with the GABA receptor complex, are not sedating, and do not cause psychomotor or cognitive impairment. Onset of therapeutic action occurs after several weeks of treatment, and there may be activation and a mild increase in anxiety when treatment is begun.

The dosage range for buspirone is 5–60 mg/day, and the average dose is 20 mg/day (Sussman 1994). Because of its relatively short half-life, the drug should be given three times per day. The most common side effects include dizziness, nausea, headache, and nervousness (Sussman 1994). Buspirone cannot be used to taper patients from benzodiazepines, and some evidence suggests that patients who were previously treated with benzodiazepines might be less responsive to azapirones (Sussman 1994).

Anticonvulsants and Mood Stabilizers

Case reports or small, uncontrolled case series advocate the use of a variety of other medications in treating anxiety symptoms, particularly the symptoms of PTSD. Lithium carbonate, carbamazepine, valproate, propranolol, and clonidine are among these allegedly useful medications (Bleich et al. 1986; Fesler 1991; Kinzie and Leung 1989; Kolb et al. 1984; Lipper et al. 1986). Each has been suggested to reduce intrusive symptoms and/or hyperarousal in PTSD (Davidson 1992). Carbamazepine may help with mood stabilization and behavioral disturbances (Cowdry and Gardner 1988; Keck et al. 1992). Carbamazepine should be started at 200 mg qhs [every night at bedtime] and, if needed, increased by 200 mg every few days. Generally, between 800 mg/day and 1,000 mg/day will be required. Therapeutic blood levels should be monitored to guard against toxicity. Valproate is started at 250 mg and should be increased to between 750 and 2,000 mg/day. Therapeutic drug monitoring should also be conducted. Therapeutic effects of either drug are not necessarily correlated with anticonvulsant levels.

Carbamazepine may cause sedation, dizziness, nausea, and vomiting. While a slight decrease in white blood count frequently occurs, a rare adverse reaction is agranulocytosis. Patients should have their complete blood count (CBC) monitored before commencing treatment and at regular intervals after that. They should be informed of the need to seek immediate physician assessment should they develop fever, sore throat, mouth ulcers, easy bruising, or petechiae.

Sodium valproate is available as either Depakene (liquid) or Depakote (capsules). The most worrisome adverse reaction is hepatic failure, which is rare and usually occurs within the first 6 months of treatment.

The most common side effects of this drug are nausea, vomiting, photosensitivity, and rash. Minor elevations of transaminase may also occur.

Women being treated with carbamazepine should be warned that the drug may change the metabolism and, consequently, the prophylactic efficacy of OCs. Carbamazepine does this by increasing cytochrome P450 isozyme activity. It may also increase metabolism of other drugs, such as antipsychotics or antidepressants (Post 1988). Valproate has little effect on cytochrome P450.

Although it is impossible to say definitively that carbamazepine is safe during pregnancy, it may be safer than other mood-stabilizing agents (Elia et al. 1987). Valproate can cause neural-tube defects and should be avoided during pregnancy (Elia et al. 1987).

Neuroleptics have shown some efficacy against flashbacks and other intrusive symptoms of PTSD; however, given the potential side effect of tardive dyskinesia, these agents are not generally recommended for PTSD patients in the absence of psychotic symptoms (Davidson 1992).

Beta-Blockers

The primary role of beta-blockers, such as propranolol and atenolol, in anxiety disorders is in the treatment of social phobia. For social phobia, choice of pharmacological intervention depends on whether one is treating "limited social phobia," including "performance anxiety," or generalized social phobia. Beta-blockers are effective for limited social phobia (Hartley et al. 1983). Propranolol differs in its rate of metabolism (oxidation and gluco-oxidation) in men and women, although large intraindividual differences in plasma levels may exceed average sex differences. Propranolol is prescribed in a dose of about 20 or 40 mg several hours before a performance, and atenolol is prescribed at either 50 or 100 mg. Both agents control peripheral symptoms of anxiety, such as tremulousness, blushing, and dry mouth. Beta-blockers may not be effective for long-term treatment of generalized social phobia (Liebowitz et al. 1992).

Summary

The frequent occurrence of anxiety disorders in women argues for the need to explore and understand certain principles of pharmacotherapy that uniquely affect women. These include dosing considerations, drug interactions (particularly with exogenous hormones), menstrual cycle effects, and modifications required during pregnancy. Future pharmacological research should take gender-related variables into consideration so that clinicians may be further guided in their care for female patients.

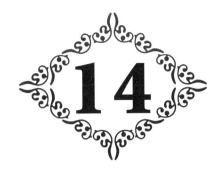

Sex Differences in Schizophrenia

Sally Szymanski, D.O.

Sex differences in first-episode and chronic schizophrenia have been reported in treatment response and relapse rates as well as in age of onset, symptom expression, course, outcome, and family history. In addition, sex effects have been observed in biological studies of schizophrenia such as neuroimaging research. Women with schizophrenia have generally had a better course of illness and treatment response than men. However, most of the studies have been performed in chronic rather than new-onset samples and much of the research is retrospective rather than prospective. Consequently, only limited information exists concerning factors underlying the sex effects in treatment response, relapse rates, and medication side effects. In this chapter I review clinical studies of sex differences in schizophrenia as a whole, with an emphasis on psychopharmacological research.

Natural History

Premorbid Adjustment

Women with schizophrenia have been observed to have better premorbid social functioning than schizophrenic men (Eaton 1975; Farina et al. 1963; Forrest and Hay 1972; Salokangas 1983; Schooler 1963; Westermeyer and Harrow 1986; Zigler and Levine 1981). Watt and Szulecka (1979) and Haas and Sweeney (1992) have reported that a steady decline in premorbid functioning was seen more often in males than in females. Childers and Harding (1990) attempted to correlate sex differences in premorbid adjustment with outcome by using findings from the Vermont Longitudinal Research Project. Female schizophrenic patients demonstrated superior premorbid adjustment and better outcome than did males in that study. However, the finding of better outcome in female versus male patients was not statistically significant.

Onset of Illness

A relatively consistent finding in the literature on schizophrenia has been an earlier age at onset or at first hospitalization in men (18–25 years) than in women (25–35 years). The more recent studies include those of Angermeyer et al. (1990), Bromet et al. (1992), Childers and Harding (1990), J. M. Goldstein (1988), Gureje (1991), Häfner et al. (1989, 1993), McCabe (1975), Salokangas (1983), Seeman (1982, 1986), Shtasel et al. (1992), and Szymanski et al. (1995). Angermeyer and Kuhn (1988) conducted a literature review of sex effects in age at first admission and found that, on the average, male schizophrenic patients were admitted at younger ages than female patients. The maximum difference between the sexes in first-admission age was 11.2 years, with the most frequent disparity being 4–5 years. In that review, men had an earlier onset of illness in a majority of the 37 studies. However, the definition of illness onset was unclear in some instances and varied between the studies.

More male than female patients are often found in new-onset studies of schizophrenia. A recent report by Iacono and Beiser (1992) suggests that the incidence of schizophrenia may be twice as great in men than in women. Using DSM-III (American Psychiatric Association 1980) diagnoses, these researchers found 1-year incidence rates of 15.76 for male subjects and 7.26 for female subjects per 100,000 population. Ring et al. (1991), in a brief review of male-to-female ratios in first-episode studies of schizophrenic patients in which sex differences in incidence rates were published, found a slightly greater percentage (1.5%) overall of males developing schizophrenia.

Lewine et al. (1984) examined the effects of criteria of six different diagnostic systems on the male-to-female ratio of schizophrenia in 387 subjects. Use of the Research Diagnostic Criteria, Taylor and Abrams' system, first-rank Schneiderian symptoms, and the flexible criteria used in the International Pilot Study of Schizophrenia produced a greater ratio of males to females diagnosed with schizophrenia. The New Haven Schizophrenia Index yielded comparable numbers of men and women. In comparison, the Feighner criteria did not diagnose any women as schizophrenic. *Consequently, the diagnostic system employed greatly affected the male-to-female ratio of schizophrenic patients.* This observation may be particularly important to note when examining studies that report sex effects.

Duration of Illness

Several investigators have studied the relationship between treatment outcome and length of untreated illness before first hospitalization. A greater duration of untreated illness before neuroleptic treatment was associated with increased relapse rates, less medication responsivity, and poorer scholastic and occupational achievement (Angrist and Schulz 1990; Crow et al. 1986; Lo and Lo 1977; May et al. 1981). Loebel et al. (1992) examined sex effects in illness duration in 70 first-episode schizophrenic and schizoaffective disorder subjects. The duration of illness from the onset of psychotic symptoms was a significant predictor of the time to treatment response, with a longer pretreatment duration associated with greater time to symptom remission. An extended duration of untreated illness was also correlated with a poorer outcome in the entire sample. Men had an earlier age at onset of psychotic symptoms—22.4 years versus 24.3 years in women. A longer duration of illness was seen in the male schizophrenic subjects (77 weeks) as compared with the female subjects (33 weeks). In another report based on that same sample (Szymanski et al. 1995), male subjects were noted to have had both a longer duration of untreated illness and a poorer outcome than female subjects.

Course and Outcome

Female schizophrenic patients have a superior course of illness and outcome compared with male schizophrenic patients. Women have fewer hospitalizations with shorter stays, and lower relapse rates. Angermeyer et al. (1990) recently reviewed outcome studies in schizophrenia that examined measures such as hospitalization variables (length of stay, number of admissions, rate of rehospitalization), relapse rate, psychiatric status at follow-up, clinical course, social adaptation, occupational status, and social integration over an average observation period of 8 years. These researchers noted that approximately 50% of the studies reported a better course of illness in women than in men, with the rest reporting no gender effect. Only six studies observed a more favorable course in men in any measure (i.e., rate of rehospitalization, clinical course, and occupational status). Furthermore, in a study of 603 schizophrenic patients, Angermeyer and colleagues (1990) found a superior outcome in the female patients, but noted no gender differences in the number of rehospitalizations. However, the lack of a gender effect in the rehospitalization data in that study suggested that a dilution of the sex differences may occur over time. Finally, on a related note, Haas et al. (1990) has documented an improved clinical outcome in symptomatology and functioning in female schizophrenic patients who received an inpatient psychoeducational family intervention, with worsening of these measures seen in male schizophrenic patients.

Symptom Expression

Symptoms in schizophrenia have been divided into two groups: positive (e.g., hallucinations, delusions) and negative (e.g., alogia, blunted affect, anhedonia). A few studies have shown that men and women with chronic schizophrenia may show different symptomatology. Female patients with chronic schizophrenia have demonstrated more dysphoria, irritability, anger, and paranoia. In contrast, male patients have exhibited more negative symptoms (J. M. Goldstein 1988; Lewine 1988). J. M. Goldstein et al. (1990) found that women with chronic schizophrenia were more likely to have dysphoria, paranoia, and a higher familial risk for schizophrenia, whereas men with schizophrenia had deficit symptoms, a poor premorbid history, a low familial risk for the disease, and a winter birth. Dworkin (1990) examined the case histories of 220 schizophrenic twins and rated them for negative symptoms and social competence. Men had greater asociality-withdrawal and poorer premorbid social competence than did women. However, no sex differences in positive symptom expression were noted.

Conflicting reports of sex differences in symptom expression in first-episode schizophrenia appear in the few published articles in this area. Häfner et al. (1993) and Haas and Sweeney (1992) recently examined gender effects in symptoms observed at first hospital admission and did not find any significant results. In contrast, Szymanski et al. (1995) reported symptom differences that reached statistical significance, with greater levels of anxiety, bizarre behavior, and inappropriate affect and less illogical thinking seen in female than in male schizophrenic patients at first admission. Finally, Ring et al. (1991) noted that women with new-onset schizophrenia had significantly lower levels of negative symptoms than did schizophrenic men with comparable positive-symptom scores.

Family History

A small number of studies have examined the sex effect of the proband on the family morbidity risk for DSM-III schizophrenia or schizophrenic spectrum illness with disparate results. Loyd et al. (1985) reported no sex effect, and Bellodi et al. (1986) noted an increased risk in the first-degree relatives of female probands. More recently, J. M. Goldstein et al. (1990) documented a higher risk among relatives of female schizophrenic patients that was significant for schizophrenia, schizophreniform, and schizoaffective disorders but not for the full spectrum of illness. In contrast, Maier et al. (1993) noted a greater rate of both schizophrenia and the spectrum disorders in relatives of female probands.

Examining the impact of gender and age at onset on the familial aggregation of schizophrenia, Pulver et al. (1990) found a relationship between the age at onset of psychosis in the male probands and the risk for schizophrenia in their relatives. The relatives of male schizophrenic probands whose onset of illness occurred when they were younger than 17 years of age was increased compared with family members of older probands. However, Maier et al. (1993) was not able to replicate that finding in a large, recently published family study.

Pharmacology

Treatment Response

Sex effects in pharmacokinetic variables such as drug absorption, bio-availability, distribution, and hepatic metabolism have been reported (Hamilton 1991; Seeman 1983; K. Wilson 1984; Yonkers et al. 1992a) that may partially underlie the differences found in medication levels. Female subjects have been reported to have higher neuroleptic levels (Ereshefsky et al. 1991; Meltzer et al. 1983; G. M. Simpson et al. 1990). In neuroleptic-refractory schizophrenic patients, sex effects have been observed in clozapine-treated patients, with women having significantly higher plasma drug concentrations (Haring et al. 1989; Szymanski et al. 1995). An improved treatment response has also been reported in female first-episode and chronic schizophrenic patients. Better response rates of typical antipsychotics are documented in female schizophrenic patients with less time and smaller dosages needed to achieve remission. Lower maintenance dosages of neuroleptics have also been seen (See-man 1982). In addition, schizophrenic women have also been found to have greater prolactin and homovanillic acid levels while on neuroleptics (Bowers et al. 1984; Halbreich et al. 1984; Meltzer et al. 1983; Szymanski et al. 1995).

Hamilton and Yonkers (Chapter 2, this volume) and Yonkers and Hamilton (Chapter 3, this volume) have noted that when sex differences in psychiatric psychopharmacological research are reported, slower clearance and greater bioavailability of medications are found in women. Consequently, unless these considerations are taken into account, drug dosages based on medication research performed in male patients could be too high for females. Hamilton and Jensvold (1991) have speculated that an increased rate of medication side effects and a greater risk of toxicity could then occur in female patients.

Medication Side Effects

Sex differences in antipsychotic medication side effects have been reported in tardive dyskinesia, extrapyramidal side effects, agranulocytosis, and neuroleptic malignant syndrome. Women (schizophrenic and nonschizophrenic) have been noted to have a greater prevalence of tardive dyskinesia with age, with a significant gender effect seen after age 70 (J. M. Smith et al. 1978). Furthermore, more severe forms of tardive dyskinesia were seen in the older women than in the older men in that study. A hypothesis proposed by Hamilton (1986) to explain the greater postmenopausal prevalence of tardive dyskinesia in schizophrenic women is that an "unmasking" of the movements occurs with diminishing levels of estrogen due to advancing age.

Reports vary concerning the incidence of extrapyramidal side effects in schizophrenic men and women. Keepers and Casey (1987) found in a retrospective chart review that young men with chronic schizophrenia develop more dystonia than do women (67% versus 32%). However, Chakos et al. (1992) reported the reverse to be true in prospectively treated first-episode women, with a 50% versus a 25% rate recorded in women and men, respectively. Akathisia and parkinsonism has been seen to occur almost twice as often in schizophrenic and nonschizophrenic women than in men (i.e., 47% versus 27% in a chart review study [Ayd 1961]). In contrast, Chakos et al. (1992) did not find a gender effect in a new-onset schizophrenic sample. Consequently, one might speculate that the stage of illness is an important consideration when examining sex effects in a schizophrenic sample.

Other medication-induced side effects also have a greater gender-specific incidence. Women over 50 years of age (schizophrenic and nonschizophrenic) manifest more neuroleptic-induced agranulocytosis than men over 50 years of age (Piscotta 1978). Likewise, women develop more clozapine-induced agranulocytosis than men, with elderly female schizophrenic patients especially at risk (Lieberman and Alvir 1992). Finally, a higher incidence of neuroleptic malignant syndrome of approximately two to one has been documented in young psychotic men as compared with women (Caroff 1980).

Neuroimaging Studies as a Biological Correlate of Sex Effects in Schizophrenia

Neuroimaging studies of schizophrenic patients have reported sex differences in ventricular size, corpus callosal size and shape, and cortical volume. These sex differences generally indicate that female patients have less neuropathology. One possible cause of the better treatment response found in female schizophrenic patients as compared with males may be the presence of less underlying brain pathology. The following represents a selective review of the research in this area.

Andreasen et al. (1982, 1990) and Flaum et al. (1990) have reported differential ventricular enlargement in schizophrenic men as compared with women in both computerized tomographic (CT) and magnetic resonance imaging (MRI) studies. Flaum et al. (1990) reviewed CT findings from four studies completed at the University of Iowa in more than 200 patients and 200 control subjects. The ventricular-brain ratio was larger in male schizophrenic patients compared with male control subjects in three of the four studies, with no differences found among the female subjects. However, a gender-by-diagnosis interaction in the data analysis was not demonstrated. Takahashi et al. (1981) have also reported a similar finding (i.e., greater left lateral ventricular abnormalities in males than in females in a CT study). Zigun et al. (1992), in a letter to the editor, criticized the control data used in the Andreasen et al. (1990) article, noting that the female control subjects had larger mean ventricular-brain ratios than the male control subjects, which is an unusual finding in the literature.

In an MRI study, Nasrallah et al. (1990) reported results indicating that schizophrenic women had smaller craniums and brains and larger lateral and third ventricles than schizophrenic men. However, they noted that the sample composition of the schizophrenic patients might have been responsible for these findings: The women in that study had an earlier onset of illness than the men, which might indicate a relatively greater severity of illness and thus explain the larger amount of structural brain abnormalities found in these female patients.

Haas et al. (1989) have reported a larger ventricular-brain ratio lateralization effect (i.e., left greater than right) in schizophrenic men but not in women. Olson et al. (1989) have observed that a family history of schizophrenia appeared to be associated with a greater ventricular size on MRI scans in men more often than in women.

Nasrallah et al. (1986) and Lewine et al. (1990) have reported data demonstrating sex differences in corpus callosal shape and size in schizophrenic patients in MRI studies. Nasrallah et al. (1986) found an increased thickness in the middle and anterior sections of the corpus callosum. Lewine et al. (1990) in a preliminary report found that schizophrenic men had a smaller corpus callosal size than control subjects but did not demonstrate a statistically significant gender effect in this measure. In contrast, Swayze et al. (1990) and Hauser et al. (1989) did not demonstrate sex differences in MRI studies in corpus callosal size or shape in their samples.

Finally, R. E. Gur et al. (1985) have reported significant sex differences in lateralization of regional blood flow in schizophrenic patients as revealed on positron-emission tomographic (PET) imaging, with males having a relatively greater lateralized left-hemispheric flow. On a related note, Kopala and colleagues (Kopala and Clark 1990; Kopala et al. 1989) studied olfactory agnosia in schizophrenic patients and found that primarily men as opposed to women demonstrated this problem. To explain their results, they have speculated that this deficit may have arisen from differences in sex hormonal effects in males and females (i.e., testosterone vs. estrogen) on the development of the orbitalfrontal cortex in the brain.

Discussion

Sex differences in schizophrenia in treatment response as well as clinical course are clearly evident, with female patients demonstrating a superior medication outcome and course of illness. Factors that could account for these results include the presence of estrogen, which may exert a "neuroleptic-like" effect (Seeman and Lang 1990); less cerebral lateralization in women, thereby conferring relatively more brain "reserve"; the lower level of structural brain abnormalities in women noted on CT and MRI studies; and the greater prenatal brain maturation in women, with a subsequent lower risk of vulnerability to the neurological sequelae of birth trauma (Seeman and Lang 1990). Finally, if the putative "gene" for schizophrenia is sex chromosome–linked, that could provide yet another explanation for the aforementioned sex differences. See Sherwin (Chapter 11, this volume) for a discussion of the effects of estrogen on neurofunctioning.

Proposed developmental models of schizophrenia that might partially explain the sex effects found in treatment response, course, and outcome include the *neurodevelopmental anomaly model* of Murray (1991). This model suggests that male schizophrenic patients may be more prone to brain damage prenatally and at birth, with a subsequent poorer course of illness and medication response than females as a consequence. Other models suggest that the brain may act as a "pathoplastic" agent (Birnbaum 1923/1974; Lewine et al. 1990) in which genetic disposition and brain morphology interact to create the schizophrenic syndrome, which could manifest differently in males and females. Or, a *stress diathesis model* may apply (Gottesman and Shields 1982; Lewine et al. 1990) in which stress acts on brain pathology to trigger the onset of the illness. A particular genetic predisposition then causes a certain type of behavior and course of illness to emerge that could also differ between the sexes.

Finally, gonadal steroids may affect neuroreceptors and thereby influence the physiological mechanism of drug action in the brain (Hamilton 1986; Hamilton and Conrad 1987; Majewska, Chapter 4, this volume; Sherwin, Chapter 11, this volume). Estrogen has been reported to increase dopamine D2 receptor density (J. H. Gordon 1980) and to enhance the neuroleptic effects of cataplexy in rat studies (J. H. Gordon 1980; Nausieda et al. 1979). Häfner et al. (1991) have also found that estradiol caused a significant reduction of dopamine agonist and antagonist activity in adult and neonatal rats, an effect that could be due to a downregulation of dopamine receptor sensitivity. The animal behavior seen in the rat studies may occur through the pituitary—possibly via prolactin, since hypophysectomy eliminates this effect (Hruska et al. 1980).

Areas of future research in schizophrenia should include further neuroimaging work, especially positron and single photon emission tomographic studies in addition to that of structural brain-imaging research (i.e., MRI) to better understand the basic sex differences in brain metabolism and neuromorphology in this illness; the possible effects of menopause, oral contraceptives, pregnancy, and the menstrual cycle on symptomology and the clinical response to typical and atypical antipsychotic and supplemental medications (i.e., anticholinergics); the use of a spectrum model of illness in which sex differences in medication responsivity and in course of schizophrenia-related disorders are investigated and the impact of aging on these sex dissimilarities in treatment responsivity and illness course assessed.

In this chapter I have reviewed sex effects on the course of schizophrenia with an emphasis on differences in treatment responsivity. The bulk of the research in this area has examined differences in onset and course of illness rather than sex effects in medication responsivity. Large, well-designed studies are needed, especially in the area of psychopharmacology. One cannot designate a particular medication "prescription" for female schizophrenic patients based on current knowledge in this area. For example, whether one particular antipsychotic medication is better than another for female patients or whether drug dosages should be adjusted on the basis of the menstrual cycle is presently unknown. It is hoped that future research will be directed toward gaining a better understanding of sex effects in the psychopharmacological treatment of schizophrenia.

Women and Substance Use Disorders

Shelly F. Greenfield, M.D., M.P.H.

It is only recently that substance use disorders in women have received any systematic attention, and even now information on the natural history, clinical presentation, physiology, and treatment of these disorders in women is quite limited. Longitudinal studies of alcohol dependence typically have used all-male samples (G. Edwards et al. 1988; Fillmore and Midanik 1984; Litt et al. 1992; Polich et al. 1981; Schuckit et al. 1993; Vaillant 1983). The reasons for past exclusion of women from such research studies include beliefs that have not been substantiated in subsequent studies, such as 1) that women are socioculturally protected from alcohol and drug problems (Jellinek 1941; Mello 1980); 2) that studying women is more logistically complicated than studying men (Hyman 1976); 3) that

This work was supported by Grants DA 07252 and DA 09400 from the National Institute on Drug Abuse and Grant AA 09881 from the National Institute on Alcohol Abuse and Alcoholism; and by the Dr. Ralph and Marian C. Falk Research Trust.

substance use disorders are the same in women and men (Lex 1991); and 4) that women with alcohol or drug problems are more socially deviant or psychologically disturbed (Ettore 1992; Lex 1991).

In addition, case finding and recruitment for clinical research may be gender biased. For example, women with drinking problems are underrepresented in alcohol-specific treatment settings but are more frequently seen in general primary care or mental health treatment facilities (Duckert 1987; Halliday et al. 1986; Weisner 1993). In one study, women seen at non–alcohol-specific treatment sites were at greater risk for problem drinking than were men seen at those same sites (Weisner 1993).

Explanations for women's underuse of alcohol and drug treatment services may include women's perception of greater social stigma associated with women's abuse of drugs and alcohol (Blume 1986; Gomberg 1988; Lex 1991; Mello 1980) as well as the fear of being formally labeled as an alcoholic or as needing treatment from an alcoholism clinic (Thom 1986).

Psychoactive substance use disorders include both abuse of, and dependence on, alcohol or drugs such as cocaine, amphetamines, opioids, marijuana, or phencyclidine (American Psychiatric Association 1994). These disorders also include abuse of, or dependence on, prescription medications such as sedatives, hypnotics, or anxiolytics. In this chapter I review what is currently known about gender differences in the epidemiology, course of illness, medical consequences, psychiatric comorbidity, and treatment outcomes for abuse of or dependence on alcohol, cocaine, and opioids. A review of gender differences in abuse of prescription medications is beyond the scope of this chapter, and readers are referred to several current reviews (Chambers and White 1980; Hohmann 1989; Williams et al. 1982), as well as earlier reviews of this topic (Cuskey et al. 1977; Fidell 1982; J. Fraser 1981; Leland 1982).

Alcohol

Epidemiology

The lifetime prevalence of alcohol use disorders in the United States is 13.8%, with a lifetime prevalence of 23.8% and 4.6% in males and females, respectively (Helzer et al. 1991). The male-to-female ratio of lifetime prevalence of alcohol use disorders in the United States, therefore, is approximately 5:1. Even though the reported prevalence of alcohol abuse and dependence is lower for women than for men, alcoholic women appear to be at greater risk of death than alcoholic men when each gender group is compared with a same-gender, nonalcoholic population (Gomberg 1989; Kilbey and Sobeck 1988). In addition, women appear to advance more rapidly from initial onset of problem drinking to development of adverse medical consequences than do men (Crawford and Ryder 1986; Orford and Keddie 1985; Piazza et al. 1989; R. B. Smith et al. 1983).

In one prospective study of 100 alcohol-dependent women admitted to psychiatric hospitals, 31% of the sample were dead at 11 years follow-up, which was four times as many deaths as expected in the general population. Most of these women died of alcohol-related causes, and their life spans were shortened by an average of 15 years (R. B. Smith et al. 1983). These mortality rates are similar to those reported in a 20-year follow-up study of 4,872 male and female hospitalized alcoholics in Stockholm, which found that when compared with the general population, women alcoholics had a fivefold greater risk of death, while alcoholic men had three times the risk of death (Lindberg and Agren 1988). There is evidence that alcohol dependence has increased in more recently born members of the population, with the greatest increases in women (Penniman and Agnew 1989; T. Reich et al. 1988). One recent study by Popkin et al. (1988) indicated that negative consequences of alcohol use, such as accidents and arrests from drunk driving, may be disproportionately greater for women than for men.

Family History and Course of Illness

Although most studies of family histories of alcoholism have focused on men, it is likely that alcohol dependence in women may be more strongly associated with a family history than in men (Lex 1992). In the 1970s, Danish adoption studies demonstrated that men with alcoholic fathers were four times as likely to develop alcohol dependence as men with no family history of alcoholism (Goodwin et al. 1973), but these studies did not find evidence for higher risk of alcoholism in women with similar family histories (Goodwin et al. 1977). The negative findings for women were attributed to the low prevalence of alcohol dependence in Danish women and small sample sizes. A more recent population-based study of 1,030 female twin pairs found strong evidence for genetic factors in the etiology of alcoholism in women and demonstrated that the heritability of vulnerability to alcoholism in women ranged from 50% to 60% (Kendler et al. 1992).

For both men and women alcoholics, a family history of alcohol dependence is associated with greater prevalence of psychopathology and more severe symptoms of alcohol dependence (V. M. Hesselbrock et al. 1982), including more loss of control over drinking behavior, more physical symptoms, and more psychosocial problems. In one study of 639 male and female alcoholics in treatment, those with alcoholic parents were characterized by more severe alcohol dependence and greater psychopathology, with the greatest levels of psychopathology found in women with alcoholic parents (Svanum and McAdoo 1991).

A number of studies have found gender differences in the course of illness (Beckman and Amaro 1986; Crawford and Ryder 1986; V. M. Hesselbrock et al. 1982; Lex 1991; Orford and Keddie 1985; Parella and Filstead 1988; Wanberg and Horn 1970). Women generally begin drinking and develop alcohol problems at a later age than men (Beckman and Amaro 1986; Crawford and Ryder 1986; V. M. Hesselbrock et al. 1982; Lex 1991; Orford and Keddie 1985; Parella and Filstead 1988). For example, in a study of 1,940 alcoholic men and women, women were significantly older when regular drunkenness began, when they realized that alcohol gave relief from withdrawal symptoms, when their alcohol problem was identified by a significant other, and when they first tried to stop drinking (Parella and Filstead 1988). For each age of first occurrence of drinking problems, women were significantly older, with men meeting any of five different criteria, on average, between the ages of 28 and 34, and women meeting these same criteria between the ages of 34 and 42 (Parella and Filstead 1988). Compared with alcoholic men, women are also thought to drink smaller quantities (Beckman and Amaro 1986); to drink alone more often (Lex 1992); and to have more regular drinking patterns, with less-frequent binge drinking (Parella and Filstead 1988). In spite of the fact that women in general consume less alcohol than men, they are also more likely to progress more rapidly from onset of drinking to the late stages of alcohol dependence with its associated severe medical sequelae—the so-called telescoping course of illness (Piazza et al. 1989).

There may also exist gender differences in the psychosocial correlates of alcohol dependence. In one study of 50 alcoholic women, employment status, number of children, and parental alcohol use had the strongest relationship with length of time from first intoxication to loss of control of drinking (Fortin and Evans 1983). A separate study found that employment within or outside the home did not predict outcome for alcoholic women, but that women working within the home drank more at baseline (Herr and Pettinati 1984).

A number of investigators have studied the relationship of menstrual cycle phase to alcohol intake in women (M. L. Griffin et al. 1987; Lex et al. 1989; Mello et al. 1990). In one prospective inpatient study of 14 women, increased drinking during the premenstruum was associated with higher scores on the Premenstrual Assessment Form (Mello et al. 1990). A study of alcohol intake across the menstrual cycle among marijuana users found that in the absence of severe premenstrual distress, menstrual cycle phase is not a good predictor of alcohol use among female social drinkers (M. L. Griffin et al. 1987).

A number of studies have found that childhood histories of experienced or witnessed domestic violence are correlated with alcohol use disorders in adulthood and poorer treatment outcomes in women (Haver 1987; Hurley 1991; B. A. Miller et al. 1987; Root 1989). Of 117 alcoholic women subjects sampled from Alcoholics Anonymous, 27.8% reported a history of childhood incest, as compared with estimated rates between 5% and 15% in the general population (Burnam et al. 1988; Winfield et al. 1990). These women were more likely than those without such a history to have experienced drinking problems at an earlier age and to have higher levels of anxiety (Kovach 1986). It may be that women with these histories represent a large subgroup with worse outcomes (Root 1989).

Medical Consequences

There is evidence that alcohol is metabolized differently by men and women (Frezza et al. 1990). Alcohol is water soluble and is metabolized primarily by alcohol dehydrogenase in the liver and gastric mucosa. After drinking comparable amounts of alcohol, women have been noted to have higher blood alcohol concentrations than men, even after allowing for differences in size and body weight (B. M. Jones and M. K. Jones 1976), although evidence has been reported that contradicts this finding (D. B. Goldstein 1992). Explanations for women's higher blood alcohol levels include a smaller total volume of distribution in women (A. W. Marshall et al. 1983); decreased alcohol metabolism by the gastric mucosa in women (so-called first-pass metabolism; Frezza et al. 1990); and influence of hormones such as estrogen. These may be some of the same mechanisms that account for the increased vulnerability of women to alcoholic liver disease (M. Y. Morgan and Sherlock 1977). Although, compared with men, women begin drinking later, consume smaller quantities, and consume excessive quantities for shorter periods of time, they are nevertheless twice as likely to develop cirrhosis of the liver (Lex 1991). Similarly, although women alcoholics show a pattern of cognitive impairment similar to that seen in alcoholic men, the impairment occurs after a markedly shorter period of drinking smaller quantities of alcohol (Crawford and Ryder 1986).

Alcoholism is associated with severe disruption in reproductive function in men, such as impotence, low testosterone levels, testicular atrophy, gynecomastia, and diminished sexual interest (Lex 1991). Similarly, alcoholism in women is associated with amenorrhea, anovulation, and luteal phase dysfunction and may also increase the risk of spontaneous abortion as well as induce early menopause (Lex 1991).

Finally, offspring of women who abuse alcohol during pregnancy may manifest one of a number of congenital abnormalities grouped under the term *fetal alcohol syndrome* (FAS). This syndrome occurs in 33% of infants born to women who drink more than 150 g of alcohol per day during pregnancy; another 33% of infants without clear FAS will be mentally retarded, and the perinatal mortality rate is 17% (Greenfield et al., in press).

Psychiatric Comorbidity

A number of studies have demonstrated gender differences in the co-occurrence of psychiatric disorders in alcohol-dependent patients. For example, women alcoholics are more frequently found to have concurrent mood (M. N. Hesselbrock et al. 1985; Rounsaville et al. 1987), anxiety, eating, and psychosexual disorders (Ross et al. 1988) than are men, whereas men more frequently have concurrent antisocial personality disorder (M. N. Hesselbrock et al. 1985; V. M. Hesselbrock et al. 1986; Rounsaville et al. 1987). However, there is inconsistent evidence about the course and prognostic significance of concurrent psychiatric diagnoses and symptoms for alcohol-dependent men and women. One study demonstrated that mood disorders predicted a poor prognosis in men and a better prognosis in women, while antisocial personality and drug abuse predicted poor outcomes in both (Rounsaville et al. 1987). However, two other studies that prospectively examined the course of depressive symptoms in women and men found that these symptoms were correlated with poorer prognoses in *both* men and women (Finney et al. 1980; Pettinati et al. 1982). Finally, although Schuckit et al. (1990) demonstrated the course and importance of anxiety symptoms in alcohol-dependent patients, their study used an all-male sample and could not assess the importance of these symptoms in women.

Treatment Outcome

Outcome studies of alcohol-dependence treatment programs are limited (Finney and Moos 1986), frequently because of methodological problems such as lack of randomization and control groups, lack of prospective design, and lack of adequate outcome measures and follow-up (M. S. Goldstein et al. 1984). Many of these studies have used all-male samples (Kilbey and Sobeck 1988), and information on gender differences in treatment outcome is therefore even more limited.

Variables that may be significant predictors of recovery in men are 1) engagement in a continuing care program, 2) ongoing counseling, 3) use of self-help groups, 4) crisis intervention, and 5) use of family treatment (Mumme 1991). Vaillant (1983) described an additional four factors that may be important in men's recovery from alcohol dependence: 1) a positive substitute dependence (such as involvement in religion, exercise, or a hobby, for example); 2) external reminders that alcohol is aversive; 3) increased unambiguous social support; and 4) a source of inspiration, hope, or enhanced self-esteem. It is not clear whether these same factors enhance recovery in women.

Women use alcohol treatment services less frequently than men (Duckert 1987) but are more likely to seek treatment for marital problems, physical illness, and emotional problems (Duckert 1987). This underutilization of alcohol treatment by women may due to women's perception of society's harsher judgment of their alcohol dependence (Sandmeier 1980); perception of greater social costs of treatment (Beckman and Amaro 1986); deficient training of health care, social service, and law enforcement professionals in identification and referral of women alcoholics (Kilbey and Sobeck 1988); and lower utilization of services by women for disorders considered incongruous with sex-role stereotypes (Beckman and Amaro 1984). In one study by Thom (1986), women were more likely than men to feel that alcohol treatment was appropriate for those who drank for the sake of drinking. However, these same women described their own drinking as a legitimate response to their personal problems and therefore thought that they did not need specific alcohol treatment.

In one treatment outcome study of 112 men and women in a community treatment center staffed by volunteers, women were more likely than men to drop out of treatment after the first visit (35% vs. 21%); only men were still attending the clinic 6 months later (Allan 1987). One explanation provided by the investigators for this discrepancy is that self-referred patients dropped out of treatment more frequently than did patients referred by shelters, employers, or the courts. In this study's sample, more women than men were self-referred and more men than women were referred by "coercive sources" (i.e., employers, shelters, or the courts).

One important predictor of poor treatment outcome is a history of childhood or recent sexual or physical assault, and such experiences appear to be more prevalent in women than in men (Haver 1987; Hurley 1991; B. A. Miller et al. 1987; Root 1989; Thom 1986). According to Thom (1986), more women than men in her sample reported having been physically assaulted in the year before treatment. In a multiple regression analysis of predictors of outcome in 44 Norwegian women alcoholics, Haver (1987) found that 11% of the variance in outcome was explained by childhood violence; an additional 14% was explained by having a violent partner; and another 9% was explained by having a concurrent personality disorder. The likelihood of having a violent partner and having a concurrent personality disorder was increased in those with childhood histories of violence. Therefore, fully 34% of the variance in outcome in these 44 women alcoholics may have been explained by the direct and indirect effects of childhood violence. These results are supported by other studies (Hurley 1991; B. A. Miller et al. 1987; Root 1989).

Duckert (1987) found that treatment programs for women had improvement rates that ranged from 20% to 60%, but it is unclear whether treatment programs specifically for women have a greater success rate than traditional programs that treat men and women together. Some authors suggest that women might do better within same-sex treatment groups (Lex 1992) and that alcoholic women would benefit most from interactions with women staff members and other recovering women with whom they might identify as role models (Connor and Babcock 1980). According to Underhill (1994), because of the social stigma associated with women's alcohol problems, alcoholic women tend to have decreased self-esteem, thus making confrontational techniques in individual and group therapy settings less likely to be productive. These and other issues of treatment techniques and efficacy deserve additional consideration and evaluation.

In spite of these issues, several clear guidelines exist for the evaluation and treatment of alcohol-dependent women. Women who come to treatment for alcohol dependence are often in a poor state of health and require a complete review of their physical health status as well as assessment of their family, work, and social environment (Popour 1983). Kilbey and Sobeck (1988) recommend a complete physical evaluation including 1) physical exam, vital signs, and appropriate blood chemistries; 2) assessment of obstetric and gynecological status, including hormonal status, yearly Pap smear, breast exam and instruction in breast self-examination, and contraception; 3) review for human immunodeficiency virus (HIV) risk factors; 4) evaluation of psychiatric status, including other co-occurring diagnoses as well as suicidality; and 5) neuropsychiatric assessment. In addition, given the high prevalence of histories of childhood sexual abuse and later sexual assault in this population, it is important to assess the presence of these factors in each woman's history (Underhill 1994). Conversely, since more women with alcohol problems are seen in non–alcohol-treatment settings, it is important for physical and mental health caregivers who see women to take a careful alcohol history from all of their patients and to be prepared to refer these patients to appropriate treatment settings when needed.

Comorbid Alcohol and Drug Abuse

According to the population-based National Institutes of Mental Health Epidemiologic Catchment Area study, 47.3% of individuals with alcohol abuse or dependence in the community will in the course of their lifetimes have a diagnosis of another drug dependence (Regier et al. 1990). In the United States, alcohol dependence confers a sevenfold increased risk of other drug dependence. Of those individuals with alcohol dependence who are seen in an alcohol, drug, or mental health treatment setting, 34% will have met criteria for another drug disorder in the 6 months before treatment (Helzer et al. 1991).

With respect to gender, alcohol dependence increases the risk of drug abuse and dependence in women more than in men (Robins and Regier 1991). According to Weisner (1993), however, important questions remain regarding the role of gender in the prevalence and natural histories of combined alcohol and drug dependence. In her comprehensive study of 685 individuals in treatment in all alcohol and drug treatment programs in one northern California county, Weisner (1993) found important distinctions between the women being treated in alcohol programs and the women in drug treatment. Women in drug treatment reported more criminal behavior than women in alcohol treatment, and women in alcohol treatment reported heavier drinking and attributed their difficulties to their comorbid drug dependence more frequently than did women in drug treatment. The study also found that the differences between the women in the two treatment systems were greater than the differences between men and women within each system (Weisner 1993). These findings suggest that caution should be used in making assumptions about the homogeneity of women with substance abuse and that greater information is needed about the diversity of this population.

Cocaine

Epidemiology

Cocaine, or benzoylmethylecgonine, is an alkaloid derived from the coca plant, *Erythroxylon coca*. In the United States, the most common routes of administration are intranasal "snorting" of cocaine hydrochloride, intravenous administration of cocaine hydrochloride dissolved in water, and smoking of alkaloidal cocaine, known as "freebase" or "crack."

The 1990 National Household Survey on Drug Abuse found that 2.0% of women and 4.3% of men reported using cocaine at least once during the previous 12 months; 0.7% of women and 1.5% of men used it 12 or more times; and 0.2% of women and 0.4% of men used it once a week or more (National Institute on Drug Abuse 1991b). This represents a decrease of 0.3% in the number of men using cocaine once a week or more between 1988 and 1990, while the percentage of women using cocaine with this frequency remained constant during the 2-year period. This finding may be consistent with earlier reports of a disproportionate rise in women callers to the cocaine hotline between 1983 and 1985 (P. G. Erickson and Murray 1989); however, gender differences in current rates of initiation and cessation of cocaine use are not clear.

Family History and Course of Illness

Studies of two groups of cocaine-dependent individuals found that most subjects had a positive family history for alcohol dependence, with at least 50% of these subjects having a first- or second-degree relative who was alcohol dependent (Khalsa et al. 1992; N. S. Miller et al. 1989). In their study of 153 men with primary cocaine dependence, Khalsa et al. (1992) found that 29% had siblings with alcohol and drug dependence and 44% had at least one parent with alcohol dependence (Khalsa et al. 1992). N. S. Miller et al. (1989) reported the results of their retrospective study of 150 patients with cocaine dependence. Among 88 men and 26 women with cocaine dependence and no other concurrent substance dependence, 47% of the men and 65% of the women had a positive family history of alcohol dependence. Among the 68 men and

10 women patients with both cocaine and alcohol dependence, 46% of the men and 90% of the women had a family history of alcohol dependence. Among the 41 men and 5 women with cocaine, alcohol, and marijuana dependence, 46% of the men and 100% of the women had a family history of alcohol dependence. Similar gender differences of slightly smaller magnitude were found in these same authors' prospective study of 113 men and women cocaine-dependent patients (N. S. Miller et al. 1989). In this study, among 48 men and 8 women with cocaine dependence only, 48% of the men and 63% of the women had a family history of alcohol dependence. Forty-eight percent of 21 men and 50% of 6 women with cocaine and alcohol dependence had a family history of alcohol dependence. Finally, in those men and women with cocaine, alcohol, and marijuana dependence, 50% of 22 men and 50% of 2 women had a family history of alcohol dependence. These results suggest that family history may be an equally strong (if not stronger) factor in the natural history of cocaine dependence in women as it is in men.

Like many other illicit drugs, the initiation of cocaine use occurs primarily in young adults. In the United States, among the household population aged 12 years and older, 11.3% had used cocaine at least once, and lifetime prevalence of use was highest (25.6%) among those aged 26–34 years (National Institute on Drug Abuse 1991b). In 1990, 40% of the population reported trying cocaine by age 27, and 9% had done so by their senior year of high school (National Institute on Drug Abuse 1991a). Approximately 3.5% of high school seniors and 5.1% of young adults had tried crack.

As with all other illicit drugs, use of cocaine by males exceeds that by females in all age groups. In the 1990 National Household Survey on Drug Abuse (National Institute on Drug Abuse 1991b), 13.8% of all males had tried cocaine, compared with 9.0% of all females. In the 26- to 34-year-old age group, 2.4% of men and 1.1% of women reported using cocaine in the month before the interview. In addition, 2.0% of all men and 0.8% of all women reported the use of crack in their lifetime. In 1990, there was an approximately equal proportion of men who had used crack in the two age groups 18–25 years and 26–34 years (1.6% and 1.5%, respectively), while the proportion of women aged 18–25 years who used crack in 1990 was more than twice the proportion of women aged 26–34 years (1.1% and 0.5%, respectively). This may suggest that women who use crack initiate drug use at an earlier age than do men. Of concern in this group is the even greater vulnerability of women crack users to increased rates of syphilis, HIV infection, and other sexually transmitted diseases (Guinan 1989).

In their study of 153 cocaine-dependent men, Khalsa et al. (1992) found that the mean age of first use was 15 years, and in the year before first cocaine use, 33% of the group used marijuana and alcohol. Sixty-nine percent of the men said that their main reason for first cocaine use was curiosity. In this sample of cocaine-dependent men, the average period of time from first cocaine use until entry into treatment was 11 years.

The natural history of cocaine dependence in women is an even more recent area of investigation. In a series of studies, Weiss et al. (1986) and M. L. Griffin et al. (1989) found that when compared with men, women had earlier initial use, younger age at first treatment, more rapid development of dependence, more frequent involvement with an addicted partner, poorer social and occupational functioning, more premorbid depression, and slower recovery from depressive symptoms during the first month of abstinence. Women most commonly reported four reasons for initiating drug use: depression, feeling unsociable, family and job pressures, and health problems (M. L. Griffin et al. 1989). In their recent prospective follow-up study of 21 male and 18 female cocaine-dependent subjects, Weiss and colleagues (R. D. Weiss, M. L. Griffin, and C. Hufford, personal communication, April 1993) found that fewer women were employed (50% vs. 65%) than men. One difference from earlier findings was that the women had used cocaine for a longer period of time than the men (9.9 years vs. 7.75 years). A greater proportion of women than men used intranasal (61.1% vs. 47.6%) and intravenous cocaine (11.1% vs. 4.8%), while more men than women smoked (47.6% vs. 27.8%).

A recent study by T. Kosten et al. (1993) of 19 women and 53 men cocaine abusers supports some of these findings. Their finding that the women had used cocaine for more years than had the men was not statistically significant. Women had histories of more years of heroin use, whereas men used alcohol for more years and had longer periods of abstinence from cocaine. In this study group, the men had proportionally more intranasal cocaine use than did the women. Clearly, additional studies are needed to investigate gender differences in the natural history of cocaine dependence and to determine whether men and women differ with respect to age of initiation of use and time elapsed between first use and dependence, as well as the process of recovery.

Medical Consequences

Cocaine exerts direct stimulatory effects on the cerebral cortex and produces feelings of excitation, restlessness, euphoria, decreased social inhibitions, increased energy, and enhanced strength and mental ability. It also causes central and peripheral sympathomimetic effects such as vasoconstriction, tachycardia, increased blood pressure and temperature, and dilated pupils (Greenfield et al. 1994). The half-life of cocaine is approximately 1 hour; the drug is metabolized by plasma and liver cholinesterases to the metabolite benzoylecgonine, which is then excreted into the urine. There is currently no clear information regarding gender differences in the metabolism of cocaine. However, there is evidence that stimulants such as dextroamphetamine may produce dysphoria in postmenopausal women while inducing elevation of mood in young men (Halbreich et al. 1981). In addition, there may be differences in adrenergic responsiveness throughout different phases of the menstrual cycle (Ghose and Turner 1977). Animal research suggests that some sex differences in sensitivity to cocaine may be related to sex-dependent differences in brain asymmetry (S. D. Glick et al. 1983; Robinson et al. 1980).

There are many medical complications associated with cocaine use. Cocaine may adversely affect most organ systems, including the cardiovascular, gastrointestinal, pulmonary, and central nervous systems (E. Brown et al. 1992; Endress et al. 1992; Perper and Van Thiel 1992). There are no current studies that report sex differences in the effects of cocaine on these organ systems. However, there are sex-specific effects of cocaine on neuroendocrine function (J. H. Mendelson et al. 1988).

Men who chronically abuse cocaine have been reported to have impotence and gynecomastia as well as persistent abnormalities in reproductive function even after cessation of cocaine use (Cocores et al. 1986;

J. H. Mendelson et al. 1988). Cocaine-dependent women may manifest derangements in menstrual cycle function, galactorrhea, amenorrhea, and infertility (Cocores et al. 1986). One possible factor implicated in these abnormalities in reproductive function is derangement in plasma prolactin levels. Decreased plasma prolactin levels were found in men and women cocaine abusers in one study (Gawin and Kleber 1985), while three other studies found elevated plasma prolactin levels (Cocores et al. 1986; Dackis and Gold 1985; J. H. Mendelson et al. 1988). In one study of 14 men and 2 women patients with cocaine abuse, 86% of the men and both of the women had hyperprolactinemia at the time of admission (J. H. Mendelson et al. 1988). In each of these patients, plasma luteinizing hormone, cortisol, and testosterone levels (in the men) were all within normal limits. It is possible that dopaminergic derangements caused by cocaine may be responsible for the selectively elevated prolactin levels in these patients.

The evidence regarding adverse cocaine-related maternal and fetal effects is conflicting. Some studies have indicated that cocaine causes physiological derangements in uterine blood flow, and that this can have an adverse effect on the fetus (Woods et al. 1987). Other studies have reported intrauterine growth retardation and congenital malformations (Chasnoff et al. 1988). However, one meta-analysis showed no increased developmental risk to the fetus (Koren and Graham 1992) and another review found evidence that cocaine use was associated with very specific adverse effects on the fetus, such as low birth weight, prematurity, and congenital anomalies of the urinary tract (Slutsker 1992).

Psychiatric Comorbidity

A large number of clinical and epidemiological studies have shown a high level of comorbidity of substance use disorders and other psychiatric disorders. According to the Epidemiologic Catchment Area study, individuals in the community who use cocaine are almost five times more likely to abuse alcohol than persons without cocaine abuse, with 84.8% of cocaine abusers having the diagnosis of alcohol abuse sometime in their lifetime (Gorelick 1992). A recent study of 298 cocaine abusers seeking inpatient or outpatient treatment revealed that 55% had received at least one concurrent psychiatric diagnosis at some time in their life (Rounsaville et al. 1991). In this study, the most frequently reported disorders were major depression, bipolar disorder, anxiety disorders, antisocial personality disorder, and a history of childhood attention-deficit disorder. These findings are consistent with earlier studies (M. L. Griffin et al. 1989; Weiss et al. 1986). In a recent study of comorbid personality disorders in cocaine dependence, 74% of 50 cocaine-dependent inpatients received a diagnosis of at least one personality disorder; 69% of these diagnoses were present both during periods of cocaine use and during abstinence (Weiss et al. 1993).

Ross et al. (1988) found sex differences in rates of psychiatric comorbidity in their study of 501 substance-dependent patients. Although women did not show higher overall rates of psychiatric disorders than men and there were no significant sex differences in rates of cognitive impairment, schizophrenia, or affective disorders, women more frequently suffered from anxiety, psychosexual disorders, and bulimia, and men more frequently were diagnosed with antisocial personality disorder. There are few studies of sex differences in the rates of psychiatric comorbidity among cocaine-dependent individuals (M. L. Griffin et al. 1989; Pettinati et al. 1991; Rounsaville et al. 1991). Pettinati et al. (1991) found that cocaine-dependent women had significantly more diagnosable personality disorders than did alcohol-dependent women. In this group, paranoid, borderline, and histrionic personality disorders were more frequent in the cocaine-dependent women. In a study of 206 men and 92 women cocaine abusers seeking treatment, Rounsaville et al. (1991) found that men had significantly more alcohol dependence and childhood attention-deficit disorders, and women had more phobias. In their study of 124 cocaine-dependent men and women inpatients, M. L. Griffin et al. (1989) found that the only statistically significant differences between men and women was the higher incidence of major depression among the women (23.5% vs. 4.2%) and the higher incidence of antisocial personality disorder among the men (22.1% vs. 0%).

Treatment Outcome

One area of consensus in the treatment of cocaine dependence is that the goal of treatment should be abstinence from cocaine and other substances of abuse, including alcohol and marijuana. Those who return to drinking alcohol or smoking marijuana have an increased risk of relapse to cocaine (Rawson et al. 1986).

Although there is no single standard treatment for cocaine dependence, as in the treatment for most other substance dependence, there are a number of psychological and pharmacological modalities available. Many individuals benefit from self-help groups that follow a 12-step model such as Cocaine Anonymous or a cognitive-behavioral model such as Rational Recovery. There have been some positive treatment results with specific psychotherapies, such as contingency contracting (Higgins et al. 1991), relapse prevention (Carroll et al. 1991), and modified psychodynamically oriented group psychotherapy (R. J. Schneider and Khantzian 1992).

Although no pharmacological treatment has gained widespread acceptance, more than 20 medications have been investigated. Treatments with desipramine, amantadine, and bromocriptine have shown mixed results (Dackis et al. 1987; Gawin et al. 1989). However, it is clear from existing studies that the substantial numbers of cocaine-dependent individuals with coexisting psychiatric disorders benefit from appropriate treatment for these conditions (Greenfield et al. 1994). In addition, one study of 124 cocaine-dependent men and women found that the remission of symptoms of depression was slower in women than in men, with women having almost twice the number of symptoms as men 4 weeks after cocaine cessation (M. L. Griffin et al. 1989). This study was conducted with inpatients during their hospital admission, and longer-term outcome was not determined.

To date, there is only one specific study of gender differences in treatment outcome among cocaine-dependent patients (T. Kosten et al. 1993). These authors investigated the results of a 6-week randomized, double-blind clinical trial of desipramine versus lithium carbonate and placebo in 19 female and 53 male cocaine abusers. There were no gender differences in the number of weeks in the study or in the proportion of male and female abstainers for at least 3 weeks during the study. However, female cocaine abusers had used significantly less cocaine than males at the 6-month follow-up, although use of other drugs or alcohol did not differ between the groups. The authors concluded from their study that although the female cocaine abusers had more severe cocaine problems, they made better use of their treatment. Further investigations are clearly needed to determine which treatments are most effective for cocaine dependence and which treatment modalities are specifically effective for men and women.

Opioids

Epidemiology

According to the National Household Survey on Drug Abuse, 0.8% of the household population over age 12 had used heroin as of 1990 (National Institute on Drug Abuse 1991b). This included 1.1% of all men and 0.5% of all women. Lifetime use was the highest among 26- to 34-year-olds and was higher among those employed full-time than among those who were employed part-time or were unemployed. According to the Epidemiologic Catchment Area study, the lifetime prevalence of opioid abuse or dependence in 1982 was 0.7% of the U.S. population (Anthony and Helzer 1991).

Family History and Course of Illness

Although the presence of a gender difference in the family histories of individuals with opioid dependence is not well studied, there is evidence of increased prevalence of substance dependence in the relatives of those with opioid abuse. In one study of 248 male chronic opioid users, both opioid and alcohol dependence clustered in the families of opioid users (Maddux and Desmond 1989). Another study of 638 opioid-dependent subjects compared those with and without parental alcohol dependence and found that those with a history of parental alcohol dependence were more likely to have alcohol dependence, depression, and antisocial personality disorder (T. R. Kosten et al. 1985). Studies of the antecedents of opioid dependence indicate that opioid abusers are a heterogeneous group. In their study of 276 male and 87 female opioid-dependent subjects in treatment, Rounsaville et al. (1982b) found that there were three distinct subgroups based on antecedents to opioid dependence: 1) those with childhood trauma whose delinquent activity and drug abuse came only after substantial disruptive childhood events; 2) those with early delinquency whose initial illicit drug abuse came after the onset of regular antisocial and criminal activities; and 3) an initial-drug-use group for whom criminal activity and disruptive events occurred after the initiation of illicit drug use. Men and women were equally represented in all three groups. Other studies have suggested that childhood sexual and physical abuse are highly prevalent among women drug abusers (Ladwig and Andersen 1989; Ryan and Popour 1983) and that heroin dependence in women is more often associated with early family problems than in men (Graeven and Schaef 1978).

In spite of the range of possible antecedents to addiction, opioid dependence confers a relatively poor prognosis. In an 11-year follow-up study of a Danish cohort of 203 male and 97 female opioid-dependent subjects, 26% were dead at 11 years' follow-up, 10% had achieved some degree of unstable abstinence, and only 24% could be classified as truly recovered (Haastrup and Jepsen 1988).

A number of gender differences have been found in the initiation of opioid use and the development of dependence (Hser et al. 1987). In a study of 567 male and female heroin-dependent subjects in methadone maintenance treatment, Hser et al. (1987) found that initial heroin use by women was highly influenced by a man who was usually a sexual partner and frequently a daily heroin user. Women were also slightly younger than men at first use and were more often unskilled than men. Women most often reported using heroin because their partner used heroin, or in order to decrease pain, while men reported initiating heroin use because of curiosity or to gain peer acceptance. Men more frequently had used alcohol and/or marijuana before initiation of narcotic use, but women reported more use of nonnarcotic drugs during the 12 months before treatment.

In a related study of the same population, Anglin et al. (1987a) found that although 25% of the subjects reported becoming addicted within 1 month after first heroin use, in general women became addicted to heroin more quickly than men and began their first treatment sooner. This finding is consistent with other studies that have reported that women become dependent on heroin more rapidly (Ellinwood et al. 1966; Rosenbaum 1981). In a separate study, Rosenbaum (1979) found that women had one of two patterns of heroin use: 1) "chipping," or intermittent use, and 2) persistent and sustained use. The key determinant in the pattern of use was availability of heroin.

After the women and men in the study became dependent on heroin, criminal activity for both men and women increased, although more men than women were involved in illegal activity and men had more incarcerations (Hser et al. 1987). Men generally had shorter periods of abstinence from heroin that were most often initiated through legal circumstances, whereas women had longer abstinences that were more frequently initiated after treatment (Hser et al. 1987).

Medical Consequences

Acute administration of opioids such as heroin produces central nervous system effects characterized by subjective feelings of an initial high followed by a sense of tranquility. Other central effects include drowsiness, lability of mood, mental clouding, apathy, motor retardation, and respiratory depression. Acute physical effects include vasodilation with resulting hypotension, pupillary constriction, constipation, and urinary hesitancy.

There are a wide variety of medical complications associated with opioid use. The majority of health problems associated with opioid abuse originate either in self-neglect or in the complications of intravenous injections. Shared needles promote infection with HIV, hepatitis B and C, staphylococcus aureus, and other agents that cause endocarditis. Poor health conditions and other infectious organisms increase the prevalence of syphilis and tuberculosis in this population as well. Approximately 25% of all cases of acquired immunodeficiency syndrome (AIDS) have occurred in intravenous drug users, with 17% occurring in those for whom intravenous drug use was the only risk factor. Increasing mortality among urban opioid abusers may be attributable to the abuse of heroin in combination with other substances, such as cocaine and alcohol, and to the rising prevalence of HIV infection in this population (Greenfield et al., in press).

Women appear to have greater medical consequences associated with their opioid dependence, according to one 12-year follow-up study of 84 female and 91 male subjects (Marsh and Simpson 1986). Women had significantly more respiratory diseases and genitourinary problems than men. In addition, significantly more women than men (30% vs. 17%, respectively) had medical problems for which they did not receive medical services. Like many other drugs of abuse, opioids cross the placenta, and approximately 75% of infants born to opioid-dependent mothers are physically dependent. Infants born to women on methadone maintenance are also at risk for neonatal opioid dependence and withdrawal. Finally, because women intravenous drug abusers and sexual partners of male intravenous drug abusers constitute the largest number of HIV-infected women of childbearing age, a further consequence of opioid dependence in women is AIDS (Greenfield et al., in press).

Psychiatric Comorbidity

The Epidemiologic Catchment Area study found that when compared with the general population, those with opioid abuse were almost seven times more likely to have a mental disorder, almost six times more likely to have a mood disorder, and almost three times more likely to have an anxiety disorder (Regier et al. 1990). A number of studies have noted increased rates of depression and anxiety among opioid-dependent subjects (Dorus and Senay 1980; T. R. Kosten and Rounsaville 1986; Rounsaville et al. 1982a). In a study of 533 opioid-dependent subjects (76% male) seeking treatment, Rounsaville et al. (1982a) found that 70% of the sample met criteria for another psychiatric diagnosis at the time of their interview, and 87% had had another psychiatric disorder at some time in their lives. This lifetime rate was considerably higher than the 17.8% general-population rate in that community. The majority of the disorders were depressive disorders, antisocial personality disorder, and alcohol dependence. The investigators also found that 68% of their subjects met criteria for at least one personality disorder. In comparing treatment-seeking opioid-dependent subjects with those in the community who were not seeking treatment, Rounsaville and Kleber (1985) found that subjects seeking treatment had more current major depression and dysphoria than did non–treatment seekers but that rates of other comorbid psychiatric disorders were comparable. Among

204 treatment-seeking individuals and 105 community subjects, 16% and 23%, respectively, had had an anxiety disorder at some time in their lives, and 15% of both groups had comorbid alcohol dependence.

Gender differences in rates of comorbid psychiatric disorders among individuals with opioid dependence are similar to those seen in alcohol- and cocaine-dependent subjects. In this same study population, Rounsaville et al. (1982a) found that women had higher lifetime rates of major depression, cyclothymic personality, bipolar disorders, panic disorders, and phobic disorders. Men were more likely to have antisocial personality disorders.

Treatment Outcome

A study by the National Institute on Drug Abuse (Anglin et al. 1987b) showed that three times as many men as women entered federally funded drug treatment programs. Several other studies reported that women had lower retention and treatment success rates than men (Cuskey et al. 1977; S. J. Levy and Doyle 1974). Some researchers have attributed such differences to the male-oriented nature of most treatment programs for opioid-dependent patients (Marsh and Simpson 1986).

However, other studies have found that women are as responsive to treatment as men (Anglin et al. 1987b; Greene and Ryser 1978; B. J. Rosenthal et al. 1979). In their study of 546 methadone maintenance patients, Anglin et al. (1987b) found that women took less time than men to enter into their first methadone maintenance treatment program; the duration for first treatment was generally shorter for women than for men; and fewer women than men were discharged involuntarily for violating program regulations. However, there were no differences between men and women in the percentage of time spent in subsequent methadone maintenance treatment, the mean number of times they entered methadone maintenance, or the average length of time on or off methadone maintenance.

A number of specific factors seem to contribute to enhanced treatment outcome for women (Anglin et al. 1987b; Eldred and Washington 1976; Ladwig and Andersen 1989; Nurco et al. 1982). Although later age of first use of marijuana and opioids and later termination of formal education appear to be predictive of better outcomes in men, this is generally not true for women. The most consistent factor reported to improve treatment outcome in women is partner support for treatment (Anglin et al. 1987b; Eldred and Washington 1976) and/or absence of an addicted partner (Nurco et al. 1982). The presence of a strong self-concept (Aron and Daily 1976) and lack of criminal involvement also appear to be associated with better treatment outcomes in women. Finally, there is evidence that increasing the focus of treatment on concerns specific to women—such as adding women's treatment groups, increasing women staff, and increasing attention to women's sexual concerns, including past histories of abuse—all improve treatment outcomes in women (Ladwig and Andersen 1989).

Conclusion

Although women with substance use disorders represent a heterogeneous group, it is clear that, in general, morbidity and mortality for women with substance use disorders equal or exceed those for men. In spite of this, women come to substance abuse treatment programs far less frequently than do men. Increased attention to substance use histories of women seen in all health care settings may help in the identification and treatment of women with substance use disorders. The precipitants of the onset of problem drinking in women, as well as the effect of other psychiatric disorders and symptoms, continue to be areas that require additional research. Furthermore, there is a paucity of information detailing differences and similarities in the process of recovery and the antecedents of relapse in women and men. Finally, further research is needed to assess the effectiveness of specific treatments for substance dependence and to determine which treatment modalities are specifically effective for women and men.

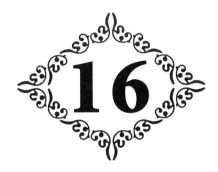

Sexual Side Effects of Psychotropic Drugs in Women and Men

Margaret F. Jensvold, M.D., Victoria C. Plaut,
Nathan Rojansky, M.D., Theresa L. Crenshaw, M.D.,
and Uriel Halbreich, M.D.

S exual side effects of psychotropic medications have become a source of increasing
concern to patients and physicians alike. Although attention to sexual
side effects is new, sexual side effects themselves are not new. Most
classes of psychotropic drugs commonly cause sexual side effects.

In this chapter we review the types, prevalences, mechanisms, management, and treatment of sexual side effects of psychotropic medica-

Modified from Rojansky N, Wang K, Halbreich U: Reproductive and sexual adverse effects of psychotropic drugs, in *Adverse Effects of Psychotropic Drugs.* Edited by Lieberman
J, Kane J. New York, Guilford, 1992, pp. 356–375. Used with permission.

tions in women and men, with an emphasis on sexual side effects in women. Previous reviews have emphasized sexual side effects in men. Rojansky et al. (1992) provides additional details about sexual side effects in men.

Limitations of the Literature
on Sexual Side Effects

The literature on sexual side effects of drugs currently has many limitations. Most information derives from single case reports or reports of small numbers of subjects. Few double-blind, placebo-controlled studies are available, although some are currently being conducted. Terms have at times been used with different meanings by different authors. For example, *impotence* most commonly refers to erectile difficulties, but sometimes also refers to ejaculatory problems and anorgasmia.

A relative lack of attention to the prevalences of sexual dysfunction in 1) healthy populations, 2) study populations before onset of illness, 3) patient populations after onset of illness but before treatment, and 4) placebo effects complicates interpretation of prevalence rates.

Few studies have compared the percentages of patients whose sexual functioning worsens due to medication and those whose sexual functioning improves. Improvement may occur either secondary to improvement in the underlying psychiatric condition with treatment or as a beneficial side effect of medication. One study that did make such a comparison was Beaumont's (1977) uncontrolled study of clomipramine treatment in 51 depressed patients, 65% of whom had prior sexual dysfunction. Among the patients who had sexual dysfunction before treatment, sexual function was improved with low-dose clomipramine treatment in 50% of patients and adversely affected in 20%.

A number of studies have documented widely divergent prevalences of sexual side effects, depending on whether the information was spontaneously reported by the patient, routinely asked about in interview, or reported in a written questionnaire. For example, DeLeo and Magni (1983) found sexual side effect prevalences of 10%, 26%, and 47% by spontaneous report, interview, and written questionnaire, respectively. Most studies do not report the method(s) by which the information was obtained.

Consequently, attempts to statistically estimate the prevalence of sexual side effects are, at best, often approximations or educated guesses, and not necessarily indicative of relative risk.

An example of an article that reported sexual side effect data well is Monteiro et al.'s (1987) placebo-controlled study of sexual side effects among 46 obsessive-compulsive disorder (OCD) patients taking clomipramine or placebo. Data for more than 12 possible sexual side effects were collected prospectively and were reported grouped 1) by sex and 2) by whether the subjects reported sexual dysfunction before starting drug or placebo. The average times of onset of sexual effects (day 3 on average), onset of benefit from the drug (days 12–14), and return to normal sexual functioning after stopping the drug (3 days) were likewise reported.

Few drug-comparative studies have been conducted. One such study is the double-blind investigation of Harrison et al. (1985). Among depressed patients treated with phenelzine or imipramine, 16% of women and 8% of men reported decreased sexual function on placebo; 57% of women and 80% of men treated with phenelzine, and 27% of women and 50% of men treated with imipramine experienced sexual dysfunction. Sexual function recovered within 1–3 weeks of stopping antidepressant medication (Harrison et al. 1985).

The current trend is toward larger studies and more placebo-controlled studies, although there is still room for small studies and case reports to be useful.

Review of Sexual Physiology

Sexual desire refers to an interest in sexual behavior. *Sexual response* refers to the body's response to sexual stimulation.

The four stages to the female sexual response are excitement, plateau, orgasm, and resolution (Masters and Johnson 1970). During the *excitement* stage, psychogenic stimuli, including either sensory or imaginative stimuli, and vasodilatory changes, including blood pressure elevation, skin flushing, and engorgement of the clitoris, vagina, and labia minora, raise the sexual tension. Lubrication is secreted from Bartholin's and Skene's glands during the *plateau* phase while continued vascular engorgement further raises the sexual tension. *Orgasm* refers to the point of maximal tension. A pleasurable climax is accompanied by pelvic and perineal muscle contractions and results in tension release. In the *resolution* phase, hemodynamic changes return to normal, with a reversal of vasocongestion, skin flush, and elevated blood pressure (Reubens 1982).

The four stages to the male sexual response are erection, plateau, orgasm, and resolution. The male *orgasmic phase* has three parts: orgasm, emission, and ejaculation. Orgasm per se, the brief, pleasurable climax resulting in release in tension, is usually automatically accompanied by ejaculation (Masters and Johnson 1970). Normal ejaculation requires three parts: seminal emission (delivery of semen from the prostate into the posterior urethra), ejaculation (delivery of semen from the posterior urethra to the urethral meatus), and bladder neck closure (to keep semen from moving into the bladder rather than through the urethral meatus). Precise neural pathways in the male are well-documented elsewhere (e.g., Buffum 1982; Rojansky et al. 1992).

Sexual functioning may be influenced at three levels: 1) peripheral, 2) hormonal, and 3) central (Meston and Gorzalka 1992). The *peripheral level* includes the sympathetic (adrenergic) and parasympathetic (cholinergic) autonomic nervous systems (ANS), which usually function in an opposed and reciprocal fashion in relation to one another. The *endocrine system* involved in sexual functioning is composed of the gonads, gonadal steroid-sensitive end organs, the pituitary, the hypothalamus, and the suprahypothalamic central nervous system (CNS). Testosterone, prolactin, and the gonadotropins affect human sexual functioning. Impulses from centers in the *cerebral cortex* travel through the *limbic system* to thoracolumbar centers affecting autonomic responses and genital functioning. Reflex spinal cord–autonomic pathways and psychogenic pathways may work in concert (Pollack et al. 1992). At the central level, serotonergic, cholinergic, adrenergic, and dopaminergic neurotransmitters are all known to affect sexual functioning.

The precise neurophysiological mechanisms and pathways of sexual response are well studied in human males. They are less studied and less completely understood in human females (Buffum 1982; Meston and Gorzalka 1992). The sexual response in males is readily measured physically using penile plethysmography. The response in females is rarely measured physically, although one elegant example of such a study is the work of G. Wagner and Levin (1980), in which changes in vaginal blood flow with orgasm and in response to medication were measured using a heat probe. In animal models, the only behavior that is measured as an indicator of female sexual response to drugs is lordosis. Lordosis has been criticized as being overly representative of reflex spinal and autonomic function and not sufficiently representative of CNS mechanisms to extrapolate well to human females (Buffum 1982).

Many researchers have equated the mechanism of erection with lubrication, and ejaculation with female orgasm; since a mechanism is proven in men (e.g., adrenergic pathways), then it must be true in women, the assumption goes. Extrapolation from documented pathways in males to presumed mechanisms in females is sometimes incorrect, however. For example, orgasm in females is a primarily cortical sensory experience rather than one involving the peripheral antiadrenergic mechanisms of emission of the male (Buffum 1982), contradicting the often-presumed equating of female orgasm and male ejaculation.

Psychotropic Drug Effects on Sexual Function: General Considerations

Psychotropic drugs may influence sexual functioning via a variety of direct or indirect effects. Table 16–1 lists possible direct sexual side effects of drugs in women and men. Indirect sexual side effects (Table 16–2) refer to the effects of drugs on other aspects of physical or emotional well-being, which in turn influence sexual desire or performance. The sexual side effects that have received by far the most research attention to date are decreased sexual desire, anorgasmia, and impaired erection and ejaculation.

While researchers and clinicians often speak in terms of global effects of drugs on sexual functioning, referring to drugs as overall facilitating or overall inhibiting sexual functioning, in fact a particular drug may facilitate one or more aspects of sexual functioning, inhibit other aspects, and have no effect on yet other aspects (Meston and Gorzalka 1992).

Few drugs have specific activity at selected receptor subtypes. Most drugs have a variety of effects involving different neurotransmitter sys-

Table 16–1.   Direct sexual side effects of psychotropic drugs

Women	
Desire	
Hyposexuality	Pain with intercourse
Inhibited sexual desire	Pain after intercourse
Aversion	**Menstrual disorders**
Hypersexuality	Dysmenorrhea
Lubrication	Menorrhagia
Orgasm	Amenorrhea
Orgasmic inhibition	**Clitoral hypertrophy**
Anorgasmia	**Infertility**
Diminished number of orgasms	**Breast disorders**
Anesthetic orgasm	Gynecomastia
Spontaneous orgasm	Galactorrhea
Dyspareunia	Breast pain/tenderness
Painful orgasm	**Paraphilia**

Men	
Desire	Orgasm without ejaculation
Hyposexuality	Retrograde ejaculation
Inhibited sexual desire	Decreased ejaculatory volume
Sexual aversion	Anaesthetic ejaculation
Hypersexuality	Spontaneous orgasm
Erection	Premature ejaculation
Inability/difficulty obtaining erection	**Dyspareunia**
	Painful ejaculation
Inability/difficulty maintaining erection	Pain with intercourse
	Pain after intercourse
Decreased quality of erection	**Infertility**
Ejaculation through flaccid or semi-erect penis	Hypogonadism
	Testicular atrophy
Painful erection	Decreased or malformed sperm atogenesis
Peyronie's disease	
Priapism	Decreased sperm motility
Decreased or absent nocturnal/ morning erections	**Breasts**
	Gynecomastia
Orgasm/Ejaculation	Galactorrhea
Ejaculatory incompetence (inability)	Breast pain/tenderness
Ejaculatory inhibition (delay)	**Paraphilia**
Ejaculation without orgasm	

Source.   Crenshaw and Goldberg 1996.

Table 16–2. Indirect sexual side effects of psychotropic drugs

Appearance/body image
Edema
Weight loss/gain
Comfort
Constipation
Dryness (skin, mouth, mucous
  membranes)
Edema
Hypothermia
Indigestion
Nausea
Pain
Rash/itching
Urinary problems (retention,
  incontinence, nocturia, cystitis)
Endocrine (hormones)
Precipitates or aggravates diabetes
Mood/mental/pleasure
Aggression
Anhedonia
Anxiety
Depression
Detachment
Irritability
Mania
Nervousness
Psychosis
	Neurological
	Analgesia
	Cognitive deficit
	Dizziness
	Fatigue
	Headache
	Movement disorder
	Neuropathy
	Pain
	Paresthesia
	Sedation
	Sleep disturbances
	Sensory loss
	Tremor
	Weakness
	Stamina/movement
	Angina
	Exercise intolerance
	Shortness of breath
	Vascular
	Arrhythmias
	Claudication
	Headache
	Peripheral
	  vasoconstriction
	  vasodilation

Source. Crenshaw and Goldberg 1996.

tems with interrelated or overlapping side effects (Meston and Gorzalka 1992), or they may act at different receptor subtypes—for example, having agonist activity at 5-hydroxytryptamine (5-HT$_{1A}$), facilitating one aspect of sexual function, and antagonist activity at the 5-HT$_2$ receptor, inhibiting another aspect of sexual function (Meston and Gorzalka 1992). Mechanisms of sexual side effects of drugs may become more clear as our understanding of roles of receptor subtypes and postreceptor effects on sexual function increases.

Known or currently suspected mechanisms of sexual side effects of psychotropic drugs are listed in Table 16–3. Some of the effects shown in this table are not consistently found, which suggests that they are not

Table 16–3.   Putative mechanisms of sexual side effects of drugs

Global sexual effects

Drug actions that may increase/facilitate sexual function:

◆ Stimulation of central dopaminergic pathways (Pollack et al. 1992)
◆ Central catecholaminergic transmission (Gessa and Tagliamonte 1974)
◆ Agonist activity at cholinergic receptors (Nestoros et al. 1981)
◆ Serotonin agonists facilitate sexual functioning (Meston and Gorzalka 1992; Pollack et al. 1992)
　◆ 5-HT$_{1A}$ agonists increase sexual functioning (Meston and Gorzalka 1992)
　◆ 5-HT$_2$ agonists (drugs that increase the density of 5-HT$_2$ receptors) increase sexual functioning (Meston and Gorzalka 1992)
◆ Testosterone/androgenic activity (increases libido and sexual activity)

Drug actions that may decrease/inhibit sexual function:

◆ Presynaptic α_2-adrenergic receptor antagonism (Kowalski et al. 1985)
◆ Blockade of central dopaminergic neurotransmission (Pollack et al. 1992)
◆ Anticholinergic effects of drugs (Nestoros et al. 1981)
◆ Serotonin antagonists inhibit sexual functioning (Meston and Gorzalka 1992; Pollack et al. 1992)
　◆ Antagonist activity at serotonin receptor subtypes 5-HT$_{1A}$ may play an inhibitory role in human sexual functioning (Meston and Gorzalka 1992)
　◆ Virtually all drugs that decrease the density of 5-HT$_2$ receptors inhibit sexual behavior (Meston and Gorzalka 1992)
◆ Hyperprolactinemia, including hyperprolactinemia secondary to dopamine receptor blockade (Arato et al. 1979)
◆ Elevated beta-endorphins hormonally (Pfaus and Gorzalka 1987a)
◆ Testosterone suppression

Specific sexual effects

Decreased sexual desire:

◆ Hyperprolactinemia (not a consistent effect) (Arato et al. 1979; Gomez 1981)
◆ Dopamine receptor blockers (either directly, or indirectly by causing hyperprolactinemia) (Arato et al. 1979; Gomez 1981)
◆ Drugs that suppress testosterone via either a gonadal (Beumont et al. 1974) or a central mechanism (Beumont et al. 1974; Brambilla et al. 1975; T. J. Smith and Talbert 1986)

(continued)

Table 16–3. Putative mechanisms of sexual side effects of drugs
(*continued*)

◆ Drugs that suppress LH and FSH (result in decreased production of testosterone)
◆ Opiates (decrease serum testosterone) (Buffum 1982)
◆ Antiandrogens (block testosterone action at end organs and may have central actions) (Buffum 1982)

Anorgasmia or delayed orgasm:
◆ Excessive sympathetic stimulation (may be central and/or peripheral effects; peripheral effects involve, in part, rerouting of blood and decreased pelvic congestion) (Buffum 1982)

Erectile difficulties:
◆ Hyperprolactinemia secondary to dopamine blockade (Arato et al. 1979)
◆ Excessive sympathetic stimulation (Buffum 1982)
◆ Decreased spinal reflexes (result in decreased erection and ejaculation) (Buffum 1982)
◆ Ganglionic-blocking agents (block sympathetic and parasympathetic ganglia, resulting in inhibition of erection and ejaculation) (Buffum 1982)

Ejaculatory difficulties:
◆ Calcium channel blockade (inhibits smooth-muscle contraction in vas deferens, interfering with contraction of ejaculatory tissue) (Pollack et al. 1992)
◆ Increased norepinephrine (hypothesized; may interfere with smooth muscle contraction; may be relevant in cases in which IMI, DMI, and protriptyline cause painful ejaculation) (Kulik and Wilbur 1982)
◆ α-sympathetic blockade
  ◆ α-adrenergic blocking agents and agents that block both α- and β-adrenergic transmission (result in decreased emission; block enervation of vas deferens, resulting in decreased movement of semen into posterior urethra; possible orgasm with dry ejaculation) (Buffum 1982)
  ◆ Retrograde ejaculation (blockade of internal urethral sphincter, resulting in incomplete closure of bladder neck) (Buffum 1982)

the sole determinants of sexual dysfunction. For example, some male patients with hyperprolactinemia due to dopamine blockade by neuroleptics develop decreased libido, impotence, and hypogonadism (Arato et al. 1979), whereas others have normal or elevated sexual activity (Gomez 1981). Some sexual effects of drugs that many authors have postulated to be peripheral effects may be due in part or completely to central neurotransmitter effects (Meston and Gorzalka 1992). Interactive effects between neurotransmitter systems may play a role. One model that has been proposed states that sexual behavior is reciprocally controlled by central serotonergic (inhibitory) and catecholaminergic/dopaminergic (stimulatory) systems (Gessa and Tagliamonte 1974).

Effects of Specific Drugs

Tables 16–4, 16–5, and 16–6 show the sexual side effects that have been found to occur with antidepressant, antipsychotic, and anxiolytic medications. Tables 16–7 and 16–8 list the drugs that have been shown to decrease or increase sexual functioning in women and men. Table 16–9 lists the drugs that have been shown to cause reproductive side effects.

Antidepressant Medications

Reported incidences of sexual dysfunction with antidepressant medication have ranged from 1.9% to 92% (Balon et al. 1993). Selective serotonin reuptake inhibitors (SSRIs), tricyclic antidepressants (TCAs), and monoamine oxidase inhibitors (MAOIs) have relatively higher prevalences—and bupropion and trazodone, lower prevalences—of adverse sexual side effects. Trazodone and bupropion have higher prevalences of beneficial sexual side effects.

Tricyclic and Tetracyclic Antidepressants

Antidepressants may augment or reduce sexual interest through their action centrally on neurotransmitters. In animal studies, decreased serotonin (5-HT) concentration appears to affect sexual functioning by enhancing testosterone effects (Hollister 1978). Thus, a potent serotonin reuptake blocker might be expected to reduce sexual functioning by increasing available serotonin. Most heterocyclic antidepressants possess

Table 16–4A. Side effects of antidepressant agents and mood stabilizers in women

Drug Generic name (brand name)	Orgasmic dysfunction	Decreased libido	Breast engorgement and galactorrhea	Menstrual disorder
Heterocyclics				
Tricyclics				
Amitriptyline (Elavil)	X	X	X	
Clomipramine (Anafranil)	X		X	X
Desipramine (Norpramin)	X	X	X	
Imipramine (Tofranil)	X	X	X	
Protriptyline (Vivactil)			X	
Tetracyclics				
Amoxapine (Asendin)	X		X	X
Maprotiline (Ludiomil)	X?	X	X	
MAOIs				
Phenelzine (Nardil)	X	X		
Isocarboxazid (Marplan)	X[a]			
Tranylcypromine (Parnate)	X[a]			
SSRIs				
Fluoxetine (Prozac)	X	X	X	
Sertraline (Zoloft)	X	X	X[b]	X
Paroxetine (Paxil)	X	X	X[c]	X[c]
Fluvoxamine (Luvox)	X[d]			X[e]
Other antidepressants				
Bupropion (Wellbutrin)				X
Trazodone (Desyrel)				X?
Nefazodone (Serzone)	X		X	X
Venlafaxine (Effexor)	X			X
Mood stabilizers				
Lithium (Eskalith, Lithobid)	X	X		X
Carbamazepine (Tegretol)				
Valproic acid (Depakote, Depakene)			X	X

Note. MAOIs = monoamine oxidase inhibitors; SSRIs = selective serotonin reuptake inhibitors. [a]Only 1 case reported. [b]Reported at 0.1%. [c]Reported at less than 1%. [d]Rare (less than 1 in 100, more than 1 in 1,000; not adjusted for sex). [e]Rare (less than 1 in 100, more than 1 in 1,000).

Table 16–4B. Side effects of antidepressant agents and mood stabilizers in men

Drug Generic name (brand name)	Erectile dysfunction	Orgasmic ejaculatory disturbances	Decreased libido	Testicular swelling	Priapism	Gynecomastia
Heterocyclics						
Tricyclics						
Amitriptyline (Elavil)	X	X	X	X	X	X
Clomipramine (Anafranil)	X	X	X			?
Desipramine (Norpramin)	X	X	X		X	X
Imipramine (Tofranil)	X	X	X			X
Protriptyline (Vivactil)	X	X	X	X		X
Tetracyclics						
Amoxapine (Asendin)	X	X	X	X		X
Maprotiline (Ludiomil)	X		X			X
MAOIs						
Phenelzine (Nardil)	X	X	X		X	
Isocarboxazid (Marplan)	X	X[a]				
Tranylcypromine (Parnate)	X		X?[a]			
SSRIs						
Fluoxetine (Prozac)	X	X	X			
Sertraline (Zoloft)	X	X	X			
Paroxetine (Paxil)	X	X	X?			
Fluvoxamine (Luvox)	X	X				

(continued)

Table 16–4B. Side effects of antidepressant agents and mood stabilizers in men *(continued)*

Drug Generic name (brand name)	Side effect					
	Erectile dysfunction	Orgasmic ejaculatory disturbances	Decreased libido	Testicular swelling	Priapism	Gynecomastia
Other antidepressants						
Bupropion (Wellbutrin)	X	X	X	X	X	X
Trazodone (Desyrel)	X	X		X	X	
Nefazodone (Serzone)	X[b]	X[b]			c	
Venlafaxine (Effexor)	X	X				
Mood stabilizers						
Lithium (Eskalith, Lithobid)	X		X		X	
Carbamazepine (Tegretol)			X		d	
Valproic acid (Depakote, Depakene)						

Note. MAOIs = monoamine oxidase inhibitors; SSRIs = selective serotonin reuptake inhibitors. [a]Very low incidence. [b]Rare (less than 1 in 100, more than 1 in 1,000). [c]Hypothesized, predicted. [d]Dose-related incidence of testicular atrophy in rats; significance to humans is not known.

prominent anticholinergic properties (Baldessarini 1985). Diversity in the sexual effects of TCAs might be related to the demonstration that those TCAs in which inhibition of serotonin reuptake predominates tend to be associated with high anticholinergic activity, whereas those in which inhibition of norepinephrine reuptake predominates are frequently associated with low anticholinergic activity. The sedation, disruption of cognition, and impaired concentration caused by some TCAs, especially at higher doses, are likely to interfere with arousal and sexual drive. Interference with the endocrine axes and with neurotransmitter receptors, centrally and peripherally, might influence arousal and

Table 16–5A. Side effects of antipsychotics in women

Drug Generic name (brand name)	Approximate equivalent dose	Breast symptoms[a]	Menstrual disorder	Orgasmic dysfunction	Decreased libido
Phenothiazines: aliphatic					
Chlorpromazine (Thorazine)	100	X		X[b]	X
Phenothiazines: piperidine					
Mesoridazine (Serentil)	50	X			
Thioridazine (Mellaril)	100	X	X	X	X
Phenothiazines: piperazine					
Fluphenazine (Prolixin)	2	X	X	X	X
Trifluoperazine (Stelazine)	5	X	X	X[b]	
Perphenazine (Trilafon)	10	X	X	X?	
Thioxanthenes					
Thiothixene (Navane)	4	X	X		
Chlorprothixene (Taractan)	100	X	X		
Butyrophenone					
Haloperidol (Haldol)	2	X	X		X
Dihydroindolone					
Molindone (Moban)	10	X	X		X
Dibenzoxazepine					
Loxapine (Loxitane)	15	X	X		
Dibenzodiazepine					
Clozapine (Clozaril)	50	X[d]	X[c]		
Benzisoxazole					
Risperidone (Risperdal)	—	X[c]	X	X	
Diphenylbutyl-piperidine					
Pimozide (Orap)	0.3–0.5	X			

Note. [a]Breast engorgement and galactorrhea. [b]Only 1 case. [c] < 1%. [d]Breast pain/discomfort < 1%.

Table 16–5B. Side effects of antipsychotics in men

Drug Generic name (brand name)	Approx. equiv. dose	Erectile dysfunction	Orgasmic ejaculatory disturbances	Decreased libido	Testicular swelling	Priapism	Gynecomastia
Phenothiazines: aliphatic							
Chlorpromazine (Thorazine)	100	X	X	X		X	X
Phenothiazines: piperidine							
Mesoridazine (Serentil)	50		X			X	X
Thioridazine (Mellaril)	100	X	X	X		X	X
Phenothiazines: piperazine							
Fluphenazine (Prolixin)	2	X	X	X	X	X	X
Trifluoperazine (Stelazine)	5	X	X			X	X
Perphenazine (Trilafon)	10	X	X			X	X
Thioxanthenes							
Thiothixene (Navane)	4	X					X
Chlorprothixene (Taractan)	100		X	X[a]			X
Butyrophenone							
Haloperidol (Haldol)	2	X	X			X	X
Dihydroindolone							
Molindone (Moban)	10					X	X
Dibenzoxazepine							
Loxapine (Loxitane)	15						X
Dibenzodiazepine							
Clozapine (Clozaril)	50	X[b]	X	X			X[b]
Benzisoxazole							
Risperidone (Risperdal)	—	X	X				X[c]
Diphenylbutyl-piperidine							
Pimozide (Orap)	0.3–0.5	X[d]				X	

Note. [a]Doubtful. [b]< 1% in frequency. [c]Rare. [d]One case.

Table 16–6A. Side effects of anxiolytics in women

Drug Generic name (brand name)	Side effect			
	Orgasmic dysfunction	Decreased libido	Breast engorgement and galactorrhea	Menstrual disorder
Benzodiazepines				
Alprazolam (Xanax)	X	X		
Chlordiazepoxide (Librium)				
Clonazepam (Klonopin)				
Diazepam (Valium)	X			
Lorazepam (Ativan)			X	X
Arylpiperazine derivative				
Buspirone (BuSpar)				

Table 16–6B. Side effects of anxiolytics in men

Drug Generic name (brand name)	Side effect					
	Erectile dysfunction	Orgasmic ejaculatory disturbances	Decreased libido	Testicular swelling	Priapism	Gynecomastia
Benzodiazepines						
Alprazolam (Xanax)		X	X			
Chlordiazepoxide (Librium)	X[a]	X[a]				
Clonazepam (Klonopin)						
Diazepam (Valium)		X	X			
Lorazepam (Ativan)			X			
Arylpiperazine derivative						
Buspirone (Buspar)						

Note. [a]One case.

sexual drive (Hollister 1978). The preexisting neuroendocrine abnormalities found in many individuals with untreated depressions complicate this area.

Amitriptyline (Elavil).   In a review of men treated with amitriptyline (100 mg/day or more), cases of ejaculatory dysfunction, impotence, and

Table 16–7.   Psychotropic drugs that may decrease sexual function

Women

Libido: amitriptyline, imipramine, desipramine, clomipramine, maprotiline, phenelzine, fluoxetine, lithium, haloperidol, fluphenazine, molindone, chlorpromazine, thioridazine, alprazolam, amphetamine

Orgasmic dysfunction: amitriptyline, imipramine, desipramine, clomipramine, amoxapine, maprotiline?, phenelzine, tranylcypromine?, isocarboxazid?, fluoxetine, sertraline, paroxetine, venlafaxine, lithium, haloperidol, perphenazine?, trifluoperazine?, chlorpromazine?, thioridazine, risperidone, alprazolam, diazepam, amphetamine

Men

Libido: amitriptyline, imipramine, protriptyline, desipramine, clomipramine, amoxapine, maprotiline, phenelzine, tranylcypromine?, fluoxetine, paroxetine?, lithium, fluphenazine, chlorpromazine, thioridazine?, clozapine, alprazolam, diazepam, lorazepam, amphetamine

Impotence: amitriptyline, imipramine, protriptyline, desipramine, clomipramine, amoxapine, maprotiline, carbamazepine, phenelzine, tranylcypromine, isocarboxazid, haloperidol, fluphenazine, perphenazine, thiothixene, trifluoperazine, chlorpromazine, thioridazine, pimozide?, risperidone, clozapine?, chlordiazepoxide?, amphetamine

Ejaculatory disturbances: amitriptyline, imipramine, protriptyline, desipramine, clomipramine, amoxapine, phenelzine, isocarboxazid?, fluoxetine, sertraline, paroxetine, venlafaxine, trazodone, haloperidol, fluphenazine, perphenazine, trifluoperazine, chlorpromazine, thioridazine, mesoridazine, chlorprothixene?, butaperazine, risperidone?, clozapine, alprazolam, chlordiazepoxide?, diazepam, amphetamine

decreased libido were found (J. E. Mitchell and Popkin 1983). Although female cases of sexual dysfunction due to amitriptyline have not been as well documented, one would expect that the drug could inhibit desire, orgasm, and lubrication and diminish sensation in women.

Amitriptyline might be expected to cause more of a decrease in libido, more lubrication/orgasmic inhibition in women, and more erection and ejaculation dysfunction in men than other TCAs due to its predominant anticholinergic properties (Snyder and Yamamura 1977), its potency to block serotonin reuptake, and its sedative properties (Hollister 1978).

Table 16–8.   Psychotropic drugs that may increase sexual function

---

Women

Libido: imipramine, desipramine, fluoxetine, clomipramine, trazodone, amphetamine, buspirone, bupropion, lorazepam, clonazepam

Other: fluoxetine (spontaneous orgasm), amphetamine and desipramine (orgasmic ability), trazodone (clitoral engorgement)

Men

Libido: imipramine, phenelzine, amphetamine, buspirone, tranylcypromine, trazodone, bupropion

Other: clomipramine (spontaneous ejaculation), trifluoperazine (spontaneous orgasm), amphetamine (spontaneous erection and increase in atypical sexual behavior), fluoxetine (spontaneous orgasms and sexual excitement), lorazepam (cured impotence)

Clomipramine (Anafranil).   Clomipramine induces sexual side effects as severe as those of amitriptyline and perhaps yields a greater incidence of negative sexual side effects in OCD patients (Crenshaw and Goldberg 1996). Estimates of incidence of sexual dysfunction during clomipramine treatment run as high as 92% (Monteiro et al. 1987). The most commonly reported sexual side effects of clomipramine in women include delayed or inhibited orgasm (Beaumont 1977). Libidinal dysfunction has also been reported (A. R. Fraser 1984).

In a carefully conducted study of clomipramine treatment of depression (Beaumont 1977), the sexual activity of 69% of the men and of 57% of the women was impaired by the depressive illness per se. Clomipramine impaired orgasm in an additional 11% of women on a low dose and 19% on a high dose. Clomipramine interfered with obtaining and maintaining an erection in about 20% of male patients and with ejaculation in about 11%.

In a double-blind, controlled study (Monteiro et al. 1987), 46 OCD patients were treated with clomipramine. Twenty-eight percent reported anorgasmia before starting clomipramine. Of the 72% of patients with previously normal orgasm, nearly all developed total or partial anorgasmia while taking clomipramine, and this effect persisted

Table 16–9.   Psychotropic medications that may cause reproductive side effects

Women

Menstrual irregularity: thioridazine, risperidone (intermenstrual bleeding at < 1%), valproic acid

Amenorrhea: clomipramine, paroxetine and risperidone (< 1%), valproic acid

Dysmenorrhea: paroxetine and risperidone and clozapine (< 1%)

Menorrhagia: paroxetine and risperidone (< 1%)

Menstrual disorders (menstrual irregularity or amenorrhea, and dysmenorrhea): clomipramine, amoxapine, sertraline, paroxetine?, venlafaxine, trazodone?, bupropion, lithium, haloperidol, fluphenazine, loxapine, molindone, perphenazine, thiothixene, trifluoperazine, thioridazine, chlorprothixene, butaperazine, risperidone, clozapine?, lorazepam

Breast enlargement or galactorrhea: amitriptyline, imipramine, protriptyline, desipramine, clomipramine, amoxapine, maprotiline, fluoxetine, sertraline?, paroxetine?, haloperidol, fluphenazine, loxapine, molindone, perphenazine, thiothixene, trifluoperazine, chlorpromazine, thioridazine, mesoridazine, chlorprothixene, butaperazine, pimozide, risperidone?, clozapine?, lorazepam, valproic acid

Men

Impotence and ejaculatory dysfunction (see Table 16–7)

Priapism: amitriptyline, desipramine, phenelzine, trazodone, lithium, haloperidol, fluphenazine, molindone, perphenazine, trifluoperazine, chlorpromazine, thioridazine, mesoridazine, chlorprothixene

Testicular swelling: amitriptyline, protriptyline, amoxapine, trazodone, fluphenazine

Gynecomastia: amitriptyline, imipramine, protriptyline, desipramine, clomipramine?, amoxapine, maprotiline, haloperidol, fluphenazine, loxapine, molindone, perphenazine, thiothixene, trifluoperazine, chlorpromazine, thioridazine, mesoridazine, chlorprothixene, butaperazine, pimozide, clozapine?

throughout the 5 months of treatment. Of the seven women taking the drug, six reported reduced or absent orgasm, three noted less-intense orgasm, three reported less satisfaction with orgasm, and six complained of increased difficulty or time to reach orgasm. None of the nine patients on placebo developed anorgasmia.

In the Clomipramine Collaborative Study Group's report of 520 patients treated for OCD for more than 10 weeks with an average dosage of 200 mg/day, 18% of the patients on clomipramine and 7% of those on placebo reported libido change (male/female not separated) (De-Veaugh-Geiss et al. 1989).

Cases have been reported of anorgasmia in female patients within 2–4 weeks of initiating treatment with 25–100 mg/day of clomipramine (Balon et al. 1993; A. R. Fraser 1984; Quirk and Einarson 1982; Riley and Riley 1986). Sexual dysfunction resolved when clomipramine was discontinued and did not recur with desipramine treatment (Quirk and Einarson 1982).

Clomipramine inhibits the reuptake of serotonin but also exhibits anticholinergic and α-adrenoceptor-antagonist activity (Riley and Riley 1986). Citing animal research literature, M. Murphy (1987) suggested that serotonin dysfunction is the best hypothesis for clomipramine-induced anorgasmia. Clomipramine has been shown to increase adrenocorticotropic hormone (ACTH), cortisol, and prolactin in humans (Golden et al. 1989). The drug may act as a blocker of the dopamine D_2 receptor, which inhibits prolactin.

Clomipramine-induced galactorrhea and amenorrhea have been reported at a dose of 75 mg bid (Anand 1985), as well as galactorrhea, breast engorgement, loss of libido, and sneezing at a dose of 50 mg/day (Fowlie and Burton 1987).

Crenshaw and Goldberg (1996) consider amitriptyline and clomipramine to be among the worst of the heterocyclics in terms of causing sexual side effects.

Desipramine (Norpramin).   Desipramine has been reported to cause changes in libido and orgasmic difficulties in women and men, and erectile and ejaculatory dysfunction and testicular retraction in men (Balon et al. 1993; Pontius 1988; Sorvino 1986; Yager 1986; Yeragani 1987). One of three women on desipramine reported sexual dysfunction, including decreased libido, increased time to reach orgasm, and difficulty reaching orgasm; however, some women on desipramine also noted increased libido and increased capacity to reach orgasm (Balon et al. 1993). Desipramine is the TCA with the least *indirect* sexual side effects (e.g., less sedation, anticholinergic activity, postural hypotension, weight gain). It has the same types of sexual side effects as other tricyclics, but these effects occur less frequently (Crenshaw and Goldberg 1996).

Anorgasmia after desipramine treatment may be due to α-adrenergic blockade or to an increase in serotonergic activity, and not to anticholinergic activity (Yeragani 1987). Desipramine may alter both 5-HT uptake and 5-HT receptor sensitivity, increasing 5-HT–mediated neuroendocrine responses (Yeragani 1987).

Imipramine (Tofranil). Imipramine has moderate anticholinergic effects as well as norepinephrine- and serotonin-blocking characteristics. Cases of imipramine-induced female anorgasmia have been reported at doses ranging from 75 to 200 mg/day (Jani and Wise 1988; Riley and Riley 1986; Segraves 1988; Sovner 1983; Steele and Howell 1986). A sexual dysfunction rate of 55% was found among patients taking imipramine (Balon et al. 1993). Women taking the drug reported decreased libido, longer time to reach orgasm, and difficulty reaching orgasm. In a double-blind study comparing the effects of phenelzine and imipramine on sexual function (Harrison et al. 1986), 3 of 11 women on imipramine reported decreased orgasm, and 2 reported decreased libido. These results were not significantly different from those of the placebo group, and sexual dysfunction was found to be greater with phenelzine.

Decreased libido may be due to serotonin reuptake blockade in the brain. Reports of reversal of imipramine-induced anorgasmia by cyproheptadine, a serotonin antagonist, suggest that imipramine may cause anorgasmia by affecting serotonin activity (Riley and Riley 1986; Steele and Howell 1986). Imipramine also exhibits anticholinergic and α-adrenoceptor-antagonist activity (Riley and Riley 1986), which may interfere with orgasm.

Paradoxical effects of imipramine have been reported, including increased libido (Balon et al. 1993). Imipramine has been found useful in treating nonparaphilic sexual addictions and paraphilias in men (Kafka 1991).

Amoxapine (Asendin). Although amoxapine was initially claimed to have a reduced potential for side effects, its pharmacological properties are quite similar to those of imipramine, and decreased libido, impotence, and painful ejaculatory inhibition have been reported (Hekimian et al. 1978). Two case reports of female orgasmic inhibition have been reported, occurring on doses ranging between 100 and 150 mg/day, and resolving when the drug was discontinued (Gross 1982; Shen 1982).

Chemically, amoxapine is a derivative of the neuroleptic drug loxapine and consequently might share some of the neuroendocrine and extrapyramidal properties of this class of drugs. The adverse effects of amoxapine are primarily anticholinergic (Lydiard and Gelenberg 1981), but the drug may also block dopamine receptors. Amoxapine can cause hyperprolactinemia and galactorrhea in depressed patients (D. S. Cooper et al. 1981; Gelenberg et al. 1979; Lydiard and Gelenberg 1981). In one woman, galactorrhea and menstrual irregularity developed within 2 weeks of starting amoxapine for unipolar depression and disappeared after discontinuation of the drug (Gelenberg et al. 1979). Dyskinetic reactions with amoxapine might interfere with sexual function, especially in elderly patients (B. M. Cohen et al. 1982).

Maprotiline (Ludiomil).   Maprotiline has been found to cause decreased libido (J. E. Mitchell and Popkin 1983; Pollack et al. 1992) and galactorrhea (Perez and Henriquez 1983).

Maprotiline is a tetracyclic antidepressant that is predominantly noradrenergic. It has a side-effect profile resembling that of the traditional TCAs. The main side effects are due to its anticholinergic properties, with a rather low incidence of adrenergic-mediated side effects. Maprotiline's overall adverse effect rate tends to be lower compared with other tricyclics.

Monoamine Oxidase Inhibitors

Antidepressant effects of the MAOIs currently marketed in the United States are related to irreversible inhibition of the catabolic enzyme, monoamine oxidase (MAO), in the brain and peripherally in many tissues, including the blood, heart, liver, and intestine. Oxidative deamination of norepinephrine, epinephrine, dopamine, and serotonin is blocked (Baldessarini 1985).

Adverse sexual effects, such as anorgasmia in women and ejaculatory-orgasmic inhibition in men, have been reported with MAOIs (Barton 1979; Lesko et al. 1982; Moss 1983) and might be related to changes in levels or synthesis of peripheral or central norepinephrine (Buffum 1982). Sexual side effects of MAOIs are more common than the better-known side effects of liver toxicity, hypotension, and hypertensive crisis (Nurnberg and Levine 1987).

Phenelzine (Nardil). A number of studies and cases reports have reported difficulty in achieving orgasm in women taking phenelzine (Barton 1979; Buigues and Vallejo 1987; Christenson 1983; A. R. Fraser 1984; Harrison et al. 1986; Jacobson 1987; Lesko et al. 1982; Moss 1983; Nurnberg and Levine 1987). Anorgasmia has occurred at doses ranging from 45 to 90 mg/day, beginning between 2 weeks and 2 months after initiating phenelzine treatment in women who had previously been orgasmic. In these cases, orgasm returned with dose reduction (new dose range, 15–45 mg/day) (Barton 1979; Jacobson 1987; Lesko et al. 1982; Moss 1983). In one case (Christenson 1983), a woman became anorgasmic and gained 40 pounds after 4 months of phenelzine treatment (45–75 mg/day). Dose reduction did not reverse the adverse effects. Two cases of female anorgasmia (after 4 weeks of 60 mg/day and after 3 weeks of 75 mg/day) resolved spontaneously at weeks 16 and 20 (Nurnberg and Levine 1987).

A sexual dysfunction rate of 16.7% was found in women in a 6-month open trial of phenelzine treatment (Buigues and Vallejo 1987). In a comparative study of side effects of phenelzine, imipramine, and tranylcypromine (Rabkin et al. 1985), 22% of patients taking phenelzine (15–90 mg/day) reported impotence/anorgasmia, which usually became evident between weeks 4 and 12. A double-blind study of phenelzine and imipramine found that a highly significant percentage of women (57%) taking phenelzine (average dose of 66 mg/day) reported orgasmic dysfunction and decreased interest, enjoyment, and arousal (Harrison et al. 1986). A case of decreased libido was reported (A. R. Fraser 1984).

The most favored explanations for the mechanism responsible for phenelzine-induced sexual dysfunction emphasize actions at the central level, specifically the inhibitory action of serotonin (Harrison et al. 1986; Meston and Gorzalka 1992; Nurnberg and Levine 1987) and discount anticholinergic and antimuscarinic effects (G. Wagner and Levin 1980). Changes in synthesis and levels of norepinephrine peripherally could possibly influence orgasm (Buffum 1982). Cyproheptadine, a serotonin antagonist, was reported to reverse phenelzine-induced anorgasmia in a male patient (Decastro 1985).

Isocarboxazid (Marplan).   A woman experienced anorgasmia while taking isocarboxazid at 30 mg/day but not at a dose of 10 mg/day (Lesko et al. 1982). The orgasmic inhibition caused by MAOIs has been used therapeutically to treat premature ejaculation with isocarboxazid 20–40 mg daily (D. Bennett 1961).

Tranylcypromine (Parnate).   Anorgasmia resulting from tranylcypromine treatment in a woman has been reported (Gross 1983). Tranylcypromine was reported to increase libido in some male patients and decrease it in others at a dose of 20 mg daily (G. M. Simpson et al. 1965). The chemical and pharmacological resemblance of this drug to amphetamines might be related to some of its sexual side effects.

Selective Serotonin Reuptake Inhibitors

The SSRIs, although structurally unrelated to one another, are all specific and potent inhibitors of presynaptic reuptake of serotonin and have essentially no effect on the reuptake of norepinephrine or other neurotransmitters. They are generally devoid of the cholinergic and adrenergic adverse side effects typical of TCAs and MAOIs.

Fluoxetine (Prozac).   Fluoxetine is well known to cause sexual dysfunction, including orgasmic difficulties and decreased libido (Balogh et al. 1992; Balon et al. 1993; Goldbloom and Kennedy 1991; F. M. Jacobsen 1992; Kline 1989; Musher 1990; Solyom et al. 1990; Zajecka et al. 1991). Cases have been reported of female anorgasmia after 5 weeks of treatment with fluoxetine 20 mg daily for OCD and major depression (Kline 1989) and after a few months of treatment for bulimia with a dose of 40–60 mg daily (Goldbloom and Kennedy 1991), and of female cases of fluoxetine-induced anorgasmia treated with amantadine (Balogh et al. 1992). Among 32 patients taking fluoxetine, 16% (5 women and 1 man) reported anorgasmia (Musher 1990). Orgasmic dysfunction occurred in 13% of 77 patients (5 women and 1 man) within 6 weeks of initiating fluoxetine treatment (Zajecka et al. 1991). Five of 9 women taking fluoxetine noted sexual dysfunction, including decreased libido, more time to reach orgasm, and difficulty reaching orgasm (Balon et al. 1993). Decreased libido and anorgasmia occurred in 4 of 10 female patients (Solyom et al. 1990), and decreased sexual desire was reported by 3 of 10 women treated with fluoxetine (Rickels and Schweizer 1990). Of 160 patients successfully treated with fluoxetine (20–40 mg/day), 34% reported onset of sexual dysfunction, including decreased sexual desire in 10%, decreased sexual response in 13%, and both problems in 11% (F. M. Jacobsen 1992). These reports contradict the low 1.9% dysfunction rate reported by the manufacturer (Crenshaw and Goldberg 1996).

Fluoxetine exerts little, if any, direct effect on adrenergic and cholinergic receptors (Zajecka et al. 1991) and therefore probably causes anorgasmia through interference with presynaptic serotonergic facilitation of sympathetic neurotransmission (Kline 1989). Zajecka et al. (1991) hypothesize that increased amounts of serotonin may work directly on central, spinal, or peripheral receptors or a combination of these to inhibit orgasm, or may exert an indirect effect on noradrenergic input or other neurotransmitter systems.

Paradoxical effects of fluoxetine have been documented in both sexes (A. J. Cohen 1992; Modell 1989). Modell (1989) reported a case of nonpainful clitoral engorgement, spontaneous orgasms without stimulation, and excessive yawning without drowsiness in a woman who was treated with fluoxetine (40 mg daily) for a major depressive episode. Such paradoxical effects may be characteristic of a drug such as fluoxetine, which exercises its effects at all of the serotonin receptor subgroups. The impact of the drug may vary according to the pharmacodynamic profile of each individual and the particular subsystems that are activated or antagonized (Meston and Gorzalka 1992). Fluoxetine's serotonin reuptake blockade effect may also indirectly stimulate or inhibit dopaminergic pathways, causing paradoxical effects such as spontaneous orgasm and yawning (A. J. Cohen 1992).

Fluoxetine has been shown to increase serum prolactin in rats after a single dose (W. W. Morgan and Herbert 1978). Studies in humans with 30 mg/day for 3 and 7 days showed no effect on basal prolactin concentrations (Meltzer et al. 1982). However, one case of elevated serum prolactin was reported on 30 mg/day fluoxetine (Meltzer et al. 1982).

Fluoxetine has been used to treat premature ejaculation, fetishes, paraphilias, and nonparaphilic sexual addictions in men (Kafka 1991).

Sertraline (Zoloft).   The manufacturer reports a 1.7% rate of sexual dysfunction in 590 women taking sertraline, compared with a rate of 0.2% in 582 women taking placebo; and a 15.5% rate of sexual dysfunction (primarily ejaculatory delay) in 271 men taking sertraline, compared with 2.2% of 271 men on placebo. The side-effect profile of this drug is similar to that of fluoxetine. However, sertraline is a more potent 5-HT uptake inhibitor than fluoxetine and thus might be expected to have more severe inhibitory sexual side effects (Crenshaw and Goldberg 1996).

The manufacturer reports a rate of menstrual disorders of 1.0% in women taking sertraline, compared with 0.5% in women taking placebo.

Paroxetine (Paxil).   This drug is a more potent serotonin reuptake inhibitor than either fluoxetine or sertraline, with more severe inhibitory sexual side effects, at least for males (Crenshaw and Goldberg 1996). In men, paroxetine has caused retarded ejaculation, lack of orgasm without ejaculatory inhibition, and decreased sensation (Peselow et al. 1989). Crenshaw and Goldberg (1996) report a relative lack of inhibition of sexual functioning among women taking paroxetine, in contrast to the severe anorgasmia seen in men. Future research will help to clarify any possible sex difference.

The manufacturer reports a 1.8% rate of genital disorders associated with paroxetine use (20–50 mg/day) in female patients, compared with a 0.0% rate with placebo in 6-week placebo-controlled trials. Premarketing assessment ($N = 4,126$) found abortion, amenorrhea, breast pain, cystitis, dysmenorrhea, dysuria, and menorrhagia to occur infrequently (1 in 100 to 1 in 1,000) (SmithKline Beecham, Paxil [paroxetine] package insert 1993).

Other Antidepressants

Bupropion (Wellbutrin).   Bupropion is an amino-ketone derivative unrelated chemically or in its pharmacological profile to any other known antidepressants. Bupropion does not inhibit MAO-A or MAO-B activity, exerts no effect on serotonin uptake, and only minimally alters the re-uptake of noradrenaline at presynaptic sites (Ferris et al. 1983). Further-more, it does not appear to exert action leading to postsynaptic, β-adrenergic downregulation, and, for this reason, it is unique among clinically useful antidepressants (Ferris et al. 1983). Although bupro-pion has minimal inhibitory effect on presynaptic dopamine uptake, this effect appears to have no causal relationship to its antidepressant action (Ferris et al. 1983). This action might at least theoretically account for the bupropion-related menstrual disorders that have been reported (Halbreich et al. 1991). Bupropion lacks the anticholinergic and antihis-taminic sedative properties that are a common problem with TCAs. The absence of such properties might at least partially explain the drug's reputation of being relatively devoid of sexual side effects (Gardner and Johnston 1985). Bupropion may act through noradrenergic pathways with minimal risk of sexual dysfunction (Gardner and Johnston 1985). Bupropion's mild to moderate blockade of dopamine reuptake may be responsible for the noted enhanced libido and sexual behavior.

Of 31 patients who switched to bupropion after experiencing flu-oxetine-associated orgasmic dysfunction, 84% reported complete reso-lution of that side effect (Gardner and Johnson 1985).

In a double-blind study of 30 female and 30 male patients with DSM-III (American Psychiatric Association 1980) diagnoses of inhib-ited sexual desire, inhibited sexual excitement, and/or inhibited orgasm, 63% of subjects (86% of men and 44% of women) reported improved sexual function on bupropion and 3% on placebo (Crenshaw et al. 1987).

Trazodone (Desyrel). Trazodone is a triazolopyridine derivative that is not related to heterocyclics, MAOIs, or any other known antidepres-sant. Trazodone has been shown not to have anticholinergic activity in in vitro and in vivo experiments. It has high affinity for α_1-adrenergic receptors, which might account for its significant sedative side effects. Trazodone may also increase oxytocin levels (Crenshaw and Goldberg 1996).

Trazodone has been known to increase sex drive and frequency of sexual behavior, to cause priapism in both sexes, and to produce para-doxical effects (Cole and Bodkin 1990; J. Erickson and Fisher 1983; Gar-trell 1986; S. D. Jones 1984; Scher et al. 1983; J. W. Thompson et al. 1990).

Increased libido has been reported to occur in 46% of female patients taking trazodone for treatment of depression (Gartrell 1986). For women whose depression did not improve with trazodone, positive sexual side effects did not occur. Some of the women who reported increased sex drive also reported more-frequent orgasm. Cole and Bodkin (1990) noted that supplemental trazodone treatment relieved phenelzine-induced anorgasmia in one woman. One case report of clitoral priapism and five cases of clitoral enlargement have been reported to trazodone's manufacturer (J. W. Thompson et al. 1990).

Conversely, trazodone may inhibit orgasm and pleasurable genital sensation in some women (Crenshaw and Goldberg 1996). Trazodone-induced anorgasmia occurred in a woman taking 50–100 mg daily for dysthymia. Orgasmic function was regained 4 days after discontinuation of trazodone treatment (Jani et al. 1988).

Cases have been reported of inhibited ejaculation in men (J. Erickson and Fisher 1983; S. D. Jones 1984). A rare, but severe adverse effect in males, necessitating surgical intervention in some cases, is priapism (Scher et al. 1983).

Nefazodone (Serzone).   Nefazodone is a phenylpiperazine antidepressant with $5\text{-}HT_2$ antagonist and 5-HT reuptake inhibitor properties. It is chemically related to trazodone. In a controlled trial, nefazodone caused fewer sexual side effects than imipramine (Rickels et al. 1994). Nefazodone is hypothesized to have the potential to assist with sexual dysfunction, with a predicted but not yet documented risk of priapism, due to its structural similarity to trazodone.

Venlafaxine (Effexor).   Venlafaxine is a structurally novel antidepressant that exerts selective inhibitory effects on serotonin and norepinephrine reuptake. The manufacturer reports (Wyeth Laboratories, Effexor [venlafaxine] package insert 1994) that the drug has no significant affinity for muscarinic, histaminergic, or adrenergic receptors, activity at which is usually associated with various cholinergic and sedative effects, including sexual side effects. Manufacturer data list abnormal ejaculation/orgasm and impotence as two of the most commonly observed adverse events associated with the use of venlafaxine. In 4- to 8-week placebo-controlled trials, involving 1,033 patients taking venlafaxine and 609 taking placebo, female patients had a 2% rate of orgasmic disturbance and a 1% incidence of menstrual disorders. Male subjects experienced a 12% incidence of abnormal ejaculation/orgasm and a 6% rate of impotence (all compared with less than 1% rates in the placebo group) at doses between 75 and 275 mg/day.

Mood Stabilizers

The mood-stabilizing medications 1) treat mania; 2) taken over time, may have a preventive effect for bipolar depression; and 3) may be used as adjuvant therapy for unipolar depression partially treated by antidepressant medication alone.

Lithium (Eskalith, Lithobid, Lithonate, Lithotabs).   Lithium may decrease inositol phosphate formation caused by various neurotransmitters, including norepinephrine, serotonin, and acetylcholine, in turn affecting second-messenger systems (Meston and Gorzalka 1992). In addition, lithium treatment appears to increase 5-HT$_{1A}$ receptors, decrease 5-HT$_{1C}$ receptors, and have no effect on 5-HT$_2$ receptors. Lithium may exert its sexual side effects via serotonergic effects (Meston and Gorzalka 1992). Sexual side effects of lithium may also be due to a decrease in testosterone secretion.

Sexual difficulties were reported by 14% of 104 bipolar patients (45 male, 59 female) treated with lithium alone and by 49% of those taking lithium plus a benzodiazepine (Ghadirian et al. 1992). Among women who were still menstruating, 35% reported menstrual disturbances, although attribution of this side effect to lithium treatment remained inconclusive. One of 10 patients on lithium for treatment of major affective disorder reported a decrease in sexual desire, and 2 of 10 patients with bipolar/unipolar depression reported a decrease in orgasmic ability with lithium (serum levels 0.5–1.0 mEq/L) (E. Kristensen and Jorgensen 1987). No effect on sexual function was found in 112 female patients treated with lithium for at least 6 months (Vestergaard et al. 1980).

Lithium was reported to cause erectile failure and decreased libido, with sexual function returning to normal when lithium was withdrawn under double-blind conditions in 33 manic-depressive patients (sex not specified) (Vinarova et al. 1972). Blood levels were reported to be 0.6–0.8 mEq/L for impaired sexual function and 1.0 mg/day for decreased libido.

Because mania can be associated with hypersexuality, a decrease in sexual function with the resolution of the manic state should be differentiated from the effect of the drug per se (Buffum 1982; Pollack et al. 1992).

Carbamazepine (Tegretol).   Carbamazepine is an anticonvulsant medication effective for treating temporal lobe and limbic seizures. It is a potent inhibitor of amygdaloid kindling and is an effective mood stabilizer. We are not aware of data about sexual side effects of carbamazepine in affective disorder patients.

Among 41 male seizure patients, carbamazepine and prolactin levels were found to be positively correlated. An increase in prolactin levels led to reversible sexual impotence (Toone et al. 1983).

Klüver-Bucy syndrome is a syndrome of bizarre behavioral disturbances, including lack of sexual inhibitions, that follows bilateral temporal lobectomy. Carbamazepine cured the nondiscriminative sexual promiscuity of a 15-year-old girl with Klüver-Bucy syndrome (Hooshmand et al. 1974). Carbamazepine helped to alleviate posttraumatic Klüver-Bucy syndrome, including symptoms of hypersexuality and sham rage attacks (marked by inappropriate sexual verbalizations), in a 20-year-old male (J. T. Stewart 1985).

Valproic acid (Depakote), divalproex (Depakene).   The manufacturer lists breast enlargement, galactorrhea, irregular menses, and secondary amenorrhea as possible side effects (prevalence rates not reported) (Abbott Laboratories, Depakote [valproic acid] package insert 1994). A computerized literature search did not find any references to sexual side effects associated with valproic acid.

Antipsychotic Drugs

In a study of drug-free and neuroleptic-treated male schizophrenic patients and healthy male control subjects, untreated schizophrenic patients experienced decreased sexual desire. Neuroleptic treatment was associated with restoration of sexual desire but caused problems with erection, orgasm, and sexual satisfaction (Aizenberg et al. 1995).

In their review of studies of sexual side effects of antipsychotic drugs, Sullivan and Lukoff (1990) concluded that these agents cause sexual side effects in 30%–60% of patients. However, fewer than 10 studies included 20 or more subjects, and only one of these studies included female subjects.

Antipsychotic drugs may interfere with sexual response and reproduction in several ways. Antipsychotic medications are known to produce varying degrees of extrapyramidal reactions, anticholinergic side effects, and sedation. Neuroleptics block central dopamine action (Baldessarini 1985), which could have an adverse effect on libido. Since dopamine acts as a prolactin-inhibiting factor, dopamine blockade also interferes with the hypothalamic-pituitary-gonadal axis through increasing prolactin secretion, which may cause gonadal hormone suppression. The resultant low testosterone level could interfere with sexual desire in both sexes. Anovulation, amenorrhea, and defective spermatogenesis may occur, contributing to reproductive failure (Arato et al. 1979; Girgis et al. 1968; Laughren et al. 1978). Also, neuroleptic-induced sedative effects and general CNS depression may cause a decrease in libido and sexual drive. Most of these drugs are also α-adrenergic-blocking agents and as such might interfere with innervation to genital organs and sexual function in both sexes (J. E. Mitchell and Popkin 1982; Shen et al. 1984).

Priapism can occur as a result of drug-induced inhibition of detumescence. Priapism has been described particularly with phenothiazines and has been attributed to their α-adrenoceptor blocking effect, which prevents constriction of the blood vessels supplying erectile tissue (J. E. Mitchell and Popkin 1983). Some of these drugs are also quite potent vasodilators and might block the erectile response in both sexes by shunting blood away from the genitals (Baldessarini 1985).

Whereas phenothiazines are known to produce such side effects, other groups of antipsychotic drugs, such as butyrophenones (e.g., haloperidol) and the diphenylbutylpiperidines (pimozide), lack the peripheral autonomic effects of the phenothiazines and rarely produce sexual dysfunction.

When evaluating the sexual side effects of antipsychotics, it is important to understand the effects of the disease process itself on sexuality. Sexual function in severely ill chronic schizophrenic patients has been found to be different from that in nonpsychiatrically ill control subjects even during the patients' premorbid state (Nestoros et al. 1980). Sexual problems of schizophrenic individuals tend to involve almost all aspects of sexuality and tend to become progressively worse with increasing age. In many cases, antipsychotics improve sexual function in individuals with schizophrenia, through "alleviation of psychotic anxiety, thought disorganization, fear of physical intimacy with potential sexual partners and other symptoms which may be expected to interfere with the patient's sexual functioning" (Nestoros et al. 1980, p. 126). This symptomatic improvement could outweigh any negative sexual effects caused by the antipsychotics.

Chlorpromazine (Thorazine).   This widely used antipsychotic has the same mode of action as—and is almost equal in sympatholytic properties in vitro to—thioridazine (Baldessarini 1985). Clinically, however, relatively few cases of sexual dysfunction have been reported with chlorpromazine compared with thioridazine. Decreased sexual desire has been associated with chlorpromazine treatment (J. E. Mitchell and Popkin 1982; Nestoros et al. 1980), as well as erectile difficulty and ejaculatory dysfunction (J. E. Mitchell and Popkin 1982; Nestoros et al. 1980). Case reports of priapism have involved patients taking chlorpromazine at a minimal daily dose of 100 mg (J. E. Mitchell and Popkin 1982). Thus, chlorpromazine and thioridazine are the two antipsychotic drugs most commonly implicated in priapism.

Few cases have been reported of sexual dysfunction in female patients. A woman receiving chlorpromazine (100 mg twice daily) reported that it produced a "pinching sensation" in her vagina that she found very uncomfortable (Degen 1982).

Thioridazine (Mellaril).   Thioridazine is one of the antipsychotics most often causing a decrease in sexual functioning. This neuroleptic drug is known for its relative lack of extrapyramidal side effects and for its marked anticholinergic activity (Baldessarini 1985). Thioridazine has been commonly associated with male sexual dysfunction, including ejaculatory-orgasmic dysfunction, with an incidence ranging from 30% to 57% (Blair and Simpson 1966; Freyhan 1961; Kotin et al. 1976; Laughren et al. 1978), erectile dysfunction (Blair and Simpson 1966; Kotin et al 1976; Yassa 1982); decreased libido; and priapism (J. E. Mitchell and Popkin 1982).

Thioridazine has also been associated with female sexual dysfunction, but this information consists primarily of isolated case reports. Decrease in sexual excitement and less-satisfying orgasms occurred in one of four female patients taking 200 mg of thioridazine; these side effects had not been noted during previous treatment with trifluoperazine or amitriptyline (Kotin et al. 1976). Inhibited female orgasm was not resolved when the daily dose was reduced from 200 to 50 mg or when the medication was switched to chlorpromazine. Symptoms resolved and did not recur when the patient was placed on depot fluphenazine 12.5 mg every 2 weeks (Degen 1982). Inhibited female orgasm developed in a woman taking thioridazine (600 mg/day). Orgasm returned 1 week after thioridazine was discontinued and loxapine (100 mg/day) substituted (Shen and Park 1982).

Thioridazine has also been associated with galactorrhea and menstrual irregularities. A 50% incidence of menstrual disorders was found among female patients taking thioridazine; normal menstrual function returned upon discontinuing the drug (Sandison et al. 1960).

Thioridazine-induced decreased libido may be due in part to severe anticholinergic and central sedative effects (Crenshaw and Goldberg 1996). Suppression of the hypothalamic-pituitary-gonadal axis, resulting in decreased testosterone, or a direct testosterone-inhibiting effect at the gonadal level are also plausible explanations (Laughren et al. 1978; Pollack et al. 1992). Lower levels of serum luteinizing hormone (LH) and testosterone were found in thioridazine-treated male patients compared with nonmedicated control subjects. The decreased LH levels would argue against a direct inhibitory effect on testosterone synthesis. Also, inhibition of erection might be due to decreased serum testosterone. Thioridazine's action on sexual function could be caused by dopaminergic effects, but thioridazine and chlorpromazine have been shown to be less potent in their ability to block D_2 receptors in comparison with chlorprothixene and haloperidol (Meston and Gorzalka 1992). Other explanations include potent α-adrenergic receptor blockade (Degen

1982; Shen and Park 1982) and stimulation of norepinephrine synthesis. Thioridazine and chlorpromazine are known to increase prolactin levels and are more potent 5-HT_2 blockers than haloperidol and trifluoperazine.

An unusual case was reported of a woman who developed severe itching and an erythematous rash on her genitals within 24 hours after sexual intercourse with her husband, who was taking thioridazine. Double-blind skin tests confirmed an allergic reaction to thioridazine in the woman. The symptoms did not recur when her husband used a condom (Sell 1985).

Trifluoperazine (Stelazine).   This drug has been associated with orgasmic dysfunction in both sexes. A schizophrenic woman experienced delayed orgasm while on trifluoperazine 15 mg/day (Degen 1982). The condition was not alleviated by reducing the dose to 5 mg/day, but orgasm reflex returned to normal 1 week after switching to loxapine.

Interference with emission and ejaculation occurred in five male patients at doses ranging from 20 to 280 mg/day and resolved a few months after discontinuing the medication (Blair and Simpson 1966). Another study, however, found no trifluoperazine effect on ejaculation (Kotin et al. 1976). Painful ejaculation has been reported at a dose of 10 mg/day.

Fluphenazine (Prolixin).   Fluphenazine, as a high-potency neuroleptic, may be one of the neuroleptics most free of systemic side effects that can cause sexual problems, such as weight gain and sedation (Crenshaw and Goldberg 1996). However, a study by Ghadirian et al. (1982) of 53 schizophrenic patients (26 male, 27 female) on long-term maintenance neuroleptic treatment showed significant rates of sexual dysfunction. Thirty-three percent of the women noted a change in quality of orgasm, 22% noted orgasmic difficulty, and 7% reported pain during orgasm. Seventy-eight percent of the women reported increased menstrual irregularity, and 78% reported change in quantity of menses. Fifty-eight percent of the men had difficulty in orgasm/ejaculation, and 40% had frequent erectile dysfunction. Most of the patients were treated with fluphenazine injections supplemented with procyclidine, an antispasmodic antiparkinsonian medication with anticholinergic properties. Other medications used included chlorpromazine, trifluoperazine, and chloprothixene. The authors offered two possible explanations for the lower rate of sexual dysfunction in women (30% versus 54% in men). First, the higher levels of estrogen in women may make dopamine receptors more tolerant, and second, the generally greater therapeutic effect of antipsychotics on female patients may result in a more rapid return to a normal sex life. Switching to fluphenazine resolved the thioridazine-induced orgasmic inhibition in one woman (Degen 1982).

Loxapine (Loxitane). A female patient's trifluoperazine-induced orgasmic inhibition returned to normal when she was switched to loxapine. Degen (1982) hypothesized that loxapine's less-potent blockade of sympathetic function accounted for this symptom resolution.

Risperidone (Risperdal). This serotonin (5-HT$_2$) and dopamine (D$_2$) antagonist drug is an antipsychotic agent belonging to a new chemical class, the benzisoxade derivatives. In premarketing studies, orgasmic, erectile, and ejaculatory dysfunction were found to be dose dependent. Among 2,607 patients in phase II and phase III studies, side effects found to occur in at least 1 in 100 women included orgasmic dysfunction, menorrhagia, and dry vagina. Adverse effects occurring in 1 in 100 to 1 in 1,000 women included nonpuerperal lactation, amenorrhea, breast pain, leukorrhea, mastitis, dysmenorrhea, perineal pain, intermenstrual bleeding, and vaginal hemorrhage. Adverse effects in men included erectile dysfunction (at least 1 in 100) and ejaculatory failure (1 in 100 to 1 in 1,000) (Janssen Pharmaceutica, Risperdal [risperidone] package insert 1994).

Clozapine (Clozaril). Clozapine is a tricyclic dibenzodiazepine derivative that appears to block dopamine receptors more selectively than other antipsychotic agents, interfering with binding of dopamine at both D$_1$ and D$_2$ receptors. Clozapine also acts as an antagonist at adrenergic, cholinergic, histaminergic, and serotonergic receptors. The drug produces little or no prolactin elevation, in contrast to more typical antipsychotic drugs. Manufacturer data shows a 1% incidence of abnormal ejaculation and the following adverse effects with a frequency of less than 1%: dysmenorrhea, impotence, breast pain/discomfort, vaginal itching, and infection (Sandoz Pharmaceuticals, Clozaril [clozapine], package insert 1994).

Antianxiety Agents

Sedatives and hypnotics (the minor tranquilizers) usually have the capability of producing widespread CNS depression, with additional effects such as muscle relaxation and anticonvulsant activity. The benzodiazepines are not general neuronal depressants, as are the barbiturates, which may also be used for general anesthesia.

Whereas the benzodiazepines tend to have similar pharmacological profiles, there are wide differences in selectivity and half-lives among drugs in the group. Benzodiazepines potentiate gamma-aminobutyric acid (GABA) inhibition. A close molecular association has been demonstrated between the sites of action of GABA and the benzodiazepines. Thus, the ability of benzodiazepines to release suppressed behaviors, as well as to produce sedation, can be ascribed in part to potentiation of GABA-ergic pathways that serve to regulate the firing of neurons containing various monamines. These neurons are known to promote arousal and sexual behavior (Baldessarini 1985).

Benzodiazepines

Alprazolam (Xanax).   This triazolobenzodiazepine derivative is marketed in the United States as an anxiolytic with antidepressant properties. In animals on chronic high doses, alprazolam has been shown to cause desensitization of adrenergic receptors. It has weak MAOI activity due to its additional triazolo ring, which might produce the antidepressant and antipanic properties. Also, anticholinergic side effects are reported by some patients taking higher doses.

Sexual and reproductive dysfunction have frequently been reported with alprazolam. Complete inhibition of orgasm and decrease in sexual enjoyment and desire occurred both times a woman was placed on alprazolam (2–7 mg/day) for borderline personality disorder (Sangal 1985). The author also noted a previous report, by the manufacturers of the drug and the U.S. Food and Drug Administration (FDA), of inhibited orgasm in a woman on 1.5–3.0 mg/day, with return to normal orgasm after the treatment was terminated. Sangal (1985) suggested that alprazolam's triazolo ring structure confers on it antidepressant properties and the ability to inhibit orgasm.

Of 32 patients treated with alprazolam for panic disorder, 57% reported decreased libido and 13% noted improved sex drive; 34% reported an unchanged ability to achieve orgasm, whereas 50% noted a worsened ability and 9% noted improvement in achieving orgasm. Separate data for men and women were not given (Lydiard et al. 1987).

In a controlled study, reversible sexual dysfunction developed in two patients being treated with alprazolam for social phobia (Uhde et al. 1988). A woman on a dose of 4.2 mg/day experienced decreased libido during the fourth week of treatment and 3 weeks later reported anorgasmia, both of which were resolved with a dose reduction to 1.4 mg/day. Similarly, a man on the same dose reported decreased erectile capacity, orgasmic dysfunction, and inability to ejaculate after 6 weeks of treatment, with return to normal sexual function when the dose was tapered.

Clonazepam (Klonopin).   Benzodiazepines have been associated with disinhibitory effects, including behavioral disinhibition during treatment with clonazepam. Sexual disinhibition occurred in one woman after a few days on clonazepam (0.5 mg tid); the woman was suffering from panic attacks, anxiety, and depression and had a history of childhood enuresis and sexual promiscuity during adolescence (Fava and Borofsky 1991). An aphrodisiac effect of this drug was reported at 1.5–6.0 mg/day in a female bipolar patient and at 2–8 mg/day in a psychotic male patient (Kubacki 1987). A preliminary hypothesis of selective inhibition by clonazepam of mesolimbic control of instinctual behavior seems plausible in accounting for this side effect (Kubacki 1987), although mania and psychosis are commonly accompanied by inappropriate sexual behavior (Fava and Borofksy 1991). It may be wise to examine patients' capacity for regulating sex drive before prescribing a benzodiazepine (Fava and Borofsky 1991).

Diazepam (Valium).   Although it has been suggested that benzodiazepines might promote sexual interest by reducing anxiety (Kaplan 1983), this effect has not been confirmed in the treatment of women with sexual unresponsiveness (Carney et al. 1978). Riley and Riley (1986) found a dose-response relationship between diazepam and orgasmic dysfunction in healthy female volunteers, including dose-related inhibition of arousability, speed of reaching orgasm, and sensation of orgasm with doses of 2 mg, 5 mg, and 10 mg/day. One woman reported anorgasmia in two of four trials. Two women experienced increased sexual function after diazepam withdrawal and flurazepam withdrawal (Nutt et al. 1986). The authors' explanation for this effect was that CNS noradrenergic activity may be increased in benzodiazepine withdrawal, especially in the locus coeruleus and other noradrenergic nuclei.

Lorazepam (Ativan).   Lorazepam was reported to cause complete loss of libido in two male patients within a month of starting treatment of anxiety with 3 mg/day (Khandelwal 1988). On the other hand, a positive influence on sexual function has also been found with lorazepam. Lorazepam was successfully used to treat premature ejaculation in a 71-year-old man (Segraves 1987b). A group of anxious, sexually dysfunctional patients benefited from 4 weeks of lorazepam treatment (3–6 mg/day), including an impotent man and a woman with vaginismus and sexual aversion (Maneshka and Harry 1975).

Nonbenzodiazepine Antianxiety Agent

Buspirone HCL (BuSpar).   This azaspirodecanedione-derivative anxiolytic agent is neither chemically nor pharmacologically related to the benzodiazepines, barbiturates, or any other sedative anxiolytic drugs. Although the mechanism of action of buspirone is not certain, it has been shown to have high affinity for serotonin (5-HT_{1A}) receptors and moderate affinity for brain D_2 dopamine receptors. It may have indirect effects on other neurotransmitter systems (Baldessarini 1985). Buspirone is less sedating than other anxiolytics and has shown no potential for abuse. No sexual and reproductive adverse effects have been reported so far with the drug. Buspirone has the disadvantage of taking 1–6 weeks to achieve its antianxiety effect; however, with regard to sexual side effects, it appears to offer a clinical advantage over existing anxiolytics, which are frequently associated with impairment of sexual function. Buspirone improved impaired sexual functioning, judging from measures of arousability, performance, and sexual contact, in 8 of 10 patients, including both men and women. The authors hypothesized that the drug may exert its effect at the highest level of the hypothalamic-pituitary-gonadal axis rather than by a local effect (Othmar and Othmar 1987).

Crenshaw and Goldberg (1996) hypothesize that buspirone probably does not adversely affect desire or drive, in part because it has no specific relaxing or sedating effect.

Management of Sexual Side Effects

Evaluation

Psychological factors, disease, and medication must all be considered as possible contributing factors in evaluating patients' reports of sexual symptoms (Crenshaw and Goldberg 1996). Sexual function should be asked about routinely before starting patients on medication and at regular intervals while on the medication. In some cases, the likely relationship of sexual side effects to medication will be clear from the temporal course of symptoms. In other cases, particularly when sexual side effects occur as late side effects (when the patient has been on the medication for months or years), the relationship may be less clear. In some cases, stopping the medication—an "on-off-on" approach—may be required to answer the question of whether a sexual symptom is due to medication.

If the sexual symptom is thought to be due to or probably due to medication, the physician should conduct a cost-benefit analysis with the patient, evaluating 1) the extent to which the side effect is bothersome or beneficial to the patient, 2) the relative advantages and disadvantages of a) stopping the medication, b) continuing the medication unchanged, c) considering other treatment options, including switching to another medication or adding supplemental medication.

Patients vary considerably in the extent to which they are bothered by sexual side effects. Among any three patients experiencing decreased sexual desire as a result of medication, one patient may not care at all that his or her sexual desire is decreased, another may be extremely distressed, and yet a third may report liking the sexual side effect due to, for example, improved relations with his or her partner because of more closely matched sex drives, leading to fewer disagreements.

Clinicians often make the mistake of presuming that because a patient does not engage in sexual intercourse, sexual function is not important to that patient. One study showed that clinicians often made the mistake of not asking their schizophrenic patients about sexual side effects because of the clinicians' assumption that sexual side effects are not important to people who do not have sexual partners.

Nonpharmacological Treatment

The traditional cornerstones of treatment of sexual side effects have been minimizing medication, improving diet and exercise, eliminating smoking and alcohol, and decreasing stress (Crenshaw and Goldberg 1996). These interventions continue as the initial focus. Treatment must also address relationships, self-esteem, depression, anxiety, and emotional issues.

Pharmacological Treatment

Until recently, pharmacological treatment of sexual side effects of drugs was conducted entirely by trial and error (Crenshaw and Goldberg 1996). Now enough information has accumulated for the approaches to be somewhat more systematized, although the information available is still, for the most part, based on small numbers of cases, and more information is needed.

There are four main approaches to pharmacological treatment of drug-induced sexual side effects: 1) the "conservative approach," 2) "drug holidays," 3) drug substitution, and 4) supplemental medication.

The "conservative approach" refers to decreasing the medication to the lowest therapeutic dose and then waiting; spontaneous remission of sexual side effects sometimes occurs. For example, in two women and one man treated with phenelzine, in whom antidepressant benefit and anorgasmia began 3 weeks into treatment, anorgasmia resolved spontaneously 3–20 weeks later while the antidepressant effect continued (Nurnberg and Levine 1987). This approach may prevent precipitous discontinuation of a drug or avoid the need to switch to or add another drug. How often and over what time period sexual side effects spontaneously remit, and with which drugs or classes of drugs, are not known. Reported cases of spontaneous remission of sexual side effects (Harrison et al. 1986) are rare; whether this is because the phenomenon is uncommon or simply underreported is not known.

"Drug holiday" refers to the practice of temporarily discontinuing the "sex-offending" medication for 24–72 hours before sexual activity. Discontinuation of medication for 72 hours has been reported to effectively decrease the sexual side effects of sertraline and paroxetine but not those of fluoxetine (Rothschild 1995). In theory, the duration of the drug holiday needed to achieve benefit would be expected to be proportionally related to the drug's half-life. Monitoring for mood changes and withdrawal symptoms is essential.

Drug substitution involves switching the medication to one less likely to cause undesirable sexual side effect(s). For example, switching from doxepin to nortriptyline, which has less anticholinergic and serotonergic and more adrenergic effects than doxepin, was found helpful (Schubert 1992). For detailed information about drug switching, see Crenshaw and Goldberg 1996.

Several possible supplemental or adjuvant medications may be added to alleviate sexual side effects (Hopkins 1992; Segraves 1992). Table 16–10 lists medications that have been shown to alleviate sexual side effects of psychotropic medications in some cases. The relative efficacies of regular dosing versus as needed (prn) dosing have not been determined.

Two antidepressant medications that have been shown to increase sexual functioning either when patients were switched to these medications or when the medications were added in a supplementary fashion are trazodone (Cole and Bodkin 1990; Gartrell 1986; Sullivan 1988) and bupropion (Crenshaw et al. 1987; Labbate and Pollack 1994; P. W. Walker et al. 1993).

Bethanechol has been reported to be without adverse effects (Gross 1982; Pollack and Rosenbaum 1987; Segraves 1987a; Sorscher and Dilsaver 1986; Yager 1986).

Side effects reported with yohimbine include anxiety, urinary infrequency, nausea, shakiness and, at higher doses, excessive sweating and insomnia (Hollander and McCarley 1992; F. M. Jacobsen 1992). Serious toxic effects of yohimbine in overdose include atrial fibrillation, peripheral vasodilation, and lowered body temperature (Hopkins 1992).

Cyproheptatine has been reported to have untoward effects, including loss of the beneficial effects of the medication, and anticholinergic crisis. Five women and three men taking fluoxetine (Feder 1991; Gold-

Table 16–10. Pharmacological treatment of sexual side effects

Treatment of sexual side effects of antidepressant medications

Agent	Dose/regimen	References
Anticholinergic agents Bethanechol (Urecholine)	10–20 mg $^1/_2$ to 2 hours before sexual activity, or 30–100 mg/day	*Effective:* Gross 1982; Pollack and Rosenbaum 1987; Segraves 1987a; Sorscher and Dilsaver 1986; Yager 1986 *Not effective:* Everett 1975
Neostigmine (Prostigmin)	7.5–15 mg $^1/_2$ hour before sexual activity	*Effective:* Kraupl Taylor 1972
α2-adrenergic blockers Yohimbine (Yocon)	5.4–16.2 mg $1^1/_2$ to 4 hours before sexual activity, or 5.4 mg tid	*Effective:* Hollander and McCarley 1992; F. M. Jacobsen 1992
Antiserotonergic agents Cyproheptadine (Periactin)[a]	4–12 mg $1^1/_2$ to 4 hours before sexual activity, or 8 mg/day	*Effective:* A. J. Cohen 1992; Decastro 1985; Goldbloom and Kennedy 1991; Kahn 1987; Pontius 1988; Riley and Riley 1986; Sovner 1984; Steele and Howell 1986; Zajecka et al. 1991 *Not effective:* Feder 1991; Goldbloom and Kennedy 1991; Price and Grunhaus 1990; Zajecka et al. 1991
Dopaminergic agents Amantadine (Symmetrel)	100–200 mg/day	*Effective:* Balogh et al. 1992

Miscellaneous

Agent	Dose/regimen	References
Trazodone (Desyrel)	Add trazodone (dose not specified)	Effective: Cole and Bodkin 1990
	Or switch to trazodone 150 mg/day +	Effective: Gartrell 1986; Sullivan 1988
Bupropion (Wellbutrin)	Add bupropion 75 mg/day	Effective: Labbate and Pollack 1994
	Or switch to bupropion	Effective: Gardner and Johnston 1985; P. W. Walker et al. 1993

Treatment of sexual side effects of neuroleptic medications

Agent	Dose/regimen	References
Prolactin-lowering agents		
Bromocriptine (Parlodel)	Add bromocriptine 2.5 mg bid or tid	Effective: Sullivan and Lukoff 1990
Drug holidays	Discontinue medication Thursday at noon; restart medication Sunday	Effective for sertraline and paroxetine; not effective for fluoxetine: Rothschild 1995

[a] Also blocks histamine H_1 receptor.

bloom and Kennedy 1991; Zajecka et al. 1991) and one man taking clomipramine (Price and Grunhaus 1990) experienced reversal of the beneficial antidepressant effect, with return of depressive symptoms occurring within 2 to 48 hours of taking cyproheptadine, and addition of cyproheptadine had no effect on anorgasmia. One woman's fluoxetine-induced anorgasmia was benefited by addition of cyproheptadine; however, the antibulimic effect was reversed (Goldbloom and Kennedy 1991). Another woman with imipramine-induced anorgasmia had benefit within hours of her first dose, but by the fifth day of taking cyproheptadine regularly, she experienced anticholinergic crisis, including dryness of mouth and eyes, weakness, increased temperature, and anxiety (Pontius 1988).

If hyperprolactinemia is documented, as occurs commonly with neuroleptics and less commonly with a number of other psychotropic medications, addition of a prolactin-lowering agent, such as bromocriptine, can be helpful. Bromocriptine has been shown to increase libido, although nausea and hypotension are common side effects and exacerbation of psychoses a less-common side effect (Sullivan and Lukoff 1990).

For impotence in men, a variety of treatment options are available in addition to the above, including injectable testosterone, self-injection of vasoactive drugs into the corpora, and, for severe cases in which less-invasive options have failed, surgical implantation of penile prostheses (Nelson 1988). Treatment of men's impotence can beneficially influence the psychological well-being and sexual functioning of their sexual partners.

One drug for which management may be different in female compared with male patients is trazodone. Trazodone increased sexual desire and activity to above premorbid levels in some female patients (Gartrell 1986). For women, increased sexual desire and activity with trazodone is not an unpleasurable or dangerous effect, whereas for men, changes in erectile function require close monitoring and possible discontinuance of the drug. Scher et al. (1983) noted that, in theory, urethral complaints in women after initiating trazodone therapy may be a sign of persistent clitoral erection, but that no case of persistent clitoral erection had been reported. In men, transient nocturnal penile tumescence may occur with trazodone and does not necessarily progress to priapism

(Cole and Bodkin 1990). True priapism is rare. However, if an erection lasts more than 1 hour, the patient should be referred to an emergency room promptly. Perfusion of the corpora cavernosa with epinephrine or norepinephrine may reduce the erection. Surgery is needed in about one-third of cases. Failure to receive adequate treatment within 24 hours may result in permanent impotence (Cole and Bodkin 1990).

Explaining the meaning of symptoms and sexual side effects to patients and providing support and reassurance can reduce medication noncompliance (Crenshaw and Goldberg 1996; Nurnberg and Levine 1987).

Summary

Although the references in this chapter have been selected with a bias toward literature on women because of the focus of this book, the available literature and research is overwhelmingly on men. Many of the studies performed with both female and male subjects concentrate on males. The male response is better known, researched, and documented. The fact that mechanisms are more difficult to study in women than in men is not a reason not to study the mechanisms in women, and does not justify simply extrapolating data from men to women. Often, what is known about males is also presumed for females without being properly documented (Crenshaw and Goldberg 1996; Meston and Gorzalka 1992).

When sexual side effect information has been collected, it often has been limited to data about impotence or ejaculation difficulties. Sexual side effect questions may be worded in such a manner that women, who do not experience erection or ejaculation, do not identify with the questions or endorse the side effects. Side-effect protocols specific for sexual side effects have been developed (Crenshaw and Goldberg 1996).

The FDA has not required collection of data on sexual side effects in drug development. However, collection of such information on both women and men should be required, "to encourage pharmaceutical companies and researchers to study sexual side effects before drugs come out. Otherwise the main method of discussing adverse effects will be considerable human suffering" (Crenshaw and Goldberg 1996).

Even so, many premarketing studies last only a few months. Because some sexual side effects emerge after a long period on medication, the percentages of sexual side effects reported from short premarketing studies will be low compared with the percentages that might be found in patients taking the medications longer.

Some researchers have claimed that women are less vulnerable to sexual side effects than men (e.g., DeLeo and Magni 1983; Kaplan 1974), although at least one researcher concluded that women were more vulnerable to such effects (A. R. Fraser 1984). We would discount any blanket assumption that men are more vulnerable to sexual side effects than women because 1) many studies design their symptom categories in a manner that automatically creates a disparity between the percentages of men and women reporting sexual side effects; 2) it is possible that men and women differ in the extent to which they spontaneously report sexual side effects, creating the misimpression that men experience more sexual side effects; and 3) sexual side effects of drugs are easier to measure physically in men (e.g., with penile plethysmography) than in women, but that does not mean that women do not experience them.

Psychotropic drugs often affect sexual functioning, with a "domino effect" on sexual partners. Inattention to sexual side effects may lead to undue distress, misunderstandings, and/or treatment noncompliance. Fortunately, research and clinical attention to sexual side effects and their treatment is growing.

Section IV
Research Methodology

17

Psychopharmacological Drug Testing in Women

Wilma Harrison, M.D.,
and Martha A. Brumfield, Ph.D.

The systematic assessment of sex- or gender-related differences in pharmacokinetic or pharmacodynamic effects of psychotherapeutic medications is a long-neglected area of research relevant to women's health. Moreover, there is a dearth of research on psychotropic drug use in female-specific conditions, such as postpartum depression and depression related to hormonal replacement therapy. The consensus of recent reviews of gender differences in the effects of psychotropic drugs is that insufficient research has been conducted to determine whether there are clinically meaningful differences related to gender or sex for most drugs (Dawkins and Potter 1991; Hamilton 1991; Yonkers et al. 1992a).

The opinions expressed in this chapter are those of the authors and do not necessarily represent the opinions of Pfizer, Inc.

Despite the paucity of formal studies, some clinically relevant gender-related pharmacological differences for psychotropic drugs have been reported (Hamilton 1991; Hamilton and Parry 1983; Preskorn and Mac 1985; Seeman 1989). Pharmacodynamic differences have also been noted. For example, Halbreich and colleagues (1981) reported a significant gender/age difference in response to dextroamphetamine challenge tests. In contrast to young men, who experienced euphoria, postmenopausal women had a dysphoric response to amphetamine (Halbreich et al. 1981).

Clinically important differences in adverse events can be missed when drugs that are studied primarily in males during early stages of testing are later used to treat disorders that predominate in women. Such a situation occurred shortly after the introduction of bupropion, when seizures were reported in bulimic women treated with this antidepressant. This finding required further study, which led to downward revision of the recommended dose for bupropion (Davidson 1989).

Several reasons for potential sex-related differences in pharmacokinetics have been proposed. These include differences in gastric emptying time and in the proportions of lean body mass and adipose tissue that can influence the volume of distribution and clearance. In addition, there may be effects on protein binding and on hepatic enzyme systems responsible for drug metabolism that are related to changing levels of endogenous ovarian hormones or use of exogenous hormones (Giudicelli and Tillement 1977; Hamilton 1991; Hamilton and Parry 1983; Hamilton and Yonkers, Chapter 2, this volume).

A major reason for the deficit in our knowledge about sex- or gender-related differences in responses to psychotropic medications is the long-standing exclusion of women from the early stages of drug testing. Of equal importance is the failure to perform subgroup by-gender analyses of data from later phase trials (when women were finally included) so as to evaluate the possibility of differences related to sex or sex and hormonal status (Merkatz et al. 1993a).

It is particularly important to conduct appropriate studies in women to determine whether there are sex- or gender-related differences for psychotherapeutic medications, given that women are the major consumers of these drugs. In 1984, women accounted for 60% of psychotherapeutic drug use, according to data derived from a pharmaceutical marketing data base, the National Disease and Therapeutic Index (NDTI) (Baum et al. 1988). A review of comparable NDTI data for 1992 demonstrated a consistent pattern, with women accounting for two-thirds of the use of psychotropic drugs.

To provide a better understanding of some of the reasons for our lack of knowledge about sex-related differences in drug effects, we first review the practices pertaining to drug testing in women and the historical basis for these practices. We then discuss the implications of two important recent government policy changes that will affect drug testing in women. Finally, we propose some recommendations for changes in methods of studying new psychotropic medications in women.

Drug Development

The majority of clinical research with medications in the United States is supported by the pharmaceutical industry and government agencies, such as the National Institutes of Health (NIH). There are substantial differences in these various types of clinical trials. Studies supported by agencies such as NIH are generally clinical trials of marketed drugs and standard medical procedures. They are designed to evaluate therapeutic utility or to compare treatments for a particular disease or medical condition. These studies have been criticized for failure to include adequate representation of women, and changes are under way to address the deficiencies.

We shall focus on studies supported by the pharmaceutical industry, which include clinical trials of investigational drugs that are conducted to obtain approval to market a new chemical entity or to expand the indications for a drug's use. These studies are intended for inclusion in a New Drug Application (NDA), which is a compilation of data supporting efficacy and safety that is submitted to the U.S. Food and Drug Administration (FDA). Other types of industry-supported drug studies include postmarketing trials to provide additional information about the drug and to support promotional materials.

To present background information that can provide a fuller understanding of the issues and controversies concerning the testing of new drugs in women, we first review the preclinical and clinical drug development process and the federal guidelines and regulations that govern that process. Before human exposure to a test drug, conventional animal toxicological testing must be completed as outlined in the 1966 FDA "Guidelines for Preclinical Toxicity Testing of Investigational Drugs for Human Use." Preclinical animal toxicity testing is generally conducted in temporal relationship to the three phases of clinical trials that provide the data for an NDA. Before each successive phase of clinical study can be initiated, animal toxicology studies of the appropriate duration must be successfully completed.

Preclinical Testing

Acute and subacute animal toxicity testing must be completed before initiation of the first phase I clinical studies (i.e., the initial exposure of humans to the drug). These initial clinical studies are limited to administration of single doses or repeated doses over a period of no more than a few days. Acute toxicity studies are conducted in three animal species, with at least one species being a nonrodent. Doses high enough to elicit frank toxicity and low enough to have no serious deleterious effect must be included in the range tested. Acute studies provide information about the magnitude of the drug's toxicity and overt effects. Information is also obtained about the rate and degree of drug absorption and about differences in toxicity due to species, sex, and age (Pharmaceutical Manufacturers Association 1977).

The duration of subacute and chronic animal toxicity studies depends on the anticipated duration of the clinical trials. Specific requirements are included in the FDA's guidelines for preclinical toxicity testing (U.S. FDA 1966). Brief studies, such as 2-week subacute animal toxicity studies in two species (one a nonrodent), are needed for phase I clinical trials, with only 1 to 3 days of treatment, for example, whereas 1-month animal studies in at least two species at several dose levels are required for up to 2 weeks of clinical treatment. A 6-month to 2-year animal toxicity study is required for a clinical trial with a duration of 6 months or longer. These toxicity studies focus on general observations of all behavioral and neurological effects, body weight and food consumption, hematology, clinical chemistry, gross and microscopic examination of body organs, and ophthalmological examinations.

Animal toxicity studies can be conducted at any point in the development program, as long as they precede the clinical study for which they provide support. Almost always, during the earliest phase of clinical studies, further animal toxicity testing is still under way. These initial clinical studies have traditionally been conducted only in male volunteer subjects. At the time that the first phase of clinical studies is initiated, animal *reproductive* toxicity studies have rarely been conducted. However, some information relevant to male reproductive toxicity risk is available from the animal toxicity studies. Histopathological examination of the gonads of male animals used in the toxicity studies provides information concerning maturation, motility, and number of sperm and abnormalities in sperm morphology (Bass 1991). In contrast, information relevant to female reproductive risk or fetal risk cannot be obtained from animal toxicology studies.

Animal Reproductive Toxicity Studies

In addition to the preclinical toxicity studies, specific animal reproductive toxicity studies are required for evaluating the safety of new drugs. These studies are usually completely separate from the standard toxicity studies discussed earlier. The animal reproductive studies are divided into three segments, with each segment focusing on a different phase of the reproductive process (Alder and Zbinden 1988; Bass 1991; Pharmaceutical Manufacturers Association 1977).

Segment I studies focus on the effects of the drug on gonadal function, estrous cycles, mating behavior, conception rates, and early stages of gestation. These studies can also provide preliminary information about teratogenicity, the later stages of gestation, and parturition and lactation. Even growth and development of immature animals can be studied with modification of conventional protocols.

Usually, segment I studies are conducted in the rat. About 20 pregnant rats per treatment group are required. Typically there are two active-dose groups and one control group. For study of the male, the animals are treated for a minimum of 60 days before mating. This allows time to evaluate potential effects on spermatogenesis. The treated males are then mated with either treated—or, more often, untreated—females. For the study of the female, the rat must be sexually mature and preferably an adult. Estrous cycles are determined by daily vaginal smears before treatment. The females are treated for 14 days and then allowed to mate with the males. Duration of gestation is then calculated. Litters are examined for size, number of stillbirths, sex ratio, and gross abnormalities. The study design and doses selected should take into account information obtained from the acute and the 2- to 13-week repeated-dose conventional toxicity studies. These will have provided histopathological examination of gonads for assessment of sperm maturation, motility, number, and abnormalities.

Segment II studies test primarily for teratogenicity. At least two species of animals are studied. Typically, the rat or mouse and the rabbit are used. Drug treatment is confined to the female. Treatment is started early enough and continued long enough to cover organogenesis of the specific species. Delivery of the fetuses by caesarean section is timed to occur 1 or 2 days before the anticipated date of parturition. The number of fetuses, their placement in the uterine horn, the number of live and dead fetuses, and the number of early and late resorptions are determined. The weight of each fetus is determined, and any external anomalies are noted. Examinations for internal anomalies with respect to the skeletal and visceral systems are also conducted.

Segment III is a perinatal and postnatal study in pregnant and lactating animals to assess drug effects on later fetal development, parturition, and lactation. Female animals are dosed for a period covering the final one-third of gestation and through lactation to weaning. Particular emphasis is placed on labor and delivery. Litter size and weight and survival of pups is determined. Continuous drug administration throughout the nursing period allows detection of adverse effects on lactation and nursing instinct. In addition, any toxic effect on the nursing pups from the drug or its metabolites secreted in maternal milk can be assessed. For evaluation of drug effects on reproductive capability in the offspring, some of the pups may be dosed until their reproductive capability is established. These studies typically require 2 years for completion (Pharmaceutical Manufacturers Association 1977).

The segmental approach to studying reproductive function has been based on the premise that the risks of human exposure to new drugs are better evaluated by studies in which drug treatment and observation are assessed during specific phases of reproduction, allowing the phase(s) at risk to be targeted. There is some suggestion that for drugs used over a long period of time, a one- or two-generation study approach may better mimic what happens in humans (Bass 1991).

The 1977 FDA guidelines, "General Considerations for the Clinical Evaluation of Drugs," clearly specified the reproductive study data needed before women of childbearing potential (WCBP) could be entered into investigational drug studies. The prerequisites were that segment II and the *female* part of segment I animal reproduction studies must have been completed and the results from these studies must have indicated no teratogenic potential. In addition, preliminary evidence of the drug's efficacy in patients must have been established. All three segments of the animal reproductive studies were to be completed before WCBP could be included in the large-scale clinical trials. In contrast, the FDA guidelines did *not* require completion of any reproductive testing before inclusion of *males* in early clinical trials.

If the long-standing policy of exclusion of fecund women from clinical trials before completion of specific animal reproductive toxicity studies were maintained, it would hinder efforts to increase the participation of WCBP in early phases of drug development. Completion of segment I and II studies requires more than a year. Therefore, it would add considerably to the lengthy development time if these reproductive studies had to be conducted before initiation of the early stages of clinical testing for all drugs. Since most new chemical entities are never marketed, overall drug development costs would also be increased. It has been estimated that only 1 of 4,000 new chemical entities are actually brought to market (C. V. Gordon and Wierenga 1991).

Clinical Phases of Drug Development

Any discussion of pharmaceutical industry policies on inclusion of women in the various stages of clinical trials requires acknowledgment of the important role that the FDA plays in these policies. The FDA is

153 218 947 1528

charged with ensuring that the safety and efficacy of new drugs has been
adequately demonstrated before they are approved for marketing, and
that the product's labeling accurately reflects what is known about the
drug. Clinical trials of new drugs conducted by pharmaceutical sponsors
are governed under the auspices of the FDA and its body of regulations
and guidelines. As a result of these regulations, the FDA has had a major
influence on policies that resulted in the exclusion of women of childbearing potential from participation in early trials of investigational
drugs during the past two decades. It has been argued that the conservative exclusionary policies resulted from a desire to avoid the tragic
consequences of teratogenicity that occurred with thalidomide (for a
more complex analysis, see Hamilton, in press b).

There are three clinical phases of drug development preparatory to
submission of an NDA. **Phase I** encompasses the first studies of the drug
in human volunteer subjects. These studies are conducted to determine
the extent of tolerability and to provide preliminary information concerning the safe dose range. The initial trials involve only single doses.
Subsequent studies include multiple doses during brief periods, usually
no more than 2–3 weeks. In addition, phase I studies include assessment
of the absorption, distribution, metabolism, and excretion of the drug
(i.e., the pharmacokinetic profile). Women of childbearing potential
have been excluded from these trials, in general, because, as noted earlier,
the animal reproductive studies have not been completed before initiation of the studies, and evidence for the drug's efficacy has not been
obtained. Since childbearing *potential* was an exclusion, most young and
middle-aged women were not eligible to participate in phase I trials. The
phase I studies were conducted in small numbers of young, healthy male
volunteer subjects. Generally, a total of less than 100 subjects participate
in phase I trials for a new drug.

In the case of drugs that will be used extensively in the treatment of
women, such as psychotropics, it is important that women be included
in phase I studies with adequate representation. However, the numbers
of subjects that would be required in order to detect modest differences
in efficacy or adverse effects between males and females is an important
consideration. Generally, phase I studies have small sample sizes so as
to limit the number of people exposed to a new compound about which
little is known. The use of small samples would preclude demonstrating

anything but very large sex- or gender-related differences. The recent revision of FDA policy on the participation of women in early trials (discussed later in this chapter) will probably result in changes in the design and scope of phase I and II trials.

Phase II psychotropic drug studies consist of relatively small double-blind placebo-controlled trials that are geared to demonstrate efficacy and that include systematic dose-response assessment. In general, several hundred patients are included in phase II trials, which compare multiple dose levels in fixed and flexible dose-titration designs. Although women of childbearing potential could have been eligible to enter these studies after the required animal reproductive studies had been completed and preliminary evidence of efficacy had been established, sponsors were required to obtain FDA approval before WCBP could be included in these trials. In effect, at this point in drug development, efficacy had rarely been adequately established. As a result, only postmenopausal or surgically sterile women were eligible for inclusion in early phase II trials (although postmenopausal women were not included in a representative way, even for cardiac drugs that are rarely used premenopausally). This meant that, as in phase I, women rarely had representative participation in phase II studies.

Phase III is an expanded phase of drug development that includes the larger controlled clinical trials conducted to corroborate and extend the efficacy results obtained in phase II and to collect further safety data to support approval of the drug. This phase of drug development also includes uncontrolled trials during which the drug is evaluated under conditions more similar to those that will prevail postmarketing. Approximately 1,000–3,000 patients are enrolled in the phase III studies. At this stage in drug development, the reproductive testing has usually been completed, and the phase II studies have established efficacy, so WCBP have been included in phase III if they were not pregnant and they were using adequate contraception. In the case of psychotropic drugs, women have generally been included in representative numbers in phase III trials. The reason that the data obtained from these trials have not been more useful in providing information about potential sex-related differences in drug effects is that the data were not generally subjected to subgroup analysis to assess possible sex differences.

Failure to conduct subgroup analyses by sex was found for most clinical trials. At the request of the Congressional Caucus for Women, the U.S. General Accounting Office (GAO) conducted a survey to assess the adequacy of participation of women in industry-sponsored clinical trials (U.S. GAO 1992). The GAO reviewed the data for new drugs approved by the FDA between January 1988 and June 1991. It was found that there were wide variations in the proportions of women included in these NDAs. However, in only 37% of the 53 drugs surveyed was the proportion of women included in the trials comparable to the proportion of women in the population with the illness studied. In the NDAs for psychotropic drugs, the proportion of women included was over 50%, which is closer to the proportion of women among patients for whom the drugs are prescribed. On the other hand, women were particularly underrepresented in trials of cardiovascular drugs. In 12 of 13 cardiovascular drugs reviewed, women were not adequately represented. In fact, the proportion of women included was rated as low (i.e., greater than 20 percentage points less than the proportion of women patients with the disease). The underinclusion of women in studies of cardiovascular drugs may have significance for the clinical management of women taking these drugs, since there are data suggesting that women metabolize some cardiovascular drugs at a slower rate than men (Walle et al. 1989).

The GAO study also found that the demographic subset analyses to assess sex differences in response to these drugs (in terms of safety and effectiveness) had been omitted in more than half of the 53 drugs surveyed, despite a 1988 FDA guideline requesting subgroup analyses. To determine whether the omission of subgroup analyses occurred because the FDA's 1988 "Guideline for the Format and Content of the Clinical and Statistical Sections of New Drug Applications" had not been available when most of these drug applications had been prepared, the FDA conducted its own internal survey. It reviewed 28 applications for "new clinical entities" submitted after July 1991. Surprisingly, its results were similar to those of the GAO survey in that only 54% of the applications included analyses by sex for safety and only 43% had analyzed efficacy by sex. The FDA noted that there was sufficient exposure of demographic subsets within these NDAs to be able to conduct the requested subgroup analyses in most cases and that the cost of providing this information would not have been significant because the data had already been collected.

Revisions of FDA Policy

Sex- or Gender-Specific Data Analyses

In a March 1993 letter, Dr. Carl Peck, the Director of the FDA's Center for Drug Evaluation and Research, requested that the President of the Pharmaceutical Manufacturers Association inform his membership that FDA reviewers had been directed to make certain that appropriate demographic subgroup analyses (including gender) were performed as required in the 1988 guidelines. The FDA reviewers were directed to indicate in their reviews the adequacy of these analyses and to include conclusions about clinical relevance, labeling implications, and need for further investigation (Peck 1993).

The FDA letter pointed out that this type of subgroup analysis could demonstrate important differences that could improve the individualization of drug treatment. It referred to data analyzed for amlodopine as an example. In the case of this new calcium channel blocker, there was a sex difference in the incidence of adverse reactions. It was found that the incidence of edema was 14.6% for 512 females but only 5.6% for 1,218 males studied. Flushing and palpitations also occurred in twice as many females as males. These sex differences in adverse events are presented in the prescribing information for amlodopine that appears in the *Physicians' Desk Reference* (1993) and in promotional materials for physicians and pharmacists.

One possible explanation for the lack of sex-related analyses in the NDA submissions was suggested in an FDA memo from the Office of Drug Evaluation. This memo pointed out that whereas the 1988 guidelines section on the Integrated Summary of Effectiveness clearly requested demographic subset analyses for gender, race, and age, the Integrated Summary of Safety section may have been unclear. It did not explicitly request analyses of adverse effects in sex and racial subsets, although this had been intended by the FDA. As a result, these guidelines are being revised so that they are more specific (Temple 1992).

We undertook a review of the FDA Summary Basis of Approval (SBA) (or equivalent documents) for the three most recently approved antidepressant medications, fluoxetine, sertraline, and paroxetine, which are all selective inhibitors of serotonin uptake. Two of these drugs, fluoxetine and sertraline, filed NDAs that were prepared before the availability of the 1988 guidelines and therefore were not expected to have included gender subset analyses. In the NDAs for both drugs, women were adequately represented in the data base, with women accounting for over half of the patients studied.

For paroxetine, the NDA was filed with the FDA on November 20, 1989, which was after the 1988 guidelines were available. Depending on the study site, women represented 31%–62% of the patients in one large multicenter study and 35%–64% in the other multicenter study. The paroxetine NDA summary provided under the Freedom of Information Act failed to include any reference to subset analyses by sex. However, a May 1993 American Psychiatric Association presentation of the paroxetine data base, analyzed for sex-specific differences, indicated an interesting difference. Women showed a significantly better response to both active drugs than to placebo but men did not, as a result of a high placebo response in males (Steiner et al. 1993). The adverse event profile for paroxetine was similar for males and females except that females had a higher incidence of nausea, somnolence, and insomnia.

Inclusion of Women in Early Phases of Clinical Drug Development

The second FDA policy change that should affect drug evaluation in women is a reversal of the ban on inclusion of WCBP in early clinical drug trials (phase I and early phase II studies). As indicated previously, phase I and early phase II studies are generally conducted before demonstration of a drug's efficacy and before completion of animal reproductive toxicity studies, so women were excluded. More than a decade has passed since Kinney et al. (1981) documented the widespread underrepresentation of woman in new drug trials. There has been growing criticism that the failure to include women in early drug trials has resulted in dosing information for most drugs that is based largely on extrapolation from data collected in young men (Hamilton 1985; Hamilton and Parry 1983). Thus, while women are more likely to suffer from depression and to be treated with antidepressants, they have been excluded from the trials that determine the doses that will be used for these drugs (Hamilton 1991). It is inappropriate to continue to assume that the data collected in young males is generalizable to women and the elderly and to ignore potential sex-, gender-, and age-related differences in pharmacokinetics and pharmacodynamics (Dresser 1992). The FDA has responded to the criticism of its policy of excluding WCBP from early clinical trials by revising the 1977 guidelines (Federal Register, July 1993).

The FDA's 1977 guidelines defined WCBP as premenopausal women *capable* of becoming pregnant. Women who had had hysterectomies or tubal ligations were not excluded from participating in early trials, but the guidelines excluded fertile women using contraception, women who were sexually inactive, lesbians not having sexual intercourse with male partners and not planning artificial insemination, and women whose partners were vasectomized. No distinction was made between the *potential* to become pregnant and the *intention* to do so. In general, this overly restrictive policy meant that women were excluded from phase I dose-finding and tolerability studies and pharmacokinetic studies as well as from the majority of phase II studies in which the range of effective doses is established.

It is difficult to recruit adequate numbers of young and middle-aged women who lack the *potential* to become pregnant. Although postmenopausal and surgically sterile women were eligible to participate in early drug trials under the 1977 guidelines, in practice they have also generally been excluded for a variety of reasons. These include some realistic concerns about including older women in very early drug trials when little is known about the tolerable dose range and the potential adverse effects.

In addition, because the early phase studies have had small sample sizes, excluding women was thought to be justified on the basis that doing so would reduce the variation and hence increase the power of the study. Potential sources of variability include effects of the menstrual cycle or of exogenous hormone use. However, it is important to have data to increase our understanding of pharmacokinetic or pharmacodynamic effects of both endogenous hormonal fluctuation and concomitant exogenous hormone administration. In fact, the newly proposed FDA "Guideline for the Study and Evaluation of Gender Differences in the Clinical Evaluation of Drugs" (Federal Register, July 1993) recommend consideration of potential pharmacokinetic effects of menstrual status and of menstrual cycle phase as well as the effect of concomitantly administered hormones. This type of assessment has clinical relevance because of potential interactions between hormones and specific hepatic cytochrome P450 isoenzymes that are responsible for the metabolism of many drugs and the widespread use of hormonal preparations (see Hamilton and Yonkers, Chapter 2, this volume). A 1987 study estimated that more than 20% of women in the age range of 15–44 years were using oral contraceptives (Mishell 1989). Evaluation of the effects of psychotropic medications on the effectiveness of oral contraceptives is also of clinical importance given that these drugs will often be used concurrently.

While the desire to protect a fetus from risk of injury is understandable, the potential risk associated with inclusion of WCBP in drug trials can be minimized, given current technological advances in pregnancy testing and contraception. Clinicians and patients can determine the timing of ovulation with a fair degree of accuracy using new techniques. This information can be used to determine relatively safe periods of drug administration (Halbreich and Carson 1989). As stated earlier, phase I dose-finding studies and pharmacokinetic studies typically involve only single doses or very brief periods of administration. These can be confined to the phase of the menstrual cycle in which there is the least chance of pregnancy. Since the phase I studies are also usually conducted while volunteers are housed "on site" for close observation, the chance of inadvertent pregnancy during drug administration can be minimized by using phase I testing centers with "unisex" housing units, and by conducting pregnancy testing before enrollment and immediately before drug administration. Using quantitative methods, it is now possible to detect elevated levels of β–human chorionic gonadotropin (β-HCG) within 1 week after implantation, so that drug administration can be terminated very early during a pregnancy. Finally, restriction of enrollment to women committed to avoiding pregnancy, who have been carefully screened, and who are well informed about general reproductive risks and the potential risk to a fetus, would further reduce the chance of inadvertent fetal exposure to an agent of undetermined potential for teratogenicity.

Acknowledging that the previous policy of exclusion of WCBP from early trials appeared "rigid and paternalistic" (Federal Register, July 1993), the FDA decided to relinquish exclusive control over the process of determining when to include WCBP in early trials and to delegate more responsibility to institutional review boards, sponsors, and investigators in this process. The revised guidelines specify that sponsors should provide results of animal reproductive toxicity studies to investigators when the studies are completed so that the informed-consent document can include this information. Alternatively, if there is no relevant information on the potential for fetal toxicity, a precautionary statement noting the potential for fetal risk will be required. The guidelines specify that the animal reproductive toxicity studies be completed before initiation of phase III studies.

The previous policy of blanket exclusion of WCBP from early drug trials ignored the issue of women's autonomy and suggested that women could not be trusted to understand the potential reproductive risks and to provide credible assurance of their intent to avoid pregnancy. Denial of women's rights to the benefits associated with participation in trials on the basis of the "potential" for becoming pregnant is probably unconstitutional and a violation of civil rights on the basis of sex discrimination, although this issue has never been tested in the courts (A. Allen 1992). It should be noted, however, that sex discrimination laws to date apply only to the employment setting.

In contrast to the restrictive policy concerning participation of fecund women in trials, there has been a tendency to ignore the reproductive risks associated with new medications in sexually active fertile males. However, it is known that a potential fetus can also be at risk from a paternal contribution, as in the case of finasteride. This is a drug used for the treatment of benign prostatic hyperplasia. Finasteride is a known teratogen. Males who wished to participate in clinical trials of finasteride were permitted to do so if they stated that they would use barrier contraception or abstain from sexual intercourse with fecund females. This example raises the question of why men should have been considered more reliable than women in making efforts to avoid potential risk to a fetus.

To reduce exposure of fecund women to drugs of undetermined teratogenic potential, phase I pharmacokinetic studies could be conducted in small numbers of women after both dose-ranging tolerability studies and pharmacokinetic studies have been completed in men. The pharmacokinetic profiles for both sexes could then be compared. If there were significant kinetic differences, then phase I dose-ranging and tolerability studies could be repeated in women. Ideally, the pharmacokinetic studies in women should be conducted in both follicular and luteal phases of the menstrual cycle.

Included in the FDA guidelines recently proposed is the suggestion that a "pharmacokinetic screen" be used to provide information about potential gender differences in pharmacokinetics. This technique involves systematic collection of a small number of steady-state plasma samples (e.g., trough samples) for all patients in most of the phase II and III studies. The large number of subjects included in these studies would permit an estimate of potentially clinically meaningful gender differences in pharmacokinetics.

It should be noted that even if pharmacokinetic studies showed no gender-related differences, this would not indicate the absence of gender-specific differences at receptor levels or of other gender-related differences (Giudicelli and Tillement 1977). As an example, in schizophrenia, gender-related differences in illness course and severity and in responsiveness to neuroleptic medications have been reported (Andia et al. 1993; Seeman 1989). Pharmacodynamic differences may influence tolerability or efficacy. They may be related to interactions of the drug with concomitant exogenous hormone administration or may reflect fluctuating levels of endogenous hormones during the menstrual cycle (Hallonquist et al. 1993; Jensvold et al. 1992; Kimmel et al. 1992). Some information of this type can be obtained from subgroup analyses by sex, age/sex, and hormonal status conducted with data collected in the large phase III trials in which women are adequately represented.

Aside from concerns about the risk to a potential fetus, the most important reasons for inadequate study of medications in women are the greater complexity and size of the studies required and the higher costs entailed (Hamilton 1985). Studying new drugs in women as well as men at the early stages of testing would require substantial increases in sample sizes (J. C. Bennett 1993). This could greatly increase the costs of new drug development if required absolutely for all medications at all stages of testing. It may be more appropriate to *target* the specific medications for which early inclusion of women is most applicable. In the case of psychotropic drugs, such as antidepressants, which will ultimately be used by twice as many women as men, women should be included in the earliest phases of testing as well as in later trials.

Higher costs of drug development could also result from the increased liability sponsors could incur as a result of fetal exposure to a teratogen and higher insurance costs related to product liability issues. Appropriate methods of dealing with issues of liability will need to be developed now that WCBP will be participating in early drug trials, particularly since participation will probably occur before animal reproductive studies have been conducted.

Recommendations

As stated earlier, there is a need for representative inclusion of women in early stages of psychopharmacological drug evaluation. This can now be accomplished because of the reversal of the previous FDA policy excluding WCBP from early phase studies. In addition, the following specific recommendations are suggested with respect to psychotropic drug testing in women:

1. Development of guidelines for early-phase psychotropic drug testing in WCBP. Thoughtful, carefully considered guidelines for inclusion of women of childbearing potential in the earliest phases of clinical trials are needed. These will be helpful in reducing the potential risk to a fetus and limiting reproductive risks to subjects in general. The challenge of developing truly useful guidelines will require the collaboration of psychopharmacologists representing industry, the federal government, and academic centers, and women should be adequately represented within this tripartite collaboration.

2. Development of specialized phase I testing centers. The specific needs for very intensive screening of female subjects and development of special procedures for education and counseling with respect to potential fetal or reproductive risks suggest that specialized

centers for phase I and early phase II psychotropic drug testing should be developed. These centers could also conduct methodological studies to address issues such as the feasibility of the use of ovulation testing in WCBP enrolled in trials (see Stern and McClintock, Chapter 18, this volume) and the optimal timing of repeated pregnancy testing before and during drug exposure. They could also establish procedures for counseling women who become pregnant during drug administration.

3. The effects of menstrual cycle phase should be determined when evaluating new psychotropic drugs. Such determination should include systematic recording of menstrual cycle phase when assessing efficacy and adverse events as well as during collection of pharmacokinetic data.

4. Similarly, the effects of concurrent exogenous hormone use (oral contraceptives and hormonal replacement therapy) on the efficacy and safety of psychotropic medications should be assessed.

5. Systematic collection of data on drug use in pregnancy are needed, and it is important that this information be readily available to clinicians.

We know that there are substantial changes during pregnancy that can significantly affect the pharmacokinetics of drugs. Gastrointestinal changes can affect absorption. There are increases in plasma volume and cardiac output, changes in regional blood flow (with increased flow to the uterus and breasts and decreased flow to skeletal muscles), and changes in serum proteins (including dilutional and other effects on albumin levels and binding capacity) that can influence protein binding of drugs. There are also effects on hepatic enzymes and renal clearance.

We need to know whether there are differences in doses or dosing intervals for specific drugs used during pregnancy. Do patterns of adverse reactions differ? Are there pharmacodynamic differences? These questions can only be addressed by systematic studies in women for whom the use of psychotropic medication cannot be avoided during pregnancy (see Wisner and Perel, Chapter 10, this volume).

Pharmacokinetic studies can be conducted in those pregnant women who cannot be managed without medication. If these women are followed up after the pregnancy, repeat studies can be conducted with those who continue on the same medication, allowing some comparison of the pharmacokinetics in the same patient without the effects of the pregnancy.

Because one aspect of the FDA's responsibilities is to determine that a drug's labeling reflects what is known about the drug, it is interesting to note the method that was developed for dealing with the paucity of data on use in pregnancy. There is a pregnancy category system to indicate in the package insert the relative safety of the use of a drug during pregnancy. The system uses categories A, B, C, D, and X. A drug is accorded category A if studies in humans have demonstrated that the drug does not increase the risk of fetal malformations. These data are rarely available for psychotropic drugs. The category B rating indicates that the animal teratogenicity studies do not indicate risk to the fetus, but that there is a lack of studies in humans. Pregnancy category C indicates that either the animal studies do show some adverse effect on the fetus but the benefit during pregnancy is believed to outweigh the potential teratogenicity or that no animal teratogenicity studies or inadequate study has been conducted. This is the case for many older drugs. Those drugs with some evidence of an adverse effect on the human fetus are accorded a D or X rating. For marketed psychotropic medications, most newer drugs are categorized as category B and older drugs as category C. There were none rated as A and none received a D or X category rating (Code of Federal Regulations 201.57 [f] [6]).

Package inserts are prepared by manufacturers in conformance with FDA requirements. They tend to be conservative in their wording with respect to use in pregnancy and generally include statements indicating that animal reproductive studies are not always predictive of human response, so that the drug should be used during pregnancy only if clearly needed. This leaves the prescribing physician in the dilemma of having little guidance about use of drugs in pregnancy. Additional post-marketing information that may have been collected on the outcomes of pregnancies during which there was in utero exposure to a particular medication is not usually added to package inserts to update the available information.

Because some pregnant woman do need to take psychotropic medications, phase IV testing should include studies in those pregnant women who must be maintained on medication. These studies should include assessment of the offspring to determine not only obvious teratogenic effects but also the presence of more subtle effects that require longer follow-up. Phase IV studies should also include tests to determine concentrations of drugs that may be excreted in breast milk.

There is no national data base for collection and dissemination of information about medication exposure during pregnancy. Data concerning pregnancy outcome after drug exposure that are provided by physicians to pharmaceutical companies during postmarketing experience can be obtained from the sponsors. Unfortunately, however, the reporting of this information to sponsors is often incomplete or the information is not provided at all. Whatever information is available is limited to pregnancy outcome and gross fetal malformations. More subtle, longer-term events that could be relevant to exposure in utero to psychotropic drugs, such as developmental delays or learning or behavioral problems, are not assessed. Special methods would have to be developed to obtain this kind of information. This type of data would, of course, be very difficult to assess. Controlling for confounding variables would be difficult, and interpretation of findings would be problematic.

Summary

It has been estimated that the current development cost for a new drug before it can be marketed is over $200 million (C. V. Gordon and Wierenga 1991). The average time for this development process is 12 years. Recommending required arbitrary inclusion of equal numbers of women—in all studies, at all stages of clinical investigation, for all new drugs—could be counterproductive, because it would further increase the costs of drug development and produce delays in clinical availability of new drugs. In the process of developing guidelines for the inclusion of women in clinical trials of new medications, it is important not to ignore the potential detrimental effect on drug development or costs that excessively rigid testing requirements could have. Significant cost increases could lead to sponsors' decisions to limit some types of new drug development. The cost of drug development is of particular relevance now, since pharmaceutical firms are addressing the need for cost containment in anticipation of health care reform changes.

However, in the case of antidepressants and other psychotropic drugs for which women are the predominant consumers, women should be included early and should be adequately represented in all phases of drug development. Such inclusion is necessary in order to determine whether there are sex-related differences in efficacy, safety, or dosage recommendations and thus optimize psychotropic drug treatment for women. Recommendations for changes in the current drug development procedures must take into consideration balancing an acceptable degree of potential risk to a fetus against the benefits of ensuring that women's special health concerns are factored into assessment of the safety and efficacy of drugs they will be taking.

It is hoped that the increased attention recently focused on women's health issues and the changes in policy at FDA and NIH will result in research that will broaden the data base with respect to all aspects of drug therapy for women. Important areas of drug evaluation in women that have been long neglected should be systematically assessed for new psychotropic drugs. The general lack of drug studies in the very elderly affects the treatment of women, because women tend to live longer than men and hence are overrepresented among the elderly. This neglected area of psychopharmacological drug evaluation should also receive more attention.

Individual Variation in Biological Rhythms

Accurate Measurement of Preovulatory LH Surge and Menstrual Cycle Phase

Kathleen N. Stern, Ph.D.,
and Martha K. McClintock, Ph.D.

Precise identification of the phases of the menstrual cycle is crucial for studying interactions among the menstrual cycle, behavior, psychological state, and the pharmacological actions of drugs. Because ovulation demarcates the transition from follicular development to formation of the corpus luteum, accurate identification of the day of ovulation is essential for precise identification of the follicular and luteal phases as well as the ovulatory phase of the cycle.

Some methods for predicting of the day of ovulation have been developed for the study and treatment of infertility (e.g., for scheduling therapeutic donor insemination [TDI], in vitro fertilization, or gamete intrafallopian transfer). Nonetheless, most of the behavioral and drug studies to date have failed to use precise indicators of menstrual cycle phase, such as identification of the day of ovulation or measurement of steroid hormone levels. Instead, they simply count forward or backward from menstruation by a specified number of days for each phase or use basal body temperature and cervical mucus, which are relatively imprecise indicators of ovulation. For example, Udry and Morris (1977) demonstrated that one could produce very different cyclic patterns with the same body of data by using these different methods for identifying day of ovulation and menstrual cycle phase.

Use of such methods represents a serious methodological shortcoming, since there are large inter- and intraindividual differences in the timing of hormonal events during the menstrual cycle. Ovulation can even occur on different days of cycles that are the same length. Moreover, variation also arises from other biological rhythms, such as circadian and seasonal changes in hormone release and the timing of ovulation. Thus, a precise method for identifying the day of ovulation must incorporate information about a variety of biological rhythms as well as compensate for individual differences in the timing of ovulation.

The preovulatory surge of luteinizing hormone (LH) is potentially the most accurate noninvasive predictor of ovulation. However, the temporal relationship between the timing of the LH surge and ovulation is itself controversial. Some investigators conclude that the LH surge occurs the day before ovulation (Billings et al. 1972; Templeton et al. 1982), while others conclude that it occurs on the same day (Etchepareborda et al. 1984; Flynn and Lynch 1976; R. H. Gray et al. 1990; Matthews et al. 1980; N. M. Morris et al. 1976). Other authors simply acknowledge this variability, reporting that the LH surge can even occur after ovulation (Depares et al. 1986; Flynn et al. 1984; R. Lloyd and Coulam 1989; Nulsen et al. 1987; Singh et al. 1984). In addition, clinicians use urine LH test results to schedule TDI, but have not significantly improved conception rates (Barratt et al. 1989; Federman et al. 1990; Kossoy et al. 1988).

A variety of other indirect indicators have also been used to predict the time of ovulation, including changes in the quality of cervical mucus, a rise in basal body temperature (BBT), and a rise in the estrogen-progesterone ratio (Baird 1983; Flynn et al. 1984; Luciano et al. 1990; Paulson et al. 1984; World Health Organization 1980, 1983). Unfortunately, the indirect indicators of ovulation often disagree, making precise prediction of ovulation difficult and at the same time raising serious questions about their validity. It is noteworthy, however, that the validity of indirect indicators is commonly assessed by using the LH surge as a reference for ovulation (Etchepareborda et al. 1984; Ferin et al. 1973; Moghissi et al. 1972; Templeton et al. 1982). Given the apparent variability in the temporal relationship between the LH surge and ovulation, it is not clear whether these other indirect indicators are inherently imprecise or whether some of the variability in their predictions reflects a problem with the measurement of the LH surge and its prediction of ovulation.

We reviewed the literature and found that most of the apparent variability in the relationship between the LH surge and ovulation is caused by systematic errors in the standard protocol for measuring the LH surge and interpreting the data to predict the day of ovulation. The protocol used most commonly by researchers and clinicians is based on a daily urine sample collected on arising in the morning (Adekunle et al. 1984; A. C. Collins et al. 1975; W. P. Collins 1983; W. P. Collins et al. 1981; Croxatto et al. 1972; Flynn et al. 1984; R. H. Gray et al. 1990; Nielsen et al. 1990; Singh et al. 1984; World Health Organization 1983). In this standard protocol, the day of ovulation is typically defined as the day after the highest LH level, the peak of the LH surge.

However, there is a second literature of detailed studies in which LH samples were collected repeatedly during the day in order to characterize the timing of the LH surge and its relationship to ovulation. The results of this second literature demonstrate that there are three important sources of error in the standard protocol: 1) the peak of the LH surge is not as good a predictor of ovulation as is its onset, 2) the LH surge has a circadian component to its timing that makes morning a suboptimal time to sample, and 3) the interval between the LH surge and ovulation is more appropriately measured in hours, not rounded to the nearest full calendar day.

In this unique review, we not only summarize the literature that points out these errors but also take the next step and present hypotheses for a revised protocol that corrects these errors, is precise, and is easy to use. This review recognizes that the menstrual rhythm is set in the context of circadian and seasonal rhythms. Although the onset of the LH surge is the best predictor of the time of ovulation, there is individual variation in the time of the onset of the LH surge. However, the variation in the time of the LH surge is not random, but rather is systematically influenced by circadian and seasonal rhythms. Our preliminary data comparing the accuracy of the revised and standard protocols indicate that the revised protocol avoids the biases inherent in other protocols and maximizes the likelihood of pinpointing the time of the LH surge, thereby enhancing the prediction of the day of ovulation.

Relationship of Onset and Peak of LH Surge to Time of Ovulation

Predictions of ovulation based on the LH surge will be in error if they do not measure the appropriate parameter of the surge. Most studies (74%, $N = 46$ studies) measure the LH peak instead of the onset of the surge (see the appendix to this chapter). However, as in vitro fertilization techniques were developed in the early 1980s, a second set of detailed studies clearly demonstrated that the onset of the LH surge is a better predictor of ovulation than its peak (see Table 18–1). These studies sampled LH in blood every 4 hours to identify when the LH surge begins and when it reaches its peak, and, in addition, used laparoscopy or ovarian biopsy to identify the time of ovulation. Thus, they measured precisely the interval between the LH surge and ovulation. Despite these impressive data, the majority of studies published in the last 10 years have been based on the peak of the LH surge.

All studies in Table 18–1 agree that there is less variation between the onset of the LH surge and the time of ovulation than there is between the LH peak and ovulation (the range of the time interval from LH onset until ovulation is approximately half that of the range of the time interval from the LH peak to ovulation). These findings are consistent with the observation that the critical biological event for triggering ovulation is the initial rise in LH, not its peaking (R. G. Edwards et al. 1980a; Garcia et al. 1981; Testart et al. 1981; World Health Organization 1981).

We conclude from these studies that ovulation usually occurs 36 hours after the onset of the LH surge (in blood), with a standard

Table 18–1. Interval between onset and peak of LH surge and ovulation (based on blood sampling every 4 hours and measurement of oocyte stage)

Study	LH onset		LH peak		
	Mean ± SD (hours)	Range (hours)	Mean ± SD (hours)	Range (hours)	Oocyte stage
Garcia et al. 1981	28.6 ± 1.2	27–31	10.0 ± 5.1	4–20	Preovulatory, unspecified
Seibel et al. 1982a	33.8 ± 3.8	28–38	22.0 ± 5.0	13–26	Metaphase II
Taymor et al. 1983	33.8 ± 3.5	28–38	20.0 ± 7.3	8–26	Metaphase II
Testart and Frydman 1982	—	34–39	—	14–31	Young corpus luteum
Taymor et al. 1983	38.3 ± 0.3	38–39	23.1 ± 4.0	18–27	Corpus luteum

Note. LH = luteinizing hormone.

deviation of only 2 hours. The most precise studies typically use as their marker of ovulation either a preovulatory follicle (stage metaphase II), which yields a slight underestimate (34 hours), or a young corpus luteum, which yields a slight overestimate (37–39 hours; see Table 18–1). This interval is similar to the 36- to 37-hour delay between an injection of human chorionic gonadotropin (HCG, an LH-like gonadotropin) and ovulation (R. G. Edwards et al. 1982; Jagiello et al. 1968; Testart and Frydman 1982). Moreover, the interval is within the ranges reported by other studies with less-precise techniques for sampling LH or identifying ovulation (Baviera et al. 1988; Ben-Aderet et al. 1977; Croxatto et al. 1980; Ferin et al. 1973; Lemay et al. 1982; Testart et al. 1981; World Health Organization 1980, 1981; Yussman and Taymor 1970).

The peak of the LH surge is not a reliable indicator of ovulation, partly because LH surges can have widely different shapes (see Figure 18–1). The peak of the surge can follow its onset by 1–29 hours (in blood samples; Baviera et al. 1988; Lemay et al. 1982; Seibel et al. 1982a; Taymor et al. 1983; Testart et al. 1981), and the surge can last between 16 and 70 hours (Baird 1983; Hoff et al. 1983; Landgren et al. 1982; Lemay et al. 1982; Thorneycroft et al. 1974). Furthermore, the LH peak

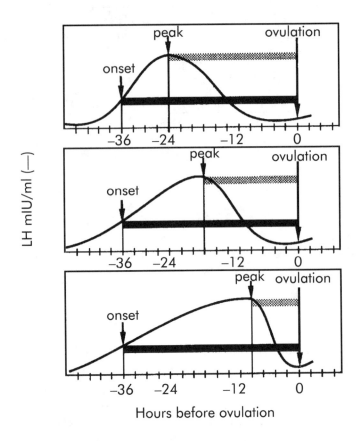

Figure 18–1. Extensive literature clearly demonstrates that the LH surge can have widely different shapes; there is less variation between the onset of the LH surge and the time of ovulation than there is between the LH peak and ovulation (Baird 1983; Baviera et al. 1988; Garcia et al. 1981; Hoff et al. 1983; Landgren et al. 1982; Lemay et al. 1982; Seibel et al. 1982a; Taymor et al. 1983; Testart and Frydman 1982; Testart et al. 1981; Thorneycroft et al. 1974). LH = luteinizing hormone.

has no consistent relationship to the stage of follicular maturation and can occur any time from 4 to 31 hours before ovulation (see Table 18–1).

Because the interval between the LH peak and ovulation is more variable than the interval between the LH onset and ovulation, studies using the LH peak have yielded variable results, especially when calendar days are used to measure the interval between the LH surge and ovulation. For example, even when sampling is conducted every 4 hours, ovulation follows the peak of the LH surge by 4–31 hours, an interval that spans 1–2 calendar days (see Table 18–1 and Figure 18–1). Thus, ovulation can occur on the same calendar day as the LH peak or on the next day. These widely different results, based only on the peak of the surge, give the impression that the temporal relationship between the LH surge and ovulation is more variable than it really is.

Although the onset of the LH surge is the best predictor of the time of ovulation, there is individual variation in the time of the onset of the LH surge. However, the variation in the time of the onset of the LH surge is not random; it is structured by circadian and annual rhythms.

Optimal Time for Daily LH Sample

The LH surge has a circadian rhythm: in blood, it usually begins in the early morning, between midnight and 8 A.M, and reaches its peak in the late afternoon or evening (in approximately 75% of cycles, LH reaches surge levels in blood before 8 A.M.; Baird 1983; Baukloh et al. 1990; Baviera et al. 1988; Testart et al. 1982). Thus, the time of day at which the LH samples are collected will affect the accuracy with which they identify the onset of the surge. Ideally, LH samples are collected every 4 hours throughout the 24-hour period, as many investigators have done (see Table 18–1). However, sampling this frequently is not always feasible, and a single daily sample is the most pragmatic method. In the 46 studies we reviewed, 50% disregard time of day either in collecting samples or in reporting results. In 37% of these studies, LH samples were collected once a day, on awakening, and in the remaining studies, LH was sampled at various other times during the day. What, then, is the optimal time of day for collecting a single daily sample with which to measure the surge onset accurately?

This question is complicated by the fact that the time of the onset of the surge has a bimodal distribution: although most LH surges begin in the morning, a small second population of surges begin in the afternoon (Casper et al. 1988; R. G. Edwards 1981; R. G. Edwards et al. 1980b;

Seibel et al. 1982b; Testart et al. 1982; cross-sectional studies of individual women). Moreover, there is a seasonal shift in this bimodal distribution. In the spring, more LH surges begin later in the day, around noon (Casper et al. 1988; R. G. Edwards et al. 1980b; Testart et al. 1982; cross-sectional studies of individual women). Thus, a *late morning blood sample* is the only way to detect the onset of these late LH surges accurately; an early morning sample would miss them altogether or would detect them a day late.

Finally, the optimal time for a daily LH sample depends on whether it is a blood or a urine sample. A blood sample taken at noon will accurately detect 80%–95% of the LH surges that begin on a given day (Seibel et al. 1982b; Testart et al. 1982). Because it requires time for LH to appear in urine, urine samples must be taken later. A *6 P.M. urine sample* will detect these typical early surges, as well as most of the second population of late surges, thus enabling accurate detection of 82%–91% of surges that begin on a given day (Casper et al. 1988; R. G. Edwards 1981; R. G. Edwards et al. 1980b).

When studies predict ovulation on the basis of the peak of the LH surge *and* detect that peak from a daily sample collected in the morning upon awakening, the two sources of error are compounded. The combination of these two errors probably explains reports that ovulation occurs anywhere from 2 days before to 4 days after the LH surge (see Table 18–2). Although biologically impossible, the report that ovulation occurs before the LH surge is probably due to LH surges of lengthy duration that have a delayed peak and therefore are detected late.

Urine samples offer several advantages over blood samples. Because the pituitary secretes LH in a pulsatile pattern, a single blood sample may not represent average hormone levels; a urine sample, on the other hand, integrates the varying levels over several hours. Additionally, urine samples are easier to collect and store.

As a result of this review of the literature, we developed a revised protocol for collecting daily LH samples. In this revised protocol a daily urine sample for LH is collected at 6 P.M. for several reasons. First, doing so minimizes the risk of missing the surges that begin in the late afternoon. Therefore, a 6 P.M. sample maximizes detection of surge levels of LH on the day that the surge actually begins. Second, 6 P.M. is close to the time the surge reaches its peak, reducing the risk of not detecting

Table 18–2. Variation in the reported relationship between ovulation (measured by ultrasound) and LH surge is associated with protocol errors made while measuring the LH surge

| Study | Percentage of cycles with ovulation on a given day Days before (−) or after (+) LH surge | | | | | | | N | Protocol errors Measured LH peak | Protocol errors Nonoptimal time for LH sample |
	−2	−1	0	+1	+2	+3	+4			
Vermesh et al. 1987				100				31	X	Not reported[a]
Depares et al. 1986		18	82					11	X	Not reported[a]
Luciano et al. 1990				6	72	21		47		Morning[a]
Flynn et al. 1984	19	28	33	10	10			21	X	First morning[b]
Singh et al. 1984		31	23	38	8			13	X	First morning[b]
Vermesh et al. 1987			54	30	10	3	3	30		First morning[b]
Vermesh et al. 1987				88	12			24		Late morning[b]

Note. LH = luteinizing hormone. [a]Blood sample. [b]Urine sample.

surge levels of LH. We can reduce variability in sample concentration by minimizing fluid intake in the afternoon. Finally, a 6 P.M. sample fits easily into most women's social schedules (i.e., at the end of the workday and before the evening meal).

Predicting the Day of Ovulation

The time of ovulation is typically predicted from LH data in terms of calendar days. One of two conflicting rules for predicting the day of ovulation is usually used. Some studies state that ovulation occurs 1 day after the peak of the LH surge, while others state that it occurs on the same day (see Table 18–3). Neither rule is universally correct because the time interval from LH peak to ovulation is so variable (4–31 hours; Table 18–1).

A correct rule needs to be based on the time of the onset of the LH surge, not the peak; ovulation occurs 36 hours after the onset in blood and 30 hours after the onset in urine (see Table 18–1 and Baviera et al. 1988; W. P. Collins et al. 1981; R. G. Edwards et al. 1980a, 1980b, 1982; Elkind-Hirsch et al. 1986; Kerin et al. 1980). Estimating this interval as 1 calendar day might be reasonable were it not for the normal and seasonal variation in the circadian timing of the surge. When the LH surge begins early in the day, as typically happens, ovulation does indeed occur 1 calendar day later. When it begins in the evening (after 6 P.M. in a urinary sample), however, ovulation occurs 2 calendar days later. For example, if the urinary LH surge begins at 9 A.M. on day 1, then ovulation will occur at approximately 3 P.M. on day 2. However, if the LH surge begins at 8 P.M. on day 1, then ovulation will occur at 2 A.M. on day 3. Thus, even when the onset of the LH surge is used, some of the apparent variation reported for the interval between the LH surge and ovulation is really an artifact of the human convention of counting calendar days beginning at midnight.

Different rules for estimating the day of ovulation have been used in most studies that assessed the validity of indirect indicators of ovulation, such as BBT or cervical mucus (see Table 18–3). In addition, these studies typically measure the peak in morning samples and do not rec-

Table 18–3. Protocol errors made in assessment of indirect indicators of ovulation: BBT and cervical mucous

Study	Measured LH peak	Nonoptimal time for LH sample	Rule for estimating day of ovulation Same day as LH peak	One day after LH peak
Billings et al. 1972	X	?		X
Moghissi et al. 1972	X	4 A.M.–5 P.M.[a]		
Flynn and Lynch 1976		?	X	X
N. M. Morris et al. 1976	X	?	X	
Lenton et al. 1977	X	?		
D. P. Wolf et al. 1977	X	?	X	
Koninckx et al. 1978	X	?		
Matthews et al. 1980	X	?	X	
Templeton et al. 1982	X	?		X
World Health Organization 1983	X	First morning[b]		
Etchepareborda et al. 1984	X	?	X	
Singh et al. 1984	X	First morning[b]	X	
Quagliarello and Arny 1986		11 A.M.–2 P.M.[b]		
Luciano et al. 1990		Morning[a]		

Note. BBT = basal body temperature; LH = luteinizing hormone. ? = Time of sampling was not reported. [a]Blood sample. [b]Urine sample.

ognize that the estimated day of ovulation is different for early and late LH surges (see Table 18–3). Not surprisingly, the conclusions of these studies are contradictory and highly questionable. In future research, we intend to use the revised protocol for sampling and interpreting LH data, and we have hypothesized that the BBT and cervical mucus indicators will be more accurate than previously reported.

Revised Protocol

In the revised protocol, a 6 P.M. urine sample is collected because then only one rule is needed to predict the day of ovulation accurately: ovulation is estimated to occur 1 day after detection of the LH surge onset (the first day of elevated LH levels). In most cases, the surge begins between midnight and 6 P.M. (82%–91%), and ovulation occurs 30 hours later, between 6 A.M. and midnight of the next calendar day (Baviera et al. 1988; Casper et al. 1988; W. P. Collins et al. 1981; R. G. Edwards 1981; R. G. Edwards et al. 1980a, 1980b, 1982; Elkind-Hirsch et al. 1986; Kerin et al. 1980). There is variation in the 30-hour interval on which this rule is based, and this variation will produce some errors (range = 15 hours; the interval between the onset of the LH surge and ovulation ranges from 20 to 35 hours [based on urine sampling for LH every 4 hours and measurement of ovulation by ultrasound or laparoscopy]; Baviera et al. 1988; R. G. Edwards et al. 1980a, 1980b, 1982; Kerin et al. 1980). This error rate, however, is negligible in comparison with that of previous methods (range = 6 days; ovulation occurs from 2 days before to 4 days after the LH surge [based on first morning urine sampling for LH and measurement of ovulation by ultrasound]; see Table 18–2).

When late surges begin after sample collection (between 6 P.M. and midnight of day 1), ovulation occurs 2 calendar days later (between midnight and 6 A.M. of day 3). Our general rule is also accurate for these late evening surges. In a cycle with a late surge, the surge will not be detected until the 6 P.M. urine sample on day 2, but applying our rule to these data predicts that ovulation occurs on day 3, which in fact will be correct.

Either home or laboratory assays for LH can be used to detect the onset of the LH surge accurately: enzyme immunoassay kits (i. e. Ovu-QUICK, OvuSTICK, or OvuKIT; Monoclonal Antibodies, Inc.) or traditional radioimmunoassays. With enzyme immunoassays, the day of the onset of the LH surge is the first day that the sample matches or exceeds the reference guide in the kit. Radioimmunoassays enable use of a ratio scale, and a typical criterion is the time when LH exceeds baseline values by 80% (Testart et al. 1981).

Comparison of Standard and Revised Protocols

In a preliminary study, we have verified the accuracy of the revised protocol for measuring the preovulatory LH surge. Subjects collected urine samples twice a day, on awakening (6–8 A.M.) and in the early evening (5–7 P.M.; $N = 18$ cycles from seven women who had regular ovulatory menstrual cycles). We used the OvuKIT (Monoclonal Antibodies, Inc.) to measure LH levels semiquantitatively, using a 5-point scale. Because two daily samples are sufficient for accurately determining the timing of the LH surge (Luciano et al. 1990), we could use these twice-a-day data to determine which day each LH surge actually began and whether it began early or late in the day (i.e., was detected first in the morning or evening sample). By sampling twice a day, the day of the onset of the LH surge was identified in all 18 cycles. These data were the standard that we used to compare the accuracy of the morning and evening samples for determining the day of the onset of the LH surge.

Data from evening samples were more accurate than those from morning samples ($P < .001$, $\chi^2 = 16.46$). Using only the evening urine samples, we correctly determined the day of the onset of the LH surge in 94% of cycles; 6% missed the LH surge. In contrast, when using only morning samples, we could correctly identify the day of the onset of the LH surge in only 22% of cycles, and the onset of the LH surge was detected 1 day late in 56% of cycles. This high error rate for data based on first morning samples is consistent with the finding that the LH surge in urine begins before 8 A.M. in only 25% of cycles (R. G. Edwards et al. 1980b). The LH surge was missed entirely in 22% of cycles. This result coincides with the report of Wilcox and colleagues (1987) that first morning sampling revealed ill-defined LH surges, or no surges at all, in 26%–32% of 260 cycles.

A series of detailed studies has repeatedly established that ovulation occurs 30 hours after the onset of the LH surge in a urine sample

(Baviera et al. 1988; W. P. Collins et al. 1981; R. G. Edwards et al. 1980a, 1980b, 1982; Elkind-Hirsch et al. 1986; Kerin et al. 1980). Using this well-established information, we can predict that ovulation occurred 1 day after the LH surge was detected in the evening urine sample. We plan to further validate our revised protocol with a larger sample size and visualization of ovulation. Nonetheless, given that our preliminary results indicate that the evening samples detect the onset of the LH surge accurately in virtually all cycles, this revised protocol is a highly promising tool for clinicians and researchers.

Menstrual Cycle Phases

To study the phases of the menstrual cycle, the revised protocol can be used to divide the menstrual cycle into hormonally distinct phases. The menstrual cycle can be divided into six hormonally distinct phases: 1) the early menses phase consists of the first 3 days of menstruation; 2) the late menses phase includes the remaining days of menstruation; 3) the follicular phase comprises the days between the late menses and LH surge phases; 4) the LH surge phase includes the LH surge onset day and the next 2 days; 5) the early luteal phase encompasses the days between the LH surge phase and the late luteal phase; and 6) the late luteal phase corresponds to the last 3 days of the cycle. The LH surge phase includes the day of the onset of the LH surge and the following 2 days, so this phase encompasses the duration of the LH surge. Because the onset of the surge is followed by ovulation on the subsequent day, this phase also includes the estimated day of ovulation plus or minus 1 day.

Conclusion

Given that our preliminary results indicate that the evening samples detect the LH surge onset accurately in virtually all cycles, this revised protocol is a highly promising tool for researchers and clinicians. The well-established data and sound logic of this review suggest that the new protocol can be used to divide the cycle into its hormonally distinct phases for research on the pharmacological, behavioral, and psychological correlates of the menstrual cycle. The revised protocol can be used to reevaluate other indirect indicators of ovulation, such as the BBT or cervical mucus, which may prove to be more accurate than previously thought.

By accurately measuring the timing of the LH surge and delineating the hormonally distinct phases of the menstrual cycle, these methods can be used to achieve a more valid, unbiased assessment of behavioral and hormonal changes in individual women during the menstrual cycle. Because endocrinological studies have established the patterns of other hormones in relation to the LH surge, researchers and clinicians can interpret the results in terms of hormonal mechanisms such as estrogens, progesterone, androgens, and adrenal hormones. Thus, the menstrual cycle can be used as a natural experiment to study the effect of these steroids on the pharmacological action of drugs, on behavior, and on psychological state.

Our protocol may also serve an important therapeutic need by improving identification of the relationship between different forms of psychopathology and the menstrual cycle. It could also improve the scheduling of TDI. In studies that have used urine LH test results to schedule TDI, none collected samples in the early evening (Barratt et al. 1989; Federman et al. 1990; Kossoy et al. 1988). Accurate prediction of the day of ovulation with our revised protocol will be a valuable tool for improving conception rates.

Finally, using the revised protocol to delineate the hormonally distinct phases of the menstrual cycle has implications for industry in terms of product development in women of childbearing potential. Product development can be conducted with specific populations of women based on the lengths of menstrual cycle phases, regular versus irregular cycles, ovulatory versus anovulatory cycles, and testing during nonfertile phases of the cycle.

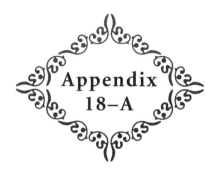

Appendix
18–A

Forty-Six Studies That Measured the Peak of the Luteinizing Hormone (LH) Surge Instead of Its Onset

Adekunle AO, Goswamy RK, Sallam HN, et al: Ultrasonic and endocrinologic monitoring of follicular growth during spontaneous and clomiphene-stimulated cycles, in Ovulation and Its Disorders (Studies in Fertility and Sterility). Edited by Thompson W, Harrison RF, Bonnar J. Boston, MA, MTP Press, 1984, pp 3–6

Barratt CLR, Cooke S, Chauhan M, et al: A prospective randomized controlled trial comparing urinary luteinizing hormone dipsticks and basal body temperature charts with time donor insemination. Fertil Steril 52:394–397, 1989

Ben-Aderet N, Potashnik G, Lunenfeld B, et al: Correlation of hormonal profile and ovarian morphologic features during the periovulatory period in humans. Fertil Steril 28:361–362, 1977

Billings EL, Brown JB, Billings JJ, et al: Symptoms and hormonal changes accompanying ovulation. Lancet 1:282–284, 1972

Brailly S, Gougeon A, Milgrom E, et al: Importance of changes in the transformation of progestin into androgen during preovulatory development and atresia of human follicles, in Follicular Maturation and Ovulation. Edited by Rolland R, Van Hall EV, Hillier SG, et al. Amsterdam, Netherlands, Excerpta Medica, 1982, pp 180–187

Collins AC, Yeager TN, Leback ME, et al: Variations in alcohol metabolism: influence of sex and age. Pharmacol Biochem Behav 3:973–978, 1975

Collins WP: Biochemical approaches to ovulation prediction and detection and the location of the fertile period in women, in Ovulation: Methods for Its Prediction and Detection (Current Topics in Reproductive Endocrinology). Edited by Jeffcoate SL. New York, Wiley, 1983, pp 49–66

Collins WP, Branch CM, Collins PO, et al: Biochemical indices of the fertile period in women. International Journal of Fertility 26:196–202, 1981

Croxatto HD, Diaz S, Fuentealba B, et al: Studies on the duration of egg transport in the human oviduct, I: the time interval between ovulation and egg recovery from the uterus in normal women. Fertil Steril 23:447–458, 1972

Depares J, Ryder REJ, Walker SM, et al: Ovarian ultrasonography highlights precision of symptoms of ovulation as markers of ovulation. BMJ 292:1562, 1986

Elkind-Hirsch K, Goldzieher JW, Gibbons WE, et al: Evaluation of the ovustick urinary luteinizing hormone kit in normal and stimulated menstrual cycles. Obstet Gynecol 67:450–452, 1986

Etchepareborda JJ, Videla L, Bortolussi S, et al: Billings natural FP method: correlation of subjective signs with ovulation and cervical mucus quality, in Research in Family Planning. Edited by Bonnar J, Thompson W, Harrison RF. Boston, MA, MTP Press, 1984, pp 17–20

Evans J: Fetal crown-rump length values in the first trimester based upon ovulation timing using the luteinizing hormone surge. Br J Obstet Gynaecol 98:48–51, 1991

Fazleabas AT, Segraves MM, Khan-Dawood FS: Evaluation of salivary and vaginal electrical resistance for determination of the time of ovulation. International Journal of Fertility 35:106–111, 1990

Federman CA, Dumesic DA, Boone WR, et al: Relative efficiency of therapeutic donor insemination using a luteinizing hormone monitor. Fertil Steril 54:489–492, 1990

Flynn AM, Lynch SS: Cervical mucus and identification of the fertile phase of the menstrual cycle. Br J Obstet Gynaecol 83:656–659, 1976

Flynn AM, Docker M, Morris R, et al: The reliability of women's subjective assessment of the fertile period relative to urinary gonadotrophins and follicular ultrasonic measurements during the menstrual cycle, in Research in Family Planning. Edited by Bonnar J, Thompson W, Harrison RF. Boston, MA, MTP Press, 1984, pp 3–11

Franks S, Van Der Spuy Z, Mason WP, et al: Luteal function after ovulation induction by pulsatile luteinizing hormone releasing hormone, in The Luteal Phase (Current Topics in Reproductive Endocrinology). Edited by Jeffcoate SL. New York, Wiley, 1985, pp 89–100

Fujimoto VY, Clifton DK, Cohen NL, et al: Variability of serum prolactin and progesterone levels in normal women: the relevance of single hormone measurements in the clinical setting. Obstet Gynecol 76:71–78, 1990

Gray RH, Campbell OM, Apelo R, et al: Risk of ovulation during lactation. Lancet 335:25–29, 1990

Grinsted J, Jacobson JD, Grinsted L, et al: Prediction of ovulation. Fertil Steril 52:388–393, 1989

Kerin JF, Edmonds DK, Warnes GM, et al: Morphological and functional relations of graafian follicle growth to ovulation in women using ultrasonic, laparoscopic and biochemical measurements. Br J Obstet Gynaecol 88:81–90, 1981

Koninckx PR, Heyns WJ, Corvelyn PA, et al: Delayed onset of luteinization as a cause of infertility. Fertil Steril 29:266–269, 1978

Kossoy LR, Hill GA, Herbert CM, et al: Therapeutic donor insemination: the impact of insemination timing with the aid of a urinary luteinizing hormone immunoassay. Fertil Steril 49:1026–1029, 1988

Lenton EA, Weston GA, Cooke ID: Problems in using basal body temperature recordings in an infertility clinic. BMJ 1:803–805, 1977

Lloyd R, Coulam CB: The accuracy of urinary luteinizing hormone testing in predicting ovulation. Am J Obstet Gynecol 160:1370–1375, 1989

Luciano AA, Peluso J, Koch EI, et al: Temporal relationship and reliability of the clinical, hormonal, and ultrasonographic indices of ovulation in infertile women. Obstet Gynecol 75:412–416, 1990

Matthews CD, Broom TJ, Black T, et al: Optimal features of basal body temperature recordings associated with conceptional cycles. International Journal of Fertility 2:319–320, 1980

Moghissi KS: Accuracy of basal body temperature for ovulation detection. Fertil Steril 27:1415–1421, 1976

Moghissi KS, Syner FN, Evans TN: A composite picture of the menstrual cycle. Am J Obstet Gynecol 114:405–418, 1972

Morishita H, Hashimoto T, Mitani H, et al: Cervical mucus and prediction of the time of ovulation. Gynecol Obstet Invest 10:157–162, 1979

Morris NM, Underwood LE, Easterling WJ: Temporal relationship between basal body temperature nadir and luteinizing hormone surge in normal women. Fertil Steril 27:780–783, 1976

Nielsen HK, Brixen K, Bouillon R, et al: Changes in biochemical markers of osteoblastic activity during the menstrual cycle. J Clin Endocrinol Metab 70:1431–1437, 1990

Nulsen J, Wheeler C, Ausmanas M, et al: Cervical mucus changes in relationship to urinary luteinizing hormone. Fertil Steril 48:783–786, 1987

Pache TD, Wladimiroff JW, De Jong FH, et al: Growth patterns of nondominant ovarian follicles during the normal menstrual cycle. Fertil Steril 54:638–642, 1990

Pauerstein CJ, Eddy CA, Croxatto HD, et al: Temporal relationship of estrogen, progesterone, and luteinizing hormone levels to ovulation in women and infrahuman primates. Am J Obstet Gynecol 130:876–886, 1978

Paz G, Yogev L, Gottreich A, et al: Determination of urinary luteinizing hormone for prediction of ovulation. Gynecol Obstet Invest 29:207–210, 1990

Prendiville W, Baker TS: The relationship between the ratio of El-3-G/Pd-3-G and the fertile period, in Research in Family Planning (Studies in Fertility and Sterility). Edited by Bonnar J, Thompson W, Harrison RF. Boston, MA, MTP Press, 1984, pp 53–54

Quagliarello J, Arny M: Inaccuracy of basal body temperature charts in predicting urinary luteinizing hormone surges. Fertil Steril 45:334–337, 1986

Reddi K, Wickings EJ, McNeilly AS, et al: Circulating bioactive follicle stimulating hormone and immunoreactive inhibin levels during the normal human menstrual cycle. Clin Endocrinol (Oxford) 33:547–557, 1990

Singh M, Saxena BB, Rathnam P: Clinical validation of enzyme immu-
    noassay of human luteinizing hormone (hLH) in the detection of the
    preovulatory luteinizing hormone (LH) surge in urine. Fertil Steril
    41:210–217, 1984

Templeton AA, Penney GC, Lees MM: Relation between the luteinizing
    hormone peak, the nadir of the basal body temperature and the cer-
    vical mucus score. Br J Obstet Gynaecol 89:985–988, 1982

Tredway DR, Chan P, Henig I, et al: Effectiveness of stimulated menstrual
    cycles and Percoll sperm penetration in intrauterine insemination.
    J Reprod Med 35:103–108, 1990

Wolf DP, Blasco L, Khan MA, et al: Human cervical mucus, II: changes
    in viscoelasticity during the ovulatory menstrual cycle. Fertil Steril
    28:47–52, 1977

Wolters-Everhardt E, Vemer H, Thomas C, et al: Ultrasound versus la-
    paroscopy in the diagnosis of the LUF syndrome, in Ovulation and
    Its Disorders (Studies in Fertility and Sterility). Edited by Thompson
    W, Harrison RF, Bonnar J. Boston, MA, MTP Press, 1984, pp 13–19

World Health Organization: Temporal relationships between indices of
    the fertile period. Fertil Steril 39:647–655, 1983

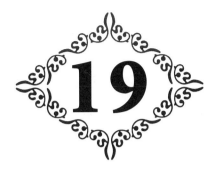

Future Research Directions

Methodological Considerations for Advancing Gender-Sensitive Pharmacology

Margaret F. Jensvold, M.D., Jean A. Hamilton, M.D., and Uriel Halbreich, M.D.

The types of studies needed to advance gender-sensitive pharmacology are often complex. In this chapter we discuss some of the methodological considerations in designing future research.

Worth noting is that sex differences in pharmacology may arise from 1) differences specific to the sexes (e.g., reproductive system differences), 2) differences in the frequency of a particular characteristic even though that characteristic could occur in persons of either sex, 3) pharmacokinetic and/or pharmacodynamic factors, and 4) gender-related factors (with gender being a complex, biopsychosocially constructed variable).

Pharmacokinetics and Pharmacodynamics

Studies of pharmacokinetics are much more common than ones of pharmacodynamics, mainly for methodological reasons. Pharmacokinetics is easier to study. Furthermore, pharmacokinetic factors must be assessed or controlled before conclusions about pharmacodynamics can be drawn. Although a number of factors make measuring effects of drugs difficult, there are many reasons why knowledge of pharmacokinetics alone is not sufficient and why an understanding of pharmacodynamics is important (Table 19–1). *Actions* of drugs are ultimately more important than plasma levels of drugs. For psychopharmacological agents, it is particularly important to measure dose–blood-level–*effect* relationships over time, rather than merely dose–blood-level relationships alone, in order to explain rationally the findings of effect and concentration measurements (Galeazzi 1985). Future research will focus on sex differences in pharmacodynamics, not just pharmacokinetics (U.S. Food and Drug Administration [FDA] 1993).

To sort out the relative contributions of pharmacokinetic (PK) and pharmacodynamic (PD) factors, dose–concentration–response curves are plotted, mathematical models applied, and actual concentrations compared with predicted concentrations (Galeazzi 1985).

Revised FDA Guidelines Encourage Informed Individualization of Treatment

Changes in FDA guidelines since 1988 (U.S. FDA 1988, 1989, 1990, 1992, 1993) have supported "informed individualization of treatment," taking into account the needs of the elderly, children, and both sexes. Table 19–2 lists the variables that the FDA's revised 1993 guidelines recommend be incorporated in drug development studies to adequately study sex differences in drugs.

Table 19–1. Pharmacokinetics versus pharmacodynamics

Reasons for popularity of pharmacokinetics studies

◆ Increasingly accurate methods have been developed to measure drug concentrations in biological fluids.

◆ Most drugs' concentrations can be measured in most patients repeatedly, making it possible to sample data many possible times.

◆ The mathematical concepts of pharmacokinetics—half-life, clearance, and "compartment"—can be conceptualized by nonmathematicians.

◆ Effects of physiological and pathological parameters on pharmacokinetic factors can be easily studied.

Factors contributing to difficulty in measuring drug effects

◆ Measurable effects show large variability, both physiological and methodological.

◆ The effects measurable in the laboratory are often not the clinically important ones.

◆ Tolerance may develop and the relationship between effect and concentration may then change.

◆ Nonevents are not measurable. If a drug is taken preventively, it may not be possible to determine whether absence of the adverse event was due to the drug or due to benign course of the disease.

◆ Mathematical formulae are difficult to conceptualize.

Reasons for measuring effects of drugs rather than simply blood levels

◆ The variability of the plasma level–effect relationship is large (this is particularly true for most antidepressant drugs).

◆ The response need not be parallel to concentrations in a measurable compartment.

◆ Diseases may have a different impact on the kinetics than on the effects.

◆ Effects may persist long after measurable concentrations of drug have disappeared.

◆ Bioavailability is usually determined by measuring blood levels and comparing areas-under-the-concentration (AUC) vs. time curves after the administration of drugs. However, it is becoming apparent that the rate of administration and the duration of certain levels are more important than AUC vs. time curve, which corresponds to total amount absorbed.

◆ Different routes of administration of the same drug may lead to different concentration-effect relationships.

Source. Galeazzi 1985.

Table 19–2.   Data analyses recommended by the FDA for studies of sex differences in drugs

Perform analyses of
A.   Effectiveness
B.   Adverse effects
C.   Dose-response
Include analyses by
1.   Demographic variables (age, race, sex)
2.   Other patient factors (body weight; renal, cardiac, and hepatic status; concomitant illnesses; concomitant use of drugs)

Generally, both sexes would be included, except in studies for which only one is appropriate (e.g., in some menstrual cycle studies, female patients and female control subjects would be adequate; in other menstrual cycle studies, a male control group would be informative).

In addition, three pharmacokinetic issues specific to women should be investigated:
1.   Menstrual status (premenopausal, postmenopausal, within-cycle change)
2.   Concomitant supplementary estrogen treatment or systemic contraception
3.   The influence of drugs on hormonal contraceptives (excretion, metabolism, and steepness of dose-response curve)

The FDA recommends reviewing data on what is known of the drug to determine whether there is any reason to suspect changes in pharmacokinetics over the course of the menstrual cycle. If so,
1.   Take measures to decrease or adjust for variability, meaning
    a.   Administer the drug at the same time in the cycle, or
    b.   Study a large number of subjects.
2.   Consider doing specific formal pharmacokinetic studies in such cases.

Pharmacokinetic studies can be performed in two ways:
1.   Pharmacokinetic screen ("troughing")
2.   Specific pharmacokinetic studies in specific subpopulations

Precautions should be taken to avoid exposure of fetuses to drugs; specifically:
1.   Require use of reliable contraception.
2.   Employ use of pregnancy testing (β–human chorionic gonadotropin [β-HCG]).
3.   Time short-duration studies to occur during or immediately after menstruation.
4.   Refer the patient to a physician knowledgeable about contraceptive methods.

Source.   FDA = U.S. Food and Drug Administration 1993.

The Menstrual Cycle in Pharmacology

Model Research Design: Repeated-Measures Study of Menstrual Cycle Phase Effects on Physiology, Pathophysiology, and Drugs

In most pharmacological research, the menstrual cycle has been over-looked as a potentially important variable. The menstrual cycle, however, clearly influences the need for or effects of drugs in some women (Hamilton and Yonkers, Chapter 2, this volume; Jensvold, Chapter 8, this volume). Among reproductive-age women with migraine headaches, asthma, seizures, and certain other conditions, some women's symptoms occur in relation to the menstrual cycle (i.e., are catamenial) and other women's symptoms occur independent of menstrual cycle phase (i.e., are noncatamenial). For example, daily spirometry ratings confirmed that asthmatic women correctly self-identified that their asthmatic symptoms did or did not vary with menstrual cycle phase (Hanley 1981). Among women with seizure disorders, menstrual cycle phase–dependent changes in blood levels of anticonvulsant medication occurred in women with catamenial seizures but not in those with noncatamenial seizures (Shavit et al. 1984) or in asymptomatic control subjects (Kumar et al. 1988). If menstrual cycle–related changes in symptoms occur in only a minority of women with a condition, the ability to recognize the menstrual cycle association may be lost in studies that pool data from all subjects. Asking women to self-report whether their symptoms vary in relation to the menstrual cycle may help in stratifying data analysis.

Certain medications—for example, nonsteroidal antiinflammatory drugs taken for treatment of dysmenorrhea—may be consumed more frequently or only during certain menstrual cycle phases. Other drugs may be taken regularly but may have varying benefit over the menstrual cycle (Conrad and Hamilton 1986; Gengo et al. 1984; Jensvold et al. 1992; Kimmel et al. 1992).

Physiological changes during the normal menstrual cycle may affect the need for or the effects of drugs. Pathophysiological processes en-trained to or deriving from the menstrual cycle may influence drugs. The mechanisms of these changes may involve PK or PD factors or both.

To distinguish among 1) the effects of physiological versus pathophysiological processes on drugs and 2) the pharmacokinetic versus pharmacodynamic effects versus expectancy, a repeated-measures research design can be applied (Figure 19–1).

With information on dose, blood levels, and effects of medication during different menstrual cycle phases, some conclusions can be drawn about phase effects and the relative contributions of PK and PD to those differences. The choice of control group(s) influences which additional variable(s) can be studied. If the patients are symptomatic regularly cycling women and the control subjects are asymptomatic regularly cycling women, conclusions can be drawn about the effects of normal menstrual cycle physiology versus pathophysiology on drugs. If a male control group is included, conclusions can be drawn about sex (male–female) differences.

Symptom ratings at baseline (before drug administration) and during or after administration of active drug and placebo allow one to dis-

		Baseline			Drug 1			Drug 2		
		P1	P2	P*n*	P1	P2	P*n*	P1	P2	P*n*
Group 1	Drug levels (*n* phases)									
	Self-ratings (*n* phases, daily)									
	Observer ratings (*n* phases)									
Group 2	Drug levels (*n* phases)									
	Self-ratings (*n* phases, daily)									
	Observer ratings (*n* phases)									

Figure 19–1. Model research design for menstrual cycle drug trials. Groups 1 and 2 = patients and asymptomatic control subjects, or patients with catamenial symptoms and patients with noncatamenial symptoms, etc. Drugs 1 and 2 = drug and placebo, or two different active drugs, etc.

tinguish among 1) presence or absence of symptomatology before drug administration, 2) menstrual cycle relationship of symptoms without drug and with drug, and 3) effects of active drug versus placebo.

The basic study design can be modified for use in studies of 1) medication taken regularly (e.g., baseline measurements × 2 cycles, active drug × 2 cycles, placebo × 2 cycles; blood levels drawn and ratings completed during two or more phases per cycle; self-ratings completed daily), or 2) bolus medication (e.g., drug infusions administered during two or more phases per cycle; ratings completed before infusion and at regular time intervals after infusions). With infusion studies, hormonal responses to the drug may also be measured; an example is growth hormone and cortisol responses to clonidine infusion during different menstrual cycle phases (Jensvold et al. 1990a, 1990b).

With a repeated-measures design, data may be analyzed by means of time-series analyses (for data measured at three or more time points) or "deltas" (difference between two points).

Although repeated-measures studies are relatively time and labor intensive, more such investigations are needed to better understand the contributions of PK and PD, physiology, and pathophysiology to studies of sex differences and phase effects with drugs.

Additional targeted studies would be needed to determine the underlying mechanisms of any PK or PD changes. Absorption, distribution, metabolism, and/or elimination may contribute to PK differences. PD mechanisms may involve changes in receptor populations, receptor-binding sensitivity, or postreceptor/intracellular effects. Basic animal research and in vitro studies may inform this process.

Several issues requiring further discussion include 1) the use of pharmacokinetic screen versus formal pharmacokinetic studies, 2) the number of menstrual cycle phases that should be studied, and 3) the role of daily ratings by study subjects.

Pharmacokinetic Screen Versus Formal Pharmacokinetic Studies

In the pharmacokinetic screen—or *troughing*—recommended by the FDA (1993; see also Harrison and Brumfield, Chapter 17, this volume), blood levels from large numbers of women taken at approximately the same times in the menstrual cycle are pooled to look for differences in average blood levels between menstrual cycle phases. With this method, large differences can theoretically be detected. The great advantage of this approach is that it can be accomplished fairly easily using a relatively small number of samples taken from each person participating in phase II and III studies, with potentially large numbers of subjects participating in the study. Data can be analyzed in a stratified manner to compare for effects of different factors, such as age, race, sex, concomitant conditions, and concurrent medications. However, changes in drug levels occurring at times in the menstrual cycle other than the time points measured will be missed. Changes occurring over the course of the menstrual cycle that are significant but that occur only in a minority of women (Smith and Lin, Chapter 7, this volume) may be obscured by pooling data. Significant changes occurring in opposite directions in subgroups of women may cancel one another out. A negative finding regarding phase differences in blood levels does not rule out pharmacodynamic differences.

The pharmacokinetic screen will provide some useful information, but formal PK studies will still be necessary to answer certain questions. Longitudinal and within-subject studies have substantial scientific advantages over studies that measure a few time points and pool results from different women. Although formal pharmacokinetic studies may be more time and labor intensive per study subject, fewer study subjects may be needed. These studies will be performed in a targeted manner rather than routinely.

During How Many Menstrual Cycle Phases Should Drug Effects Be Studied?

Due to differences in cycle length, the number of days from the beginning of the menstrual cycle does not necessarily correspond to the same phase in all women. Consequently, care must be taken to ensure that the samples pooled in fact represent the same menstrual cycle phase.

Stern and McClintock recommend a method by which the menstrual cycle is divided into six hormonally distinct phases (see Stern and McClintock, Chapter 18, this volume).

In 1986, the Society for Menstrual Cycle Research (SMCR) recommended that data in menstrual cycle studies be divided into five phases: *menses, premenstrual phase* (defined as the 7 days preceding menses; this covers the entire period of estrogen and progesterone decline), *ovulation* (defined as 5 days, the day of ovulation and the 2 days on both sides; this covers the entire period of ovulatory change), *postmenses* (of variable length, from the end of menses to the ovulatory phase), and *postovulatory period* (of variable length, from the end of the ovulatory phase to the beginning of the premenstrual phase). The premenstrual phase can be divided into two subphases: *early premenses* (covering the early, slow decline of estrogen and progesterone) and *late premenses* (covering the late, precipitous decline in estrogen and progesterone levels) (SMCR 1986a, 1986b; see also Stern and McClintock, Chapter 18, this volume).

The major differences between the SMCR method and the Stern and McClintock method are that 1) the former counts premenses as one phase, whereas the latter delineates an early menses phase and a late menses phase; and 2) the luteinizing hormone (LH) surge/ovulation phase is shorter (3 days) in the Stern and McClintock method than in the SMCR's 1986 recommendation (5 days) because Stern and McClintock's protocol for timing ovulation is more accurate than previous commonly used methods.

How Many Measurements During the Menstrual Cycle Are Sufficient?

The greater the number of time points measured, the more sophisticated the conclusions that can be drawn. Measurement of drug levels at two time points may allow for comparisons of drug levels at times when hormone levels measured in the periphery are high versus low. However, measuring at only two time points may miss key events happening at other times in the cycle. The cycle is, after all, a continuous event, with change occurring at all times. Frequency of blood sampling is important with periodic phenomena. For example, sampling at 1- to 4-minute intervals was needed before the high-frequency pulsatility of LH could be detected. It was missed altogether as long as LH levels were measured only every 20 minutes (Veldhuis et al. 1984). A study that examined anticonvulsant drug levels daily over nine menstrual cycles in six women found a significant drop in drug levels between days 27 and 28 of the menstrual cycle, corresponding with worsening of symptoms at that time. Measurements twice per cycle could not have detected the drop between days 27 and 28. Also, comparing blood levels and effects at only two time points presumes that effects correlate with current blood levels. This assumption disregards the possibility that effects may be influenced by blood levels or physiological events occurring a number of days earlier (Rojansky et al. 1991).

Many studies examine drug levels at only two points in the menstrual cycle. The most frequently studied phase pairs are the early follicular + midluteal phases and midfollicular + late luteal phases. Those paired time points contrast times of high versus low blood levels of estrogen and/or progesterone.

Dye (1990) concluded that drug levels drawn twice in the menstrual cycle are "entirely inadequate." Four test sessions have been considered to be the minimum necessary by some authors (Bruguerolle 1986; Dye 1990; Jensvold, Chapter 8, this volume). A group proposing policy changes recommended that blood levels be drawn in "at least two and possibly three menstrual cycle phases, luteal, follicular and during menses" (Hamilton 1991, p. 25). The number of measurements needed depends on the questions being asked. Fewer time points in more study subjects will answer certain questions. More time points in fewer subjects will answer other questions.

It is worth noting that among women who report "premenstrual symptoms," the length of the symptomatic phase is quite variable, ranging from 1 day to the entire luteal phase (Halbreich and Endicott 1985a). Onset of symptoms at different times (e.g., during the early, middle, or late luteal phase or during menses) may represent different mechanisms of symptoms.

Drug levels should be drawn at approximately the same time of day to control for an interactive effect of circadian rhythms with circamenstrual rhythms (Bruguerolle 1986; Dye 1990).

The day of ovulation should be determined whenever possible. An accurate and practical method for assessing the time of ovulation is described by Stern and McClintock (Chapter 18, this volume): Collect urine samples daily at 6 P.M. and measure urine LH levels. Ovulation is estimated to occur 1 day after onset of the LH surge (which is the first day of elevated LH levels). More precise timing of ovulation results in improved accuracy of assignment of data to particular menstrual cycle phases, significantly increasing comparability of data across menstrual cycles.

Daily ratings. Daily ratings serve different purposes in research and clinical arenas. For research, symptoms must be recorded to be quantified and to allow comparisons to be made over time. When medication is taken on a regular basis, ratings should be made daily. In bolus studies, ratings should be made before and at regular intervals after administration of the drug.

Research subjects may either 1) record the number and severity of discrete events—such as seizures, migraine headaches, or panic attacks—in a daily diary or 2) complete rating scales—such as analog or digital scales of mood or anxiety symptoms—daily or at specified times.

In clinical care settings, daily ratings may help the patient and the clinician to better understand the pattern of the patient's symptoms, thus assisting the patient in coping strategies and aiding the clinician in designing treatment strategies.

However, a major assumption among most premenstrual syndrome investigators—that daily ratings are always the "gold standard" of diagnosis and that they automatically take precedence over the patient's retrospective self-report of usual presence or absence of premenstrual syndrome (PMS)—has been challenged by some. It has been reported that women reporting PMS, women reporting absence of PMS, and men all might meet certain criteria for PMS based on daily ratings. What has been reported to distinguish the groups was not simply the presence or severity of symptoms, but also the degree to which there was self-identification as experiencing PMS (Gallant et al. 1992a, 1992b).

For clinical and research purposes, categorizing patients based on their self-reports and daily ratings as *concordant positive* (the patient reports having menstrual cycle–related symptoms and daily ratings confirm this), *concordant negative* (the patient reports *not* having menstrual cycle–related symptoms and daily ratings confirm this), or *discordant* (+ self-report/– daily rating or – self-report/ + daily rating) might be both more accurate and more helpful to the clinician and the patient in trying to understand the patient's experiences and beliefs (Jensvold 1993a). Assessing the possible reasons for discordance may be helpful to both the clinician and the patient. Patients, whether they fit into concordant or discordant subtypes, often can be helped significantly.

Some women's menstrual cycle–related symptoms may be so severe (e.g., suicidality) that it may be unethical to require them to complete daily ratings for two or more cycles before initiating treatment. Many women's symptoms can be helped significantly by medication, and they may prefer not to wait two or more cycles before embarking on treatment. Starting treatment without 2 months of daily ratings untreated disqualifies these patients from receiving a definitive diagnosis of premenstrual dysphoric disorder by DSM-IV (American Psychiatric Association 1994) criteria.

Gender Effects in Pharmacology

Model Study: Sex, Gender, and Hormonal Effects on Over-the-Counter Appetite Suppressants

Few studies have examined gender effects in psychopharmacology as opposed to sex differences. One study that in many ways might provide a model for the research needed to advance *gender*-sensitive psychopharmacology is a study of phenylpropanolamine (PPA). In this section we briefly describe a study of sex, gender, and hormonal effects on PPA and explain the rationale for the study.

PPA is the main ingredient in over-the-counter (OTC), nonprescription appetite suppressants. In reviewing all published studies of PPA in humans, Gallant et al. (S. J. Gallant, C. R. Lake, and J. A. Hamilton, "Sex, Stress, and Responses to Phenylpropanolamine and Caffeine" [revised unpublished manuscript], Uniformed Services University of the Health Sciences, Medical Psychology Department, Bethesda, MD, July 1989) documented that cardiovascular and psychological health effects of PPA have not been adequately studied for women. Despite the 9:1 excess usage of this medication in women, Gallant and colleagues found that experimental investigations of PPA's effects on blood pressure have often been conducted only in males, and that studies including females either contained only very small numbers of female subjects or did not present summary results by sex, making sex differences impossible to assess.

What makes this observation so striking is that PPA is the major ingredient in nonprescription diet medications, and women are the primary consumers of PPA diet aids (Vener and Krupka 1985). Of special concern are case reports of stroke in young women using PPA (Lake et al. 1990).

Although PPA is generally considered safe and is widely available, concerns have been raised about possible dose-related or interactive effects with other medications that may increase risk for clinically significant elevations of blood pressure (S. J. Gallant, C. R. Lake, and J. A. Hamilton, "Sex, Stress, and Responses to Phenylpropanololamine and Caffeine" [revised unpublished manuscript], Uniformed Services University of the Health Sciences, Medical Psychology Department, Bethesda, MD, July 1989; Lake et al. 1988). PPA is a sympathomimetic agent, with a structure similar to that of amphetamine. Other sympathomimetics are known to elevate blood pressure.

The rationale for conducting sex-related studies of PPA derives in part from a variety of basic science findings. Sex-steroid hormones modulate the neurochemical substrate for PPA action (J. A. Hamilton, unpublished data, June 1989). Estrogen affects arteriolar contractile responses to sympathomimetics similar to PPA (e.g., norepinephrine and phenylephrine). PPA has a weak inhibitory effect on monoamine oxidase (Lasagna 1988) that appears to vary with menstrual cycle phase (Belmaker et al. 1974). Sex steroids affect central biogenic amines, and PPA effects will be enhanced by gonadal steroids.

Another reason that a study of PPA use in women would be of high interest is that the drug's connection to dieting highlights the role of gender in pharmacology as a partly socially constructed variable. As one example, women seek diet aids such as PPA partly because of social pressures for thinness. These pressures may lead women to take higher dosages than are recommended.

In addition, the ecological context in which drug use actually occurs in women, as well as in men, is of interest. Some women in natural settings undoubtedly consume PPA along with caffeine and oral contraceptives. Caffeine and oral contraceptives can independently have blood pressure–elevating effects, so it is reasonable to wonder whether there may be additive or interactive effects with PPA. Because the half-life of caffeine is doubled in oral contraceptive users, it is suggested that any potentiating effects on responses to PPA may be prolonged (S. J. Gallant, C. R. Lake, and J. A. Hamilton, "Sex, Stress, and Responses to Phenyl-propanololamine and Caffeine" [revised unpublished manuscript], Uniformed Services University of the Health Sciences, Medical Psychology Department, Bethesda, MD, July 1989).

Sex, gender, and hormone effects on PPA could be studied in a two-part experimental design using double-blind, randomized, placebo-controlled trials.

In the first part of the study, the effects of 1) usual-dose or 2) higher-dose PPA, or of 3) PPA and caffeine on blood pressure would be tested in males and females, with the latter tested during the early follicular cycle phase (when hormones are at their lowest levels), and with some women 4) also taking oral contraceptives. In addition, a subgroup of women would be tested at two points in the menstrual cycle: early follicular and midluteal.

In the second part of the study, responses to various stressors would be assessed in males and females with and without a family history of hypertension. Because stress may enhance PPA-induced blood pressure elevation, effects would be studied under differing conditions of stress. In addition, because males and females do not find laboratory stressors to be equally salient, a variety of stressors must be used to characterize stress reactivity in males and females.

Another issue deserving attention in future psychopharmacology research is the need for better documentation of study subjects in journal articles. This includes identification of the study subjects' sex and premenopausal or postmenopausal status and of whether they are taking hormonal contraceptives, hormone replacement therapy, or neither. Better identification of study subjects will assist with the meta-analysis of data.

Conclusion

More and better designed research is needed to improve our understanding of the important effects of sex and gender on psychopharmacology. Types of studies needed include investigations of factors unique to or more salient in women (for example, menstrual cycle research); multivariate studies examining interactions of biological, psychological, and social factors (such as the phenylpropanololamine [PPA] study described in this chapter); and meta-analyses of numerous studies already conducted (such as the meta-analysis of sex differences in response to imipramine described in Chapter 12). Such research, if pursued, can be expected to contribute significantly to the growth of a more gender-sensitive psychopharmacology, both refining research methodologies in this area and yielding knowledge whose application will result in improved clinical care not only for women but for all patients.

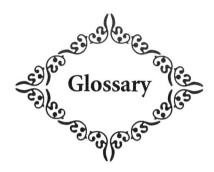

Glossary

absorption The uptake of substances into or across tissues (e.g., skin, intestine, and kidney tubules).

acid Any of a large class of chemical substances defined by three chemical concepts of increasing generality: 1) a substance that lowers the pH (increases the ion concentration) when added to an aqueous solution; 2) a species that acts as a proton donor in solution; 3) a species that can accept a pair of electrons to form a covalent bond.

acidity The quality of being acid or sour; containing acid (hydrogen ions).

amino acid Any organic compound containing an amino and a carboxyl group. *See also* protein.

antagonist A substance that tends to nullify the action of another, as a drug that binds to a cell receptor without eliciting a biological response.

antisense DNA In molecular genetics, the strand of a double-stranded DNA that is complementary to the *sense* (q.v.) strand. *See* sense DNA.

assay Determination of the amount of a particular constituent of a mixture, or of the biological or pharmacological potency of a drug.

Sources:

1. *Dorland's Medical Dictionary,* 28th Edition. Philadelphia, PA, WB Saunders, 1994.
2. *Stedman's Medical Dictionary,* 25th Edition. Baltimore, MD, Williams & Wilkins, 1990.
3. Segen JC (ed): *The Dictionary of Modern Medicine.* Park Ridge, NJ, Parthenon, 1992.
4. *International Dictionary of Medicine and Biology.* New York, Wiley, 1986.

autoinduction   A drug may increase its own metabolism by inducing the liver to produce the enzymes that metabolize the drug. *See also* microsomal enzymes.

base   In chemistry, the nonacid part of a salt; a substance that combines with acids to form salts; a substance that dissociates to give hydroxide ions in aqueous solutions; a substance with a molecular ion that can combine with a proton (hydrogen ion); a substance capable of donating a pair of electrons (to an acid) for the formation of a covalent bond.

> **purine bases and pyrimidine bases**   Groups of compounds in which purines or pyrimidines, respectively, are the bases. Common constituents of nucleic acids. *See* deoxyribonucleic acid; *see also* ribonucleic acid.

binding protein   Any of a number of plasma proteins that bind to hormones of low solubility (chiefly the thyroid and steroid hormones), thus providing a transport system for them. Some binding proteins are specific for particular hormones, while others bind to any sparingly soluble hormones. Also called *carrier protein* and *transport protein*.

bioavailability   The degree to which a drug or other substance becomes available to the target tissue after administration.

biotransformation   The series of chemical alterations of a compound (e.g., a drug) that occur within the body as by enzymatic activity.

capacity   1. Power or ability to hold, retain, or contain, or the ability to absorb. 2. Maximum ability to do a task (e.g., drug-metabolizing capacity).

chain, side   *See* side chain.

chronobiology   The scientific study of the effect of time on living systems.

clearance   1. The process of clearing; the rate at which a substance is removed from the blood; 2. A quantitative measure of the rate at which a substance is removed from the blood; the volume of plasma that is completely cleared of the substance per unit time. *See also* creatinine clearance.

conjugated protein   *See* protein.

conjugation   In chemistry, the act of joining together of two compounds to produce another compound, such as the combination of a toxic product with some substance in the body to form a detoxified product that can then be eliminated.

creatinine   The cyclic anhydride of creatine, produced as the final product of decomposition of phosphocreatine and excreted in the urine. *See also* creatinine clearance.

creatinine clearance   The renal clearance of exogenous creatinine, a commonly used clinical measurement that closely estimates the glomerular filtration rate (GFR). Measurements of excretion rates of creatinine are used as diagnostic indicators of kidney function and muscle mass and can be used to simplify other clinical assays.

cyclic   In chemistry, having a molecular structure containing one or more rings.

> **heterocyclic**   Having or pertaining to a closed chain or ring formation that includes atoms of different elements.
>
> **tetracyclic**   Containing four fused rings or closed chains in the molecular structure.
>
> **tricyclic**   Containing three fused rings or closed chains in the molecular structure.

cytochrome   Any electron transfer hemoprotein having a mode of action in which the transfer of a single electron is effected by a reversible valence charge of the central iron atom of the heme prosthetic group between the +2 and +3 oxidation states; classified as *cytochromes a* when the heme contains a formyl side chain, *cytochromes b* when protoheme (or a closely similar heme) is not covalently bound to the protein, *cytochromes c* when the protoheme or other heme is covalently bound to the protein, and *cytochromes d* when the iron-tetra-pyrrole has fewer conjugated double bonds than the hemes have. Well-known cytochromes have been numbered within groups and are designated by subscripts (beginning with no subscript; e.g., cytochromes c, c_1, c_2, ...). New cytochromes are named according to the wavelength in nanometers of the absorption maximum of the alpha (α)-band of the iron (II) form in pyridine.

> **cytochrome P450, P450**   Trivial name (P for pigment, 450 nm for the absorption maximum of the carbon monoxide derivative) for a cytochrome occurring in most tissues and containing a protoheme IX prosthetic group. It serves as the oxygenating

catalyst in a wide variety of reactions catalyzed by monooxygenases (e.g., hydroxylation of steroid hormones and oxidations involved in the detoxification of many drugs). Cytochrome P450 activates molecular oxygen for an attack on the substrate.

demethylation Removal of a methyl group.

deoxyribonuclease DNAse, any nuclease specifically catalyzing the cleavage of phosphate ester linkages in deoxyribonucleic acids.

deoxyribonucleic acid (DNA) The nucleic acid in which the sugar is deoxyribose, constituting the primary genetic material of all cellular organisms and the DNA viruses, and occurring predominantly in the nucleus. It is a linear or a circular polymer with a backbone composed of deoxyribose moieties that are linked by phosphate groups attached to their 5′ and 3′ hydroxyls, with side chains composed of purine (adenine, guanine) and pyrimidine (cytosine, thymine) bases attached to the sugars. In double-stranded DNA, adenine forms two hydrogen bonds with thymine, and cytosine forms three with guanine; these are complementary base pairs. The strands are twisted to form a double helix and are antiparallel. DNA is duplicated by replication, and it serves as a template for synthesis of ribonucleic acid (transcription), from which, in turn, polypeptide chains (proteins) are synthesized (translation).

DNA *See* deoxyribonucleic acid.

DNAse *See* deoxyribonuclease.

efficacy In pharmacology, the ability of a drug to produce the desired therapeutic effect; it is independent of *potency,* which expresses the amount of the drug necessary to achieve the desired effect.

electrolyte *See* ion.

electrophoresis The separation of ionic solutes based on differences in their rates of migration in an applied electric field.

　　gel electrophoresis A type of electrophoresis in which the support medium is a gel, in the form of tubes or in a thin slab; it is usually composed of agarose, polyacrylamide, or starch and is so named. Specific types are used to separate certain classes of molecules on the basis of charge, size, or both. Also called *electrophoretic mobility shift assay.*

electrophoretic mobility shift assay *See* electrophoresis.

element   A simple or fundamental component of a more complex entity (e.g., estrogen response element).

> **transposable element**   Any piece of duplex DNA capable of moving from one location in a genome to another, such as a transposon in bacteria.

elimination   The act of expulsion or of extrusion, especially expulsion from the body. *Compare with* excretion.

estrus   The recurrent, restricted period of sexual receptivity in female mammals other than human females, marked by intense sexual urge. *See also* estrus cycle.

estrus cycle   The recurring periods of heat, or estrus, in the adult female of most mammals and the correlated changes in the reproductive tract from one period to the next. Includes estrus, metestrus, diestrus, and proestrus phases. Also known as *estrous cycle.*

excrete   To throw off or eliminate, as waste matter, by a normal discharge.

excretion   1. The act, process, or function of excreting. 2. Material that is excreted. *Compare with* elimination.

factor   An agent or element that contributes to the production of a result, such as a chemical compound that is essential to a reaction (e.g., a transcription factor).

filtration   The passage of a liquid through a filter, accomplished by gravity, pressure, vacuum, or suction.

> **glomerular filtration**   Passage of uriniferous liquid through the glomerular tubuli of the kidney.

first-pass elimination   Presystemic elimination. The rate at which circulating drugs are metabolized as they traverse the liver; first-pass elimination kinetics assume the amount of parent drug arriving at the liver is proportional to its concentration in the circulation, and further assumes there is optimal blood flow, uncompromised hepatic function, free access of the drug to the liver's metabolic "machinery," and appropriate transportation by carrier molecules.

first-pass metabolism   Presystemic metabolism; the rate at which circulating drugs are metabolized as they traverse the liver. *See also* first-pass elimination.

follicle, ovarian   The egg-containing, fluid-filled sphere that develops in the ovary and ruptures at ovulation to liberate the ovum. It is also an endocrine gland, producing estrogens and giving rise after ovulation to the corpus luteum. The egg and its encasing cells, at any stage of its development.

follicular phase The first half of the menstrual cycle, lasting from the onset of menses until ovulation. During the follicular phase, the oocyte develops in the primordial follicle, ending when the follicle ruptures at ovulation, releasing the oocyte.

gender The complex of attitudes, expectations, and the like, that a society or individual attaches to the male and female roles; *see* sex, psychological and sex, social. A culturally, socially, or biopsychosocially defined variable (Deaux 1993).

gene A segment of a DNA molecule that contains all of the information required for synthesis of a product (polypeptide chain or RNA molecule), including both coding and noncoding sequences. It is the biological unit of heredity, self-reproducing, and transmitted from parent to progeny. Each gene has a specific position *(locus)* on the chromosome map. From the standpoint of function, genes are conceived of as structural, operational, and regulatory genes.

glomerulus, renal Globular tuft of capillaries, projecting into the expanded end or capsule of each of the uriniferous tubules of the kidney, which together with the kidney's surrounding capsule (glomerular capsule) constitute the renal corpuscle. Plural, glomeruli.

half-life $(t^1/_2)$ The time taken for the concentration of a substance to fall to half of its initial value, either by catabolism (biological half-life), or by elimination in a system (elimination half-life), or by degradation and/or decay (radioactive half-life). This time is independent of the initial concentration in many processes—as, for example, in radioactive decay—and approximately so for others—as in the elimination of many foreign substances from the body.

hepatic microsomal drug-metabolizing systems *See* microsomal enzymes.

heterocyclic *See* cyclic.

hybridization The act or process of producing hybrids.

> **in situ hybridization** Molecular hybridization in which a known nucleic acid, single stranded and usually labeled with radioactivity or fluorescence, is applied to prepared cells or histologic sections and annealing occurs in situ; performed to analyze

the intracellular or intrachromosomal distribution, transcription, or other characteristics of the nucleic acids.

molecular hybridization In molecular biology, formation of a partially or wholly complementary nucleic acid duplex by association of single strands, usually between DNA and RNA strands or previously unassociated DNA strands, and also between RNA strands; used to detect and isolate sequences, measure homology, or define other characteristics of one or both strands.

hydrosoluble Soluble in water.

hypersensitivity A state of altered reactivity in which the body reacts with an exaggerated response; exhibiting abnormally increased sensitivity. *See also* sensitivity.

hypersensitization The process of rendering or condition of being abnormally sensitive.

index, therapeutic *See* therapeutic index.

induction The act or process of inducing or causing to occur.

enzyme induction Increased synthesis of an enzyme in response to an inducer or other stimulus.

inhibin A nonsteroid, gonad-derived inhibitor of pituitary follicle-stimulating hormone (FSH) secretion.

in situ In the natural or normal place; confined to the site of origin without invasion of neighboring tissues.

in situ hybridization *See* hybridization, in situ.

intron, or intronic sequence A noncoding intervening sequence in a gene; almost all eukaryotic genes contain several introns separating the coding sequences (exons). After the 5′ cap and polyA tail are added to a primary mRNA transcript, the introns are removed and the exons spliced together by enzymes that recognize short sequences that identify exon-intron junctions, resulting in a mature mRNA that is ready for translation (protein synthesis). Also called *intervening sequence.*

in vitro Within a glass; observable in a test tube; in an artificial environment.

in vivo Within the living body.

ion An atom or radical having a charge of positive (cation) or negative (anion) electricity owing to the loss (positive) or gain (negative) of one or more electrons. Substances that form ions are called *electrolytes.*

ionization Any process by which a neutral atom gains or loses electrons, thus acquiring a net charge, as the dissociation of a substance in solution into ions.

ionize To separate into ions.

lipophilic 1. Having an affinity for fat; pertaining to or characterized by lipophilia. 2. Absorbing, dissolving, or being dissolved in lipids.

luteal 1. Pertaining to or having the properties of the corpus luteum or its active principle. 2. Of or related to the luteal phase of the menstrual cycle.

luteal phase The phase of the menstrual cycle lasting from ovulation until onset of menses. Named for the corpus luteum, or yellow body, which is the sac that remains after the follicle ruptures at ovulation and the oocyte is released from the ovary.

menstrual cycle The period of the regularly recurring physiologic changes in the endometrium that culminate in its shedding (menstruation).

messenger An information carrier; the mediator of an effect (e.g., a hormone secreted in one part of an organism and having an effect on distant cells, sometimes operating via a second messenger).

> **second messenger** Any of several classes of intracellular signals acting at or situated within the plasma membrane that translate electrical or chemical messages from the environment into cellular responses; such messengers include changes in membrane potential, calcium ions, cyclic nucleotides, including cyclic AMP, and products of phosphatidylinositol turnover.

messenger RNA mRNA, designating the RNA that carries the information encoded in a DNA sequence to the site of protein synthesis, where it specifies the order of amino-acid residues.

meta-analysis Any systemic method that uses statistical analysis to integrate the data from a number of independent studies.

metabolism 1. The sum of all the physical and chemical processes by which living organized substance is produced and maintained (anabolism), and also the transformation by which energy is made available for the uses of the organism (catabolism). 2. Biotransformation.

> **drug metabolism** Biotransformation of drugs.

metabolite Any substance produced by metabolism or by a metabolic process.

methyl The chemical group or radical CH_3-.

methylation Treatment with a reagent to add a methyl group to a compound.

microsomal enzymes A group of enzymes on the smooth endoplasmic reticulum, within cells. Microsomal enzymes are abundant in the liver, are present in the kidneys and gastrointestinal tract, and are divided into 1) glucuronyl transferases and 2) mixed-function oxidases (MFOs). Microsomal MFOs catabolize endogenous substances (e.g., corticosteroids) by hydroxylation and are the major pathway for catabolizing exogenous substances (e.g., detoxification of various drugs) involving many reactions: N-, O- and S-dealkylation, aromatic or aliphatic hydroxylation, N- or S-oxidation, deamination or desulfuration and epoxidation (an *epoxide* is a cyclic ether composed of an O_2 molecule bound to two different carbons). Usually, microsomal enzymes operate by first-order kinetics (catabolism at the first pass through the system) and only rarely by zero-order kinetics, which are reactions limited by substrate kinetics, as would be competition. Many substances can induce hyperplasia of the microsomal enzyme system. MFO can be induced by at least two classes of compounds: 1) phenobarbital and related molecules and 2) polycyclic hydrocarbons (e.g., 3,4 benzpyrene).

microsome Any of the vesicular fragments of endoplasmic reticulum formed after disruption and centrifugation of cells.

mixed function oxidases MFO; *see* oxidase, mixed function; *see also* microsomal enzymes.

neural plasticity *See* plasticity.

neurotransmitter Any of a group of substances that are released on excitation from the axon terminal of a presynaptic neuron of the central or peripheral nervous system and travel across the synaptic cleft to either excite or inhibit the target cell.

nitroreduction *See* reduction.

nuclear receptor *See* receptor, nuclear.

nuclease An enzyme or group of enzymes that split nucleic acid into mononucleotides and other products. They are present as digestive enzymes in the intestinal tract and as autolytic enzymes in many cells. Some are specific for RNA (ribonuclease) and others for DNA (deoxyribonuclease).

osmosis   The passage of pure solvent from a solution of lesser to one of greater solute concentration when the two solutions are separated by a membrane that selectively prevents the passage of solute molecules, but is permeable to the solvent.

osmotic pressure   The pressure required to stop osmosis through a semipermeable membrane between a solution and pure solvent; it is proportional to the osmolality of the solution.

oxidase   A term used in the recommended names of some oxidoreductases to denote those in which molecular oxygen is the hydrogen acceptor.

    mixed-function oxidase   Monooxygenase. *See* oxygenase; *see also* microsomal enzymes.

oxidation   The act of oxidizing or state of being oxidized. Chemically it consists of the increase in positive charges on an atom or the loss of negative charges. Most biological oxidations are accomplished by the removal of a pair of hydrogen atoms (dehydrogenation) from a molecule. Such oxidations must be accompanied by reduction of an acceptor molecule. Univalent oxidation = indicates loss of one electron; divalent oxidation = the loss of two electrons.

oxidation-reduction   The chemical reaction whereby electrons are removed (oxidation) from atoms of the substance being oxidized and transferred to atoms being reduced (reduction). Also called *redox.*

oxidize   To combine or cause to combine with oxygen, or to lose electrons.

oxygenase   Any member of a subclass of enzymes of the oxidoreductase class that catalyze the oxidation of a single substrate (hydrogen donor) with incorporation of one or both atoms of oxygen from molecular oxygen into the substance oxidized.

P450 cytochrome oxygenases   *See* cytochrome P450; *see also* oxygenases.

pathway   A sequence of reactions by which one substance is converted into another.

    metabolic pathway   The series of consecutive reactions by which a substance is transformed in a living organism, such as the glycolytic pathway from carbohydrate to lactate or ethanol.

pharmacodynamics   The field of study of the action of drugs in the animal organism.

pharmacokinetics   Pertains to the delivery of drugs to and removal of drugs from their sites of action.

plasticity   The capability of being molded.

neural plasticity   The capability of neural tissue of being molded. *See* synaptic plasticity.

synaptic plasticity   The ability of synapses to change as circumstances require. They may alter function, such as increasing or decreasing their sensitivity; or they may increase or decrease in actual numbers. This phenomenon is thought to be the main source of the overall plasticity of nervous system pathways.

polymorphism   The quality or character of occurring in several different forms.

genetic polymorphism   The occurrence together in the same population of two or more genetically determined phenotypes in such proportions that the rarest of them cannot be maintained merely by recurrent mutation.

proestrus   The period of heightened follicular activity preceding estrus in female mammals.

progestational agents   A group of hormones secreted by the corpus luteum and placenta, and in small amounts by the adrenal cortex, including progesterone, that induce the formation of a secretory endometrium. Preparations having progestational activity are also produced synthetically. Also called *gestogens, progestins, progestational hormones,* and *progestogens.*

progestin   The name originally given (Corner and Allen 1929) to the crude hormone of the corpora lutea. The term is now used for synthetic and naturally occurring progestational agents. *See* progestational agents.

proliferative phase   The early or preovulatory half of the menstrual cycle, initiated by the small peak in follicle-stimulating hormone; this phase, also known as the follicular phase, begins in the late luteal phase of the previous menstrual cycle under the influence of ovarian estrogen; the endometrium undergoes regeneration in preparation for implantation of an egg, if it becomes fertilized; during proliferation, the cervix becomes more vascularized, the os widens and the cervical mucus increases in volume and elasticity and undergoes arborization.

prophylactic   1. Tending to ward off disease; pertaining to prophylaxis. 2. An agent that tends to ward off disease.

prophylaxis   The prevention of disease; preventive treatment.

promoter   A segment of DNA usually occurring upstream from a gene coding region and acting as a controlling element in the expression of that gene; it serves as a recognition signal for an RNA polymerase and marks the site of initiation of transcription. Also called *promoter region.*

protein   Any of a group of complex organic compounds that contain carbon, hydrogen, oxygen, nitrogen, and usually sulfur, the characteristic element being nitrogen, and that are widely distributed in plants and animals. Proteins, the principal constituents of the protoplasm of all cells, are of high molecular weight and consist essentially of combinations of a-amino acids in peptide linkages. Twenty different amino acids are commonly found in proteins, and each protein has a unique, genetically defined amino acid sequence that determines its specific shape and function. Proteins serve as enzymes, structural elements, hormones, immunoglobulins, and so forth. Proteins may be classified as follows: 1) Simple or globular proteins, including most of the proteins in the body, are generally soluble in water or in salt solution and yield only a-amino acids on complete hydrolysis. Based mainly on their chemical properties, this class includes albumins, globulins, histones, and protamines. 2) Fibrous or fibrillar proteins, the principle structural proteins of the body, are generally insoluble. The major types of this class are collagens, elastins, keratins, and actin and myosis. 3) Conjugated or compound proteins are those in which the protein molecule is united with a nonprotein molecule or molecules (the prosthetic group) other than a salt. They include nucleoproteins, mucoproteins, lipoproteins, chromoproteins, phosphoproteins, and metalloproteins. *See also* binding protein.

protein bound   *See* binding protein.

receptor   A molecular structure within a cell or on the surface characterized by 1) selective binding of a specific substance and 2) a specific physiologic effect that accompanies the binding (e.g., cell-surface receptors for peptide hormones, neurotransmitters, antigens, complement fragments, and immunoglobulins and cytoplasmic receptors for steroid hormones).

adrenergic receptors Postulated sites on effector organs innervated by postganglionic adrenergic fibers of the sympathetic nervous system, classified as α-adrenergic and β-adrenergic receptors according to their reaction to norepinephrine and epinephrine, respectively, and to certain blocking and stimulating agents. Also called *adrenoceptor* and *adrenoreceptor.*

α-adrenergic receptors Adrenergic receptors that respond to norepinephrine and to such blocking agents as phenoxybenzamine and phentolamine.

β-adrenergic receptors Adrenergic receptors that respond to epinephrine and to such blocking agents as propranolol; they are of two types, β_1 (lipolysis and cardiostimulation) and β_2 (bronchodilation and vasodilation).

cholinergic receptors Cell-surface receptor molecules that bind the neurotransmitter acetylcholine and mediate its action on postjunctional cells, including parasympathetic autonomic ganglion cells, striated muscle, and certain central neurons. Commonly divided into two classes, muscarinic receptors and nicotinic receptors. Also called *cholinoceptors.*

estrogen receptors A cellular regulatory protein that binds estrogenic hormones, found on nearly all cell types, but particularly in estrogen-sensitive tissues such as the uterus and breast. Cytoplasmic levels are measured in surgically removed breast carcinoma; high levels indicate that a positive response to endocrine therapy is likely.

muscarinic receptors Cholinergic receptors that are stimulated by the alkaloid muscarine and blocked by atropine; they are found on autonomic effector cells and on central neurons in the thalamus and cerebral cortex. Three types may be distinguished on the basis of pharmacologic specificity and five types on the basis of molecular structure; a number of differing nomenclatures have been applied to these types.

nicotinic receptors Cholinergic receptors that are stimulated initially and blocked at high doses by the alkaloid nicotine and

blocked by tubocurarine; they are found on autonomic ganglion cells, on striated muscle, and on spinal central neurons.

nuclear receptors   Receptors located in the cell nucleus. These include receptors for steroid hormones.

opiate receptors   Any of a number of types of receptors for opiates
and opioids; at least seven different types are postulated at different locations in the body, grouped according to the specific
substances they bind and to the specific physiological effect(s)
(e.g., analgesia, respiratory depression, or a psychotomimetic
effect) that binding causes or inhibits.

reduction   In chemistry, the addition of hydrogen to a substance, or
more generally, the gain of electrons.

nitroreduction   The addition of hydrogen, or gain of electrons, to
a nitrogen atom or nitrogen containing compound.

renal tubule   One of the minute, reabsorptive, secretory, and collecting
canals, made up of basement membrane lined with epithelium, that
form the substance of the kidneys.

reporter gene   A gene, the phenotype of which is relatively easy to
monitor, that may be used to study promoter activity at different
points in an organism's development; in recombinant DNA technology, reporter genes may be attached to a promoter region of interest.

reproduction   1. The production of offspring by organized bodies.
2. The creation of a similar object or situation; duplication; replication.

reproductive   Subserving or pertaining to the production of offspring.

ribonucleic acid   RNA, the nucleic acid in which the sugar is ribose,
playing a role in the flow of genetic information and constituting
the genetic material in the RNA viruses. Ribosyl moieties are linked
via phosphate groups attached to their 5′ and 3′ hydroxyl groups to
form the backbone of a linear polymer, with purine and pyrimidine
bases attached to the sugars as side chains. The characteristic bases
adenine (A), uracil (U), cytosine (C), and guanine (G) are specified
by the presence of thymine (T), A, G, and C, respectively, in the gene
being transcribed. Many RNA molecules contain bases modified by
posttranscriptional processing (methylation, deamination, isomeri-
zation), and some contain secondary structure such as base-pairing

between self-complementary sequences, which stabilizes specific conformations.

second messenger   *See* messenger, second.

secretory phase   The latter half of the menstrual cycle, also known as the luteal phase.

sense DNA   In molecular genetics, referring to the strand of a double-stranded DNA that is transcribed and specifies a product (RNA or protein). *Compare with* antisense.

sensitivity   1. The state or quality of being sensitive; often used to denote a state of abnormal responsiveness to stimulation, or of responding quickly and acutely. 2. Analytical sensitivity, the smallest concentration of a substance that can be reliably measured by a particular analytic method. 3. Diagnostic sensitivity; the conditional probability that a person having a disease will be correctly identified by a clinical test (i.e., the number of true negative results).

sex   1. The fundamental distinction, found in most species of animals and plants, based on the type of gametes produced by the individual or category into which the individual fits on the basis of that criterion; ova, or macrogametes, are produced by the female; and spermatozoa, or microgametes, are produced by the male, the union of these distinctive germ cells being the natural prerequisite for the production of a new individual in sexual reproduction. 2. The category to which an individual is assigned on the basis of sex.

> **chromosomal sex**   Sex as determined by the presence of the XX (female) or the XY (male) genotype in somatic cells, and without regard to phenotypic manifestations. Also called *genetic sex.*

> **endocrinologic sex**   Sex determined by gender-specific hormonal patterns.

> **gonadal sex**   The sex as determined on the basis of the morphology of the external genitals.

> **nuclear sex**   The sex as determined on the basis of the presence or absence of sex chromatin in somatic cells, its presence normally indicating the XX (female) genotype, and its absence the XY (male) genotype.

> **phenotypic sex**   The phenotypic manifestations of sex determined by endocrine influences, such as breast development in the female, phallic enlargement in the male.

psychological sex   The self-image of the gender role of an individual.

social sex   The complex of attitudes, expectations, and the like, that a society attaches to the male and female roles.

sex differences   Differences related to sex, gender, sexuality, and/or reproductive function.

sexual   1. Pertaining to sex. 2. A person considered in his or her sexual relations.

sexuality   1. The characteristic quality of the male and female reproductive elements. 2. The constitution of an individual in relation to sexual attitudes or activity.

side chain   A chain of atoms attached to a larger chain or to a ring.

side effect   A consequence other than the one(s) for which an agent or measure is used, as the adverse effects produced by a drug, especially on a tissue or an organ system other than the one sought to be benefited by its administration.

therapeutic index   Originally, the ratio of the maximum tolerated dose to the minimum curative dose; now defined, so as to account for the variability of individual response, as the ratio of the median lethal dose (LD_{50}) to the median effective dose (ED_{50}). It is used in assessing the safety of a drug. Also called *chemotherapeutic index*.

therapy   The treatment of disease.

transcription   The process by which a single-stranded RNA with a base sequence complementary to one strand of a double-stranded DNA is synthesized. The enzymes involved are called *DNA-dependent RNA polymerases*.

translation   In genetics, the process by which polypeptide chains are synthesized, the amino acid sequence being completely determined by the sequence of bases in a messenger RNA (mRNA), which in turn is determined by the sequence of bases in the RNA of the gene from with it was transcribed.

tricyclic   *See* cyclic.

vector   A carrier, especially the animal that transfers an infective agent from one host to another.

viral vector   A plasmid or viral chromosome into whose genome a fragment of foreign DNA is inserted; used to introduce the foreign DNA into a host cell in the cloning of DNA.

volume of distribution (Vd)   A dilution method for determining the volume of fluids (e.g., plasma, a body fluid compartment). A solute (e.g., insulin) is injected into the compartment and, after it is equally distributed, a sample is taken. Then the quantity of solute removed (as by metabolism, excretion, and so forth) is subtracted from the quantity administered, and the result is divided by the concentration per milliliter in the sample.

References

Aarskog D: Association between maternal intake of diazepam and oral clefts (letter). Lancet 2:921, 1975

Abdu-Aguye L, Dunlop D, Patel P, et al: Propranolol pharmacokinetics during the menstrual cycle. Postgrad Med J 62:1093–1095, 1986

Abernethy DR, Greenblatt DJ, Arendt R, et al: Impairment of diazepam metabolism by low-dose estrogen-containing oral-contraceptive steroids. N Engl J Med 306:791–792, 1982a

Abernethy DR, Divoll M, Ochs HR, et al: Increased metabolic clearance of acetaminophen with oral contraceptive use. Obstet Gynecol 60:338–341, 1982b

Abernethy DR, Greenblatt DJ, Ochs HR, et al: Lorazepam and oxazepam kinetics in women on low-dose oral contraceptives. Clin Pharmacol Ther 33:628–632, 1983

Abernethy DR, Greenblatt DJ, Shader RI: Imipramine disposition in users of oral contraceptive steroids. Clin Pharmacol Ther 35:792–797, 1984

Abraham GE: Ovarian and adrenal contributions to peripheral androgens during the menstrual cycle. J Clin Endocrinol Metab 39:340–346, 1974

Abraham HC, Kanter VB, Rosen I, et al: A controlled clinical trial of imipramine (Tofranil) with outpatients. Br J Psychiatry 109:286–293, 1963

Adams JB, Wacher A: Specific changes in the glycoprotein components of seromucoid in pregnancy. Clin Chem Acta 21:155–157, 1968

Adekunle AO, Goswamy RK, Sallam HN, et al: Ultrasonic and endocrinologic monitoring of follicular growth during spontaneous and clomiphene-stimulated cycles, in Ovulation and Its Disorders (Studies in Fertility and Sterility). Edited by Thompson W, Harrison RF, Bonnar J. Boston, MA, MTP Press, 1984, pp 3–6

Agarwal DP, Goedde HW: Alcohol Metabolism, Alcohol Intolerance and Alcoholism. Berlin, Springer-Verlag, 1990

Agarwal DP, Hafer G, Harada S, et al: Studies on aldehyde dehydrogenase and aldehyde reductase in human brain, in Enzymology of Carbonyl Metabolism: Aldehyde Dehydrogenase and Aldo-Keto Reductase. Edited by Weiner H, Flynn TG. New York, Alan R Liss, 1982, pp 319–328

Aizenberg D, Zemishlany Z, Dorfman-Etrog P, et al: Sexual dysfunction in male schizophrenic patients. Am J Psychiatry 56:137–141, 1995

Alder S, Zbinden G: National and International Drug Safety Guidelines. MTC Verlag Zolliken, 1988, pp 164–173

Allan CA: Seeking help for drinking problems from a community-based voluntary agency: patterns of compliance amongst men and women. British Journal of Addiction 82:1143–1147, 1987

Allen A: Oral presentation. Presented at Women in Clinical Trials of FDA-Regulated Products meeting, Washington, DC, Food and Law Institute, October 1992

Allen LA, Richey MF, Chai YM, et al: Sex differences in the corpus callosum of the living human being. J Neurosci 11:933–942, 1991

Allen LS, Gorski RA: Sexual orientation and the size of the anterior commissure in the human brain. Proc Natl Acad Sci U S A 89:7199–7202, 1992

Allen LS, Hines M, Shryne JE, et al: Two sexually dimorphic cell groups in the human brain. J Neurosci 9:497–506, 1989

Allen MD, Greenblatt DJ, Harmatz JS, et al: Desmethyldiazepam kinetics in the elderly after oral prazepam. Clin Pharmacol Ther 28:196–202, 1980

Altshuler L, Burt VK, McMullen M, et al: Breast feeding and sertraline: a twenty-four-hour analysis. J Clin Psychiatry 56:243–245, 1995

Altura BM: Sex and estrogens and responsiveness of terminal arterioles to neurohypophyseal hormones and catecholamines. J Pharmacol Exp Ther 193:403–412, 1975

American College of Obstetricians and Gynecologists: Oral contraceptives (ACOG Technical Bulletin No 106). Washington, DC, ACOG, July 1987

American Hospital Formulary Service: AHFS Drug Information 93. Bethesda, MD, American Society of Hospital Pharmacists, 1993

American Medical Association: Drug interactions and adverse drug reactions, in AMA Drug Evaluations. Chicago, IL, American Medical Association Press, 1983, pp 31–44

American Psychiatric Association: Diagnostic and Statistical Manual of Mental Disorders, 3rd Edition. Washington, DC, American Psychiatric Association, 1980

American Psychiatric Association: Diagnostic and Statistical Manual of Mental Disorders, 3rd Edition, Revised. Washington, DC, American Psychiatric Association, 1987

American Psychiatric Association: Practice guidelines for major depressive disorders in adults. Am J Psychiatry 150 (suppl):1–26, 1993

American Psychiatric Association: Diagnostic and Statistical Manual of Mental Disorders, 4th Edition. Washington, DC, American Psychiatric Association, 1994

Anand VS: Clomipramine-induced galactorrhoea and amenorrhoea. Br J Psychiatry 147:87–88, 1985

Ananth J, Pecknold JC, Van Der Steen N, et al: Double blind comparative study of clomipramine and amitriptyline in obsessive neurosis. Prog Neuropsychopharmacol Biol Psychiatry 5:257–262, 1981

Andersch B, Hahm L, Andersson M, et al: Body water and weight in patients with premenstrual tension. Br J Obstet Gynaecol 85:546–550, 1978

Anderson E, Hamburger S, Liu JG, et al: Characteristics of menopausal women receiving assistance. Am J Obstet Gynecol 156:428–433, 1987

Andia AM, Zisook S, Braff DL, et al: Gender differences in schizophrenia. Paper presented at the 146th annual meeting of the American Psychiatric Association, San Francisco, CA, May 22–27, 1993

Andreasen NC, Smith MR, Jacoby CG, et al: Ventricular enlargement in schizophrenia: definition and prevalence. Am J Psychiatry 139:292–296, 1982

Andreasen NC, Swayze VW, Flaum M, et al: Ventricular enlargement in schizophrenia evaluated with computerized tomographic scanning. Arch Gen Psychiatry 47:1008–1015, 1990

Angermeyer MC, Kuhn L: Gender differences in age at onset of schizophrenia. European Archives of Psychiatry and Neurological Sciences 237:351–364, 1988

Angermeyer MC, Kuhn L, Goldstein JM: Gender in the course of schizophrenia: differences in treated outcomes. Schizophr Bull 16:293–306, 1990

Anglin MD, Hser Y, McGlothin WH: Sex differences in addict careers, II: becoming addicted. Am J Drug Alcohol Abuse 13:59–71, 1987a

Anglin MD, Hser Y, Booth MW: Sex differences in addict careers, IV: treatment. Am J Drug Alcohol Abuse 13:253–280, 1987b

Angrist B, Schulz SC: Introduction, in The Neuroleptic-Nonresponsive Patient: Characterization and Treatment. Edited by Angrist B, Schulz SC. Washington, DC, American Psychiatric Press, 1990, pp xvii–xxviii

Angst J, Baumann U, Hippius H, et al: Clinical aspects of resistance to imipramine therapy. Pharmakopsychiatrie Neuro-Psychopharmakologie (Stuttgart) 7:211–216, 1974

Anthony JC, Helzer JE: Syndromes of drug abuse and dependence, in Psychiatric Disorders in America. Edited by Robins LN, Regier DA. New York, Free Press, 1991, pp 116–154

Arafat ES, Hargrove JT, Maxson WS, et al: Sedative and hypnotic effects of oral administration of micronized progesterone may be mediated through its metabolites. Am J Obstet Gynecol 159:1203–1209, 1988

Arato M, Erdos A, Polgar M: Endocrinological changes in patients with sexual dysfunction under long-term neuroleptic treatment. Pharmakopsychatrie Neuropsychopharmakologie 12:426–431, 1979

Arato M, Frecska E, Tekes K, et al: Serotonergic interhemispheric asymmetry: gender difference in the orbital cortex. Acta Psychiatr Scand 84:110–111, 1991

Arias TD, Jorge D, Lee MD, et al: The oxidative metabolism of sparteine in the Cuna Amerindians of Panama: absence of evidence for deficient metabolizers. Clin Pharmacol Ther 43:456–465, 1988

Aron WS, Daily DW: Graduates and splitees from therapeutic community drug treatment programs: a comparison. Int J Addict 11:1–18, 1976

Arvela P, Kirjarinta M, Kirjarinta M, et al: Polymorphism of debriso-quine hydroxylation among Finns and Lapps. Br J Clin Pharmacol 26:601–603, 1988

Astrand P-O, Cuddy TE, Saltin B, et al: Cardiac output during submaxi-mal work. J Appl Physiol 19:268–274, 1964

Atallah AN, Guimaraes JAG, Gebara M, et al: Progesterone increases glomerular filtration rate, urinary kallikrein excretion and uric acid clearance in normal women. Braz J Med Biol Res 21:71–74, 1988

Athinarayanan P, Pierog SH, Nigam S, et al: Chlordiazepoxide with-drawal in the neonate. Am J Obstet Gynecol 124:212–213, 1976

Atkinson HC, Begg EJ, Darlow BA: Drugs in human milk: clinical phar-macokinetic considerations. Clin Pharmacokinet 14:217–240, 1988

Attella MJ, Nattinville A, Stein DG: Hormonal state affects recovery from frontal cortex lesions in adult female rats. Behavioral and Neural Bi-ology 48:352–367, 1987

Avis NE, Kaufert PA, Lock M, et al: The evolution of menopausal symp-toms. Clinics in Endocrinology and Metabolism 7:17–32, 1993

Ayd FJ: A survey of drug-induced extrapyramidal reactions. JAMA 175:1054–1060, 1961

Aylward M: Plasma tryptophan levels and mental depression in post-menopausal subjects: effects of oral piperazine-oestrone sulphate. IRCS Journal of Medical Science 1:30–34, 1973

Aylward M: Estrogens, plasma tryptophan levels in perimenopausal pa-tients, in The Management of the Menopause and Post-Menopausal Years. Edited by Campbell S. Baltimore, MD, University Park Press, 1976, pp 135–147

Bachevalier J, Hagger C: Sex differences in the development of learning abilities in primates. Psychoneuroendocrinology 16:177–188, 1991

Back D, Orme M: Pharmacokinetic drug interactions with oral contra-ceptives. Clin Pharmacokinet 18:472–484, 1990

Bäckström T: Epilepsy in women: oestrogen and progesterone plasma levels. Experientia 32:248–249, 1976

Bäckström T: Estrogen and progesterone in relation to different activi-ties in the central nervous system. Acta Obstet Gynecol Scand 66:1–17, 1977

Bäckström T, Jorpes P: Serum phenytoin, phenobarbital, carbamazepine, albumin and plasma estradiol and progesterone concentration during the menstrual cycle in women with epilepsy. Acta Neurol Scand 50:63–71, 1979

Bader TF, Newman K: Amitriptyline in human breast milk and the nursing infant's serum. Am J Psychiatry 137:855–856, 1980

Baird DT: Prediction of ovulation: biophysical, physiological and biochemical coordinates, in Ovulation: Methods for Its Prediction and Detection (Current Topics in Reproductive Endocrinology). Edited by Jeffcoate SL. New York, Wiley, 1983, pp 1–17

Baird DT: Amenorrhea, anovulation, and dysfunctional uterine bleeding, in Endocrinology. Edited by DeGroot L, Besser G, Marshall J, et al. Philadelphia, PA, WB Saunders, 1989, pp 1950–1968

Baldessarini RJ: Chemotherapy in Psychiatry. Cambridge, MA, Harvard University Press, 1979

Baldessarini RJ: Drugs and the treatment of psychiatric disorders, in The Pharmacological Basis of Therapeutics, 7th Edition. Edited by Goodman L, Gilman A. New York, Macmillan, 1985, pp 387–445

Balestrieri M, Ruggeri M, Bellantuono C: Drug treatment of panic disorder—a critical review of controlled clinical trials. Psychiatric Developments 4:337–350, 1989

Ballenger JC: The use of anticonvulsants in manic-depressive illness. J Clin Psychiatry 49 (suppl):21–24, 1988

Ballenger JC: Efficacy of benzodiazepines in panic disorder and agoraphobia. J Psychiatr Res 24 (suppl 2):15–25, 1990

Ballinger CB: Psychiatric morbidity and the menopause: screening of general population sample. BMJ 3:344–346, 1975

Balogh S, Hendricks SE, Kang J: Treatment of fluoxetine-induced anorgasmia with amantadine. J Clin Psychiatry 53:212–213, 1992

Balon R, Yeragani VK, Pohl R, et al: Sexual dysfunction during antidepressant treatment. J Clin Psychiatry 54:209–212, 1993

Balter MB, Levine L, Manheimer DI: Cross-national study of the extent of anti-anxiety/sedative drug use. N Engl J Med 290:769–774, 1974

Bancroft J, Boyle H, Warner P, et al: The use of an LHRH agonist, buserelin, in the long-term management of premenstrual syndromes. Clin Endocrinol (Oxford) 27:171–181, 1987

Barbeau A, Cloutier T, Roy M, et al: Ecogenetics of Parkinson's disease: 4-hydroxylation of debrisoquine. Lancet 2:1213–1215, 1985

Bardenstein KK, McGlashan TH: Gender differences in affective, schizoactive, and schizophrenic disorders. Schizophr Res 3:159–172, 1990

Barlow SM, Knight AF, Sullivan FM: Prevention by diazepam of adverse effects of maternal restraint stress on postnatal development and learning in the rat. Teratology 19:105–110, 1979

Barratt CLR, Cooke S, Chauhan M, et al: A prospective randomized controlled trial comparing urinary luteinizing hormone dipsticks and basal body temperature charts with time donor insemination. Fertil Steril 52:394–397, 1989

Barrett-Connor E, Kritz-Silverstein D: Estrogen replacement therapy and cognitive function in older women. JAMA 269:2637–2641, 1993

Barton JL: Orgasmic inhibition by phenelzine. Am J Psychiatry 136:1616–1617, 1979

Bass R: Guideline on detection of toxicity to reproduction for medicinal products. First International Conference on Harmonization, July 1991

Baukloh V, Fischer R, Naether O, et al: Patterns of serum-luteinizing hormone surges in stimulated cycles in relation to injections of human chorionic gonadotropin. Fertil Steril 53:69–75, 1990

Baulieu EE, Robel P, Vatier O, et al: Neurosteroids: pregnenolone and dehydroepiandrosterone in the rat brain, in Receptor-Receptor Interactions: A New Intramembrane Integrative Mechanism. Edited by Fuxe K, Agnati LF. New York, Macmillan–Basingstoke, 1987, pp 89–104

Baum C, Kennedy DL, Knapp DE, et al: Prescription drug use in 1984 and changes over time. Med Care 26:105–114, 1988

Baumann P, Eap CB: Alpha$_1$-Acid Glycoprotein Genetics, Biochemistry, Physiological Functions, and Pharmacology. New York, Alan R Liss, 1988

Baumann P, Eap CB: Plasma monitoring of antidepressants: clinical relevance of the pharmacogenetics of metabolism and of 1-acid glycoprotein binding (abstract). Biol Psychiatry 29 (suppl):116S, 1991

Baviera G, Rigano A, Sfameni F: Four-hour urinary and serum immunofluorimetric assay for luteinizing hormone to detect onset of preovulatory LH surge. Acta Eur Fertil 19:25–28, 1988

Beaumont G: Side effects of clomipramine. J Int Med Res 5:37–44, 1977

Becker JB: Estrogen rapidly potentiates amphetamine-induced striatal dopamine release and rotational behavior during microdialysis. Neurosci Lett 118:169–171, 1990

Becker JB, Cha JH: Estrous cycle-dependent variation in amphetamine-induced behaviors and striatal dopamine assessed with microdialysis. Behav Brain Res 35:117–125, 1989

Becklake MR, Frank H, Dagenais GR, et al: Influence of age and sex on exercise cardiac output. J Appl Physiol 20:938–947, 1965

Beckman LJ, Amaro H: Patterns of women's use of alcohol treatment agencies, in Alcohol Problems in Women. Edited by Wilsnack S, Beckman L. New York, Guilford, 1984, pp 319–348

Beckman LJ, Amaro H: Personal and social difficulties faced by women and men entering alcoholism treatment. J Stud Alcohol 47:135–145, 1986

Beckmann H, Goodwin FK: Antidepressant response to tricyclics and urinary MHPG in unipolar patients: clinical response to imipramine or amitriptyline. Arch Gen Psychiatry 32:17–21, 1975

Bedard P, Langelier P, Villeneuve A: Oestrogens and extrapyramidal system (letter). Lancet 2:1367, 1977

Behrman RE, Vaughan VC: Nelson Textbook of Pediatrics, 13th Edition. Philadelphia, PA, WB Saunders, 1987

Bellodi L, Bussoleni C, Scorza-Smeraldi R: Family study of schizophrenia: exploratory analysis for relevant factors. Schizophr Bull 12:120–128, 1986

Belmaker RH, Murphy DL, Wyatt RJ, et al: Human platelet monoamine oxidase changes during the menstrual cycle. Arch Gen Psychiatry 31:553–556, 1974

Ben-Aderet N, Potashnik G, Lunenfeld B, et al: Correlation of hormonal profile and ovarian morphologic features during the periovulatory period in humans. Fertil Steril 28:361–362, 1977

Benitez J, Llerena A, Cobaleda J: Debrisoquin oxidation polymorphism in a Spanish population. Clin Pharmacol Ther 44:74–77, 1988

Bennett D: Treatment of ejaculation praecox with monoamine oxidase inhibitors (letter). Lancet 2:1309, 1961

Bennett JC: Inclusion of women in clinical trials—policies for population subgroups. N Engl J Med 329:288–292, 1993

Bergman A, Brenner PF: Alterations in the urogenital system, in Menopause: Physiology and Pharmacology. Edited by Mishel DR. Chicago, IL, Year Book Medical, 1987, pp 67–75

Berkow R (ed): The Merck Manual, 14th Edition. Rahway, NJ, Merck Sharp & Dome, 1982

Berlin CM: Pharmacologic considerations of drug use in the lactating mother. Obstet Gynecol 58 (suppl):17S–23S, 1981

Berlin F, Bergey G, Money J: Periodic psychosis of puberty: a case report. Am J Psychiatry 139:119–120, 1982

Bertilsson L, Aberg-Wistedt A: The debrisoquine hydroxylation test predicts steady-state plasma levels of desipramine. Br J Clin Pharmacol 15:388–390, 1983

Bertilsson L, Eichelbaum M, Mellstrom B, et al: Nortriptyline and antipyrine clearance in relation to debrisoquine hydroxylation in man. Life Sciences 27:1673–1677, 1980

Bertilsson L, Alm C, DeLas Carreras C, et al: Debrisoquine hydroxylation polymorphism and personality (letter). Lancet 1:555, 1989

Best NR, Rees MP, Barlow DH, et al: Effect of estradiol implant on noradrenergic function and mood in menopausal subjects. Psychoneuroendocrinology 17:87–93, 1992

Beumont PV, Corker CS, Friesen HG, et al: The effects of phenothiazines on endocrine function, II: effects in men and postmenopausal women. Br J Psychiatry 124:420–430, 1974

Biegon A, McEwen BS: Modulation by estradiol of serotonin receptors in brain. J Neurosci 2:199–205, 1982

Biegon A, Bercovitz H, Samuel D: Serotonin receptor concentration during the estrous cycle in the rat. Brain Res 187:221–225, 1980

Biegon A, Reches A, Snyder L, et al: Serotonergic and noradrenergic receptors in the rat brain: modulation by chronic exposure to ovarian hormones. Life Sciences 32:2015–2021, 1983

Billings EL, Brown JB, Billings JJ, et al: Symptoms and hormonal changes accompanying ovulation. Lancet 1:282–284, 1972

Birnbaum K: The making of a psychosis: the principles of structural analysis in psychiatry (1923), in Themes and Variations in European Psychiatry. Edited by Hirsch SR, Shepherd MS. Bristol, UK, J Wright, 1974, pp 199–238

Bitar MS, Ota M, Linnoila M, et al: Modification of gonadectomy-induced increases in brain monamine metabolism by steroid hormones in male and female rats. Psychoneuroendocrinology 16:547–557, 1991

Bjerkedal T, Czeizel A, Goujard J, et al: Valproic acid and spina bifida (letter). Lancet 2:1096, 1982

Bjerre M, Gram F, Kragh-Sorensen P, et al: Dose-dependent kinetics of imipramine in elderly patients. Psychopharmacology (Berl) 75:354–357, 1981

Blain PG, Mucklow JC, Rawlins MD, et al: Determinants of plasma a-1-acid glycoprotein (AAG) concentrations in health. Br J Clin Pharmacol 20:500–502, 1985

Blair J, Simpson G: Effect of antipsychotic drugs on reproductive functions. Diseases of the Nervous System 27:645–647, 1966

Bland RC, Orn H, Newman SC: Lifetime prevalence of psychiatric disorders in Edmonton. Acta Psychiatr Scand 77 (suppl):24–32, 1988

Bleich A, Siegel B, Garb R, et al: Post traumatic stress disorder following combat exposure: clinical features and psychopharmacological response. Br J Psychiatry 149:365–369, 1986

Blume S: Women and alcohol: a review. JAMA 256:1467–1470, 1986

Blumer D, Heilbronn M: Antidepressant treatment for chronic pain: treatment outcome of 1,000 patients with the pain-prone disorder. Psychiatric Annals 14:796–800, 1984

Bogerts B, Meertz E, Sconfeldt-Bausch R: Basal ganglia and limbic system pathology in schizophrenia. Arch Gen Psychiatry 42:784–791, 1985

Booth M, Hunt JN, Miles JM, et al: Comparison of gastric emptying and secretion in men and women with reference to prevalence of duodenal ulcer in each sex. Lancet 1:657–659, 1957

Borga O, Piafsky KM, Nilsen OG: Plasma protein binding of basic drugs, I: selective displacement from alpha$_1$-acid glycoprotein by tris (2-butoxyethyl) phosphate. Clin Pharmacol Ther 22:539–544, 1977

Bottiger LE, Furhoff AK, Holmberg L: Fatal reactions to drugs. Acta Medica Scandinavica 205:451–456, 1979

Bourdon KH, Boyd JH, Rae DS, et al: Gender differences in phobias: results of the ECA community survey. Journal of Anxiety Disorders 2:227–241, 1988

Bowers MB, Swigar ME, Jatlow PI, et al: Plasma catecholamine metabolites and early response to haloperidol. J Clin Psychiatry 45:248–251, 1984

Bracken MB, Holford TR: Exposure to prescribed drugs in pregnancy and association with congenital malformations. Obstet Gynecol 58:336–343, 1981

Brailly S, Gougeon A, Milgrom E, et al: Importance of changes in the transformation of progestin into androgen during preovulatory development and atresia of human follicles, in Follicular Maturation and Ovulation. Edited by Rolland R, Van Hall EV, Hillier SG, et al. Amsterdam, the Netherlands, Excerpta Medica, 1982, pp 180–187

Brambilla F, Gaustalla A, Rovere C, et al: Neuroendocrine effects of haloperidol therapy in chronic schizophrenia. Psychopharmacologia (Berl) 44:17–22, 1975

Brann DW, Zamorano PL, Putnam-Roberts CD, et al: Gamma-aminobutyric acid-opioid interactions in the regulation of gonadotropin secretion in the immature female rat. Neuroendocrinology 56:445–452, 1992

Braun P, Greenberg D, Dasberg H, et al: Core symptoms of posttraumatic stress disorder unimproved by alprazolam treatment. J Clin Psychiatry 51:236–238, 1990

Brenner PF: The menopausal syndrome. Obstet Gynecol 72 (suppl):6–11, 1988

Breslau N, Davis GC, Andreski P: Traumatic events and traumatic stress disorder in an urban population of young adults. Arch Gen Psychiatry 48:218–222, 1990

Bressler R: Adverse drug reactions, in Drug Therapy for the Elderly. Edited by Conrad KA, Bressler R. St. Louis, MO, CV Mosby, 1982, pp 64–85

Brick J, Nathan PE, Westrick E, et al: The effect of menstrual cycle on blood alcohol levels and behavior. J Stud Alcohol 47:472–477, 1986

Briggs M, Briggs M: Relationship between monoamine oxidase activity and sex hormone concentration in human blood plasma. J Reprod Fertil 29:447–450, 1972

Brixen-Rasmussen L, Halgrener J, Jorgensen A: Amitriptyline and nortriptyline excretion in human breast milk. Psychopharmacology (Berl) 76:94–95, 1982

Brochner-Mortensen J, Paaby P, Fjeldborg P, et al: Renal haemodynamics and extracellular homeostasis during the menstrual cycle. Scand J Clin Lab Invest 47:829–835, 1987

Brockington I, Kelly A, Hall P, et al: Premenstrual relapse of puerperal psychosis. Journal of Affective Disorders 14:287–292, 1988

Bromet EJ, Schwartz JE, Fennig S, et al: The epidemiology of psychosis: the Suffolk County mental health project. Schizophr Bull 28:243–255, 1992

Brooks PJ, Funabashi T, Kleopoulos, et al: Widespread expression and estrogen regulation of preproenkephalin intron A–like nuclear RNA in rat brain (abstract 202.2). Society for Neuroscience Abstracts 19:483, 1993

Brosen K, Gram LF, Klysner R, et al: Steady-state levels of imipramine and its metabolites: significance of dose-dependent kinetics. Eur J Clin Pharmacol 30:43–49, 1986

Brown CS, Rakel RE, Wells BG, et al: A practical update on anxiety disorders and their pharmacologic treatment. Arch Intern Med 151:873–884, 1991

Brown E, Prager J, Lee HY, et al: CNS complications of cocaine abuse: prevalence, pathophysiology, and neuroradiology. American Journal of Roentgenology 159:137–147, 1992

Bruce J, Russell GFM: Premenstrual tension: a study of weight changes and balances of water, sodium and potassium. Lancet 2:267–271, 1962

Bruguerolle B: Modifications de la pharmacocinetique des médicaments au cours du cycle menstruel. Thérapie 41:11–17, 1986

Buffum J: Pharmacosexology: the effects of drugs on sexual function—a review. J Psychoactive Drugs 14:5–34, 1982

Buigues J, Vallejo J: Therapeutic response to phenelzine in patients with panic disorders and agoraphobia with panic attacks. J Clin Psychiatry 48:55–59, 1987

Bungay GT, Vessey MP, McPherson CK: Study of symptoms in middle-life with special reference to the menopause. BMJ 2:181–183, 1980

Bunt JC, Lohman TG, Boileau RA: Impact of total body water fluctuations on estimation of body fat from body density. Med Sci Sports Exerc 21:96–100, 1989

Burger HG, Hailes J, Menelaus M, et al: The management of persistent menopausal symptoms with oestradiol-testosterone implants: clinical lipid and hormonal results. Maturitas 6:351–358, 1984

Burnam MA, Stein JA, Golding JM, et al: Sexual assault and mental disorders in a community population. J Consult Clin Psychol 56:843–850, 1988

Byrd PJ, Thomas TR: Hydrostatic weighing during different stages of the menstrual cycle. Res Q Exerc Sport 54:296–298, 1983

Cameron OG, Kuttesch D, McPhee K, et al: Menstrual fluctuation in the symptoms of panic anxiety. Journal of Affective Disorders 15:169–174, 1988

Camp DM, Robinson TE: Susceptibility to sensitization, I: sex differences in the enduring effects of chronic D-amphetamine treatment on locomotion, stereotyped behavior and brain monamines. Behav Brain Res 30:55–68, 1988a

Camp DM, Robinson TE: Susceptibility to sensitization, II: the influence of gonadal hormones on enduring changes in brain monoamines and behavior produced by the repeated administration of D-amphetamine on restraint stress. Behav Brain Res 30:69–88, 1988b

Campbell S, Whitehead M: Oestrogen therapy and the menopausal syndrome. Clin Obstet Gynecol 4:31–47, 1977

Carlsson M, Carlsson A: A regional study of sex differences in rat brain serotonin. Prog Neuropsychopharmacol Biol Psychiatry 12:53–61, 1988

Carney A, Bancroft J, Mathews A: Combination of hormonal and psychological treatment for female sexual unresponsiveness. Br J Psychiatry 132:339–346, 1978

Caroff SN: The neuroleptic malignant syndrome. J Clin Psychiatry 41:79–83, 1980

Carr B, Wilson J: Disorders of the ovary and female reproductive tract, in Harrison's Principles of Internal Medicine. Edited by Brunwald E, Isselbacher K, Petersdorf R, et al: New York, McGraw-Hill, 1989, pp 1818–1825

Carroll KM, Rounsaville BJ, Keller DS: Relapse prevention strategies for the treatment of cocaine abuse. Am J Drug Alcohol Abuse 17:249–265, 1991

Casper RF, Erskine HJ, Armstrong DT, et al: In vitro fertilization: diurnal and seasonal variation in luteinizing hormone surge onset and pregnancy rates. Fertil Steril 49:644–647, 1988

Casson P, Hahn PM, van Vugt DA, et al: Lasting response to ovariectomy in severe intractable premenstrual syndrome. Am J Obstet Gynecol 162:99–105, 1990

Chakos MH, Mayerhoff DI, Loebel AD, et al: Incidence and correlates of acute extrapyramidal symptoms in first episode of schizophrenia. Psychopharmacol Bull 28:81–86, 1992

Chakravarti S, Collins WF, Newton JR, et al: Endocrine changes and symptomatology after oophorectomy in premenopausal women. Br J Obstet Gynaecol 84:769–775, 1977

Chamberlain S, Hahn PM, Casson P, et al: Effect of menstrual cycle phase and oral contraceptive use on serum lithium levels after a loading dose of lithium in normal women. Am J Psychiatry 147:907–909, 1990

Chambers CD, White OZ: Characteristics of high-frequency consumers of prescription psychoactive drugs. Chemical Dependencies: Behavioral and Biomedical Issues 4:33–46, 1980

Chambless DL, Mason J: Sex, sex-role stereotyping and agoraphobia. Behav Res Ther 24:231–235, 1986

Chamness GC, King TW, Sheridan PJ: Androgen receptor in the rat brain—assays and properties. Brain Res 161:267–276, 1979

Charette L, Tate DL, Wilson A: Alcohol consumption and menstrual distress in women at higher and lower risk for alcoholism. Alcohol Clin Exp Res 14:152–157, 1990

Charney DS, Heninger GR: Serotonin function in panic disorders: the effect of intravenous tryptophan in healthy subjects and patients with panic disorder before and during alprazolam treatment. Arch Gen Psychiatry 43:1059–1065, 1986

Charney DS, Deutch AY, Krystal JH, et al: Psychobiologic mechanisms of posttraumatic stress disorder. Arch Gen Psychiatry 50:295–305, 1993

Chasnoff I, MacGregor S, Chisum G: Cocaine use during pregnancy: adverse perinatal outcome (abstract), in Problems of Drug Dependence, 1987: Proceedings of the 49th Annual Scientific Meeting, Committee on Problems of Drug Dependence, Philadelphia, PA, June 1987 (NIDA Research Monograph 81). Rockville, MD, NIDA, 1988, p 265

Chevillard C, Barden N, Saavedra JM: Estradiol treatment decreases type A and increases type B monoamine oxidase in specific brain stem areas and cerebellum of ovariectomized rats. Brain Res 221:177–181, 1981

Childers SE, Harding CM: Gender, premorbid social functioning, and long-term outcome in DSM-III schizophrenia. Schizophr Bull 18:309–318, 1990

Chiodo LA, Caggiula AR: Substantia nigra dopamine neurons: alterations in basal discharge rates and autoreceptor sensitivity induced by estrogen. Neuropharmacology 22:593–599, 1983

Christenson R: MAOIs, anorgasmia, and weight gain (letter). Am J Psychiatry 140:1260, 1983

Christy NP, Shaver JC: Estrogens and the kidney. Kidney Int 6:366–376, 1974

Clark DM: A cognitive approach to panic. Behav Res Ther 24:461–470, 1986

Clark WG, Brater DG, Johnson AR (eds): Goth's Medical Pharmacology, 12th Edition. St. Louis, MO, CV Mosby, 1988

Clarke WP, Goldfarb J: Estrogen enhances a 5-HT$_{1A}$ response in hippocampal slices from female rats. Eur J Pharmacol 160:195–197, 1989

Clarke WP, Maayani S: Estrogen effects on 5-HT$_{1A}$ receptors in hippocampus membranes from ovariectomized rats: functional and binding studies. Brain Res 518:287–291, 1990

Cleary MF: Fluphenazine decanoate during pregnancy. Am J Psychiatry 134:815–816, 1977

Clemens LG, Barr P, Dohanich GP: Cholinergic regulation of female sexual behavior in rats demonstrated by manipulation of endogenous acetylcholine. Physiol Behav 45:437–442, 1989

Cockcroft DW, Gault MH: Prediction of creatinine clearance from serum creatinine. Nephron 16:31–41, 1976

Cocores JA, Dackis CA, Gold MS: Sexual dysfunction secondary to cocaine abuse in two patients. J Clin Psychiatry 47:384–385, 1986

Cohen AJ: Fluoxetine-induced yawning and anorgasmia reversed by cyproheptadine treatment (letter). J Clin Psychiatry 53:174, 1992

Cohen BM, Harris PQ, Atterman RI, et al: Amoxapine: neuroleptic as well as antidepressant? Am J Psychiatry 139:1165–1167, 1982

Cohen J: A power primer. Psychol Bull 112:155–159, 1992

Cohen LS, Rosenbaum JF, Heller VL: Panic attack–associated placental abruption: a case report. J Clin Psychiatry 50:266–267, 1989

Cohen LS, Friedman JM, Jefferson JW, et al: A reevaluation of risk of in utero exposure to lithium. JAMA 271:146–150, 1994

Cole J, Bodkin JA: Antidepressant drug side effects. J Clin Psychiatry 51 (suppl 1):21–26, 1990

Cole-Harding S, Wilson JR: Ethanol metabolism in men and women. J Stud Alcohol 48:380–387, 1987

Collins AC, Yeager TN, Leback ME, et al: Variations in alcohol metabolism: influence of sex and age. Pharmacol Biochem Behav 3:973–978, 1975

Collins WP: Biochemical approaches to ovulation prediction and detection and the location of the fertile period in women, in Ovulation: Methods for Its Prediction and Detection (Current Topics in Reproductive Endocrinology). Edited by Jeffcoate SL. New York, Wiley, 1983, pp 49–66

Collins WP, Branch CM, Collins PO, et al: Biochemical indices of the fertile period in women. International Journal of Fertility 26:196–202, 1981

Comas-Diaz L, Jacobsen FM: Psychopharmacology for women of color: an empowering approach, in Psychopharmacology From a Feminist Perspective: Women and Therapy. Edited by Hamilton JA, Jensvold MF, Rothblum E, et al. New York, Haworth, 1995, pp 85–112

Connelly CE, Davenport YB, Nurnberger JI Jr: Adherence to treatment regimen in a lithium carbonate clinic. Arch Gen Psychiatry 39:585–588, 1982

Conney AH, Pantuck EJ, Hsiao KC, et al: Regulation of drug metabolism in man by environments and diet. Federation Proceedings 36:1647–1652, 1977

Connor B, Babcock M: The impact of feminist psychotherapy on the treatment of women alcoholics: focus on women. Journal on Addiction and Health 2:72–92, 1980

Conrad CD, Hamilton JA: Recurrent premenstrual decline in lithium concentration: clinical correlates and treatment implications. Journal of the American Academy of Child Psychiatry 26:852–853, 1986

Conte HR, Karasu TB: A review of treatment studies of minor depression: 1980–1991. Am J Psychother 46:58–74, 1992

Cook BL, Noyes R, Garvey MJ, et al: Anxiety and the menstrual cycle in panic disorder. Journal of Affective Disorders 19:221–226, 1990

Cooper DS, Gelenberg AJ, Wojeck TC, et al: The effect of amoxapine and imipramine on serum prolactin levels. Arch Intern Med 14:1023–1025, 1981

Cooper HM, Rosenthal R: Statistical versus traditional procedures for summarizing research findings. Psychol Bull 87:442–449, 1980

Coppen A, Wood K: Tryptophan and depressive illness. Psychol Med 8:49–57, 1978

Corner GW, Allen WM: Production of a special uterine reaction (progestational proliferation) by extracts of the corpus luteum. Am J Physiol 88:326–339, 1929

Costa D, Predescu V, Visan-Ionescu I, et al: Endogenous depression and imipramine levels in the blood. Psychopharmacology (Berl) 70:291–294, 1980

Cotton P: Is there still too much extrapolation from data on middle-aged white men? JAMA 263:1049–1050, 1990

Cowdry RW, Gardner DL: Pharmacotherapy of borderline personality disorder: alprazolam, carbamazepine, trifluoperazine, and tranylcypromine. Arch Gen Psychiatry 45:111–119, 1988

Cowe L, Lloyd DJ, Dawling S: Neonatal convulsions caused by withdrawal from maternal clomipramine. BMJ 284:1837–1838, 1982

Crabtree BL, Jann MW, Pitts WM: Alpha$_1$ acid glycoprotein levels in patients with schizophrenia: effect of treatment with haloperidol. Biol Psychiatry 29 (suppl):43A–185A, 1991

Cramer JL, Scott B, Rolfe B: Metabolism of [^{14}C]imipramine, II: urinary metabolites in man. Psychopharmacologia 15:207–225, 1969

Cramer OM, Parker CR, Porter JC: Estrogen inhibition of dopamine release into hypophyseal blood. Endocrinology 104:419–421, 1979

Crawford S, Ryder D: A study of sex differences in cognitive impairment in alcoholics using traditional and computer based tests. Drug Alcohol Depend 18:369–375, 1986

Crenshaw TL, Goldberg JP: Sexual Pharmacology: Drugs That Affect Sexual Function. New York, Norton, 1996

Crenshaw TL, Goldberg JP, Stern WC: Pharmacologic modification of psychosexual dysfunction. J Sex Marital Ther 13:239–252, 1987

Crombie DL, Pinsent RJ, Fleming D: Imipramine and pregnancy (letter). BMJ 2:745, 1972

Cromer B, Smith D, Blair J, et al: Depo-Provera: effectiveness, side effects and satisfaction in adolescents. Paper presented at NASPAG 7th Annual Meeting, Colorado Springs, CO, April 16–18, 1993, as reported in Contraception and Adolescents, in the Contraception Report 4:4–10, Grimes DA (ed), 1993

Croughan JL, Secunda SK, Katz MM, et al: Sociodemographic and prior clinical course characteristics associated with treatment response in depressed patients. J Psychiatr Res 22:222–237, 1988

Crow TJ, MacMillan JF, Johnson AL, et al: A randomized controlled trial of prophylactic neuroleptic treatment. Br J Psychiatry 148:120–127, 1986

Croxatto HD, Diaz S, Fuentealba B, et al: Studies on the duration of egg transport in the human oviduct, I: the time interval between ovulation and egg recovery from the uterus in normal women. Fertil Steril 23:447–458, 1972

Croxatto HD, Ortiz ME, Croxatto HB: Correlation between histologic dating of human corpus luteum and the luteinizing hormone peak–biopsy interval. Am J Obstet Gynecol 136:667–670, 1980

Cruz AF, Garcia JV, Domingo CM: La influencia de la foliculina y luteina sobre el rendimiento digestivo del estómago: secreción y evacuación. Archivos de Medicina Experimental 14:103–119, 1951

Cullberg J: Mood changes and menstrual symptoms with different gestagen/estrogen combinations: a double-blind comparison with a placebo. Acta Psychiatr Scand 236:1–86, 1972

Cupit GC, Rotmensch HH: Principles of drug therapy in pregnancy, in Principles of Medical Therapy in Pregnancy. Edited by Gleicher N. New York, Plenum, 1985, pp 77–90

Cuskey WR, Berger LH, Densen-Gerber J: Issues in the treatment of female addiction: a review and critique of the literature. Contemporary Drug Problems 6:307–371, 1977

Cyr MG, Moulton AW: The physician's role in prevention, detection, and treatment of alcohol abuse in women. Psychiatric Annals 23:454–462, 1993

Dackis CA, Gold MS: New concepts in cocaine addiction: the dopamine depletion hypothesis. Neurosci Biobehav Rev 9:460–477, 1985

Dackis CA, Gold MS, Sweeney DR, et al: Single-dose bromocriptine reverses cocaine craving. Psychiatry Res 20:261–264, 1987

Dahl-Puustinen ML, Liden A, Alm C, et al: Disposition of perphenazine is related to polymorphic debrisoquine hydroxylation in human beings. Clin Pharmacol Ther 46:78–81, 1989

Dalton K: The Premenstrual Syndrome. London, Heinemann, 1964

Dalton K: Ante-natal progesterone and intelligence. J Psychiatry 114:1377–1382, 1968

Dalton K: The Premenstrual Syndrome and Progesterone Therapy. Chicago, IL, Year Book Medical, 1977

D'Angelo EJ: Security of attachment in infants with schizophrenic, depressed and unaffected mothers. J Gen Psychol 147:421–422, 1986

Daniluk JC, Fluker M: Fertility drugs and the reproductive imperative: assisting the fertile woman, in Psychopharmacology From a Feminist Perspective. Edited by Hamilton JA, Jensvold MF, Rothblum E, et al. New York, Haworth, 1995, pp 31–48

Dannan GH, Guengerich FP, Waxman DJ: Hormonal regulation of rat liver microsomal enzymes: role of gonadal steroids in programming, maintenance, and suppression steroid-5a-reductase, flavin containing monoxygenase, and sex-specific cytochromes P450. Biol Chem 261:10728–10735, 1986

Datz FL, Christian PE, Moore JG: Gender-related differences in gastric emptying. J Nucl Med 28:1204–1207, 1987a

Datz FL, Christian PE, Moore JG: Differences in gastric emptying rates between menstruating and postmenopausal women (abstract). J Nucl Med 28:604–605, 1987b

Davidson JRT: Seizures and bupropion: a review. J Clin Psychiatry 50:256–260, 1989

Davidson JRT: Drug therapy of post-traumatic stress disorder. Br J Psychiatry 160:309–314, 1992

Davidson JRT, Pelton S: Forms of atypical depression and their response to antidepressant drugs. Psychiatry Res 17:87–95, 1986

Davidson JRT, Giller EL, Zisook S, et al: An efficacy study of isocarboxazid and placebo in depression, and its relationship to depressive nosology. Arch Gen Psychiatry 45:120–127, 1988

Davidson JRT, Kudler H, Smith R, et al: Treatment of posttraumatic stress disorder with amitriptyline and placebo. Arch Gen Psychiatry 47:259–266, 1990

Davies GJ, Crowder M, Reid B, et al: Bowel function measurements of individuals with different eating patterns. Gut 27:164–169, 1986

Davison JM, Noble MCB: Serial changes in 24 hour creatinine clearance during normal menstrual cycles and the first trimester of pregnancy. Br J Obstet Gynaecol 88:10–17, 1981

Dawkins K, Potter WZ: Gender differences in pharmacokinetics and pharmacodynamics of psychotropics: focus on women. Psychopharmacol Bull 27:417–421, 1991

de Lacoste MC, Adesanya T, Woodward DJ: Measure of gender differences in the human brain and their relationship to brain weight. Biol Psychiatry 28:931–942, 1990

Dean AL, Abels JC, Taylor HC: Effects of certain hormones on renal function of man. J Urol 53:647–653, 1945

Dean M, Stock B, Patterson RJ, et al: Serum protein binding of drugs during and after pregnancy in humans. Clin Pharmacol Ther 28:253–261, 1980

Deaux K: Commentary: Sex or gender? Psychological Science 4:125–126, 1993

Debrovner D: Of mice and men. American Druggist 207:28–34, 1993

Decastro RM: Reversal of MAOI-induced anorgasmia with cyproheptadine (letter). Am J Psychiatry 142:783, 1985

Degen K: Sexual dysfunction in women using major tranquilizers. Psychosomatics 23:959–961, 1982

Delaney AG: Anesthesia in the pregnant woman. Clin Obstet Gynecol 26:795–800, 1983

DeLeo D, Magni G: Sexual side effects of antidepressant drugs. Psychosomatics 24:1076–1082, 1983

DeLeve LD, Piafsky KM: Clinical significance of plasma binding of basic drugs. Trends Pharmacol Sci 2:283–284, 1981

DeLisi L, Dauphinais ID, Hauser P: Gender differences in the brain: are they relevant to the pathogenesis of schizophrenia? Compr Psychiatry 30:197–208, 1989

Dennerstein L, Burrows GD, Hyman GJ, et al: Hormone therapy and affect. Maturitas 1:247–259, 1979

Depares J, Ryder REJ, Walker SM, et al: Ovarian ultrasonography highlights precision of symptoms of ovulation as markers of ovulation. BMJ 292:1562, 1986

Desmond M, Rudolph AJ, Hill RM, et al: Behavioral alterations in infants born to mothers on psychoactive medication during pregnancy, in Congenital Mental Retardation. Edited by Farrell G. Austin, TX, University of Texas Press, 1967, pp 235–241

Deurenberg P, Westrate JA, Paymans I, et al: Factors affecting bioelectrical impedance measurements in humans. Eur J Clin Nutr 42:1017–1022, 1988

DeVeaugh-Geiss J, Landau P, Katz R: Preliminary results from a multicenter trial of clomipramine in obsessive-compulsive disorder. Psychopharmacol Bull 25:36–40, 1989

Diamond MC: Hormonal effects on the development of cerebral lateralization. Psychoneuroendocrinology 16:121–129, 1991

Diamond S, Rubinstein A, Dunner D, et al: Menstrual problems in women with primary affective illness. Compr Psychiatry 17:541–548, 1976

Dickenson RG, Harland PC, Lynn PK, et al: Transmission of valproic acid (Depakene) across the placenta: half-life of the drug in mother and baby. J Pediatr 94:832–835, 1979

Dickey R: Medical approaches to reproductive regulation: the pill. American College of Obstetricians and Gynecologists (ACOG) Seminars in Family Planning, 1974

Dickey R: Managing Contraceptive Pill Patients, 4th Edition. Durant, OK, Creative Infomatics, 1984

Dignam WS, Voskian J, Assali NS: Effects of estrogens on renal hemodynamics and excretion of electrolytes in human subjects. Journal of Clinical Endocrinology 16:1032–1042, 1956

Dilsaver SC, Coffman JA: Cholinergic hypothesis of depression: a reappraisal. J Clin Psychopharmacol 9:173–179, 1989

Dilsaver SC, Kronfol Z, Sackellares JC, et al: Antidepressant withdrawal syndromes: evidence supporting the cholinergic overdrive hypothesis. J Clin Psychopharmacol 3:157–164, 1983

Dinan TG, Barry S, Yatham LN, et al: The reproducibility of the prolactin response to buspirone: relationship to the menstrual cycle. Int Clin Psychopharmacol 5:119–123, 1990

Ditkoff EC, Crary WG, Cristo M, et al: Estrogen improves psychological function in asymptomatic postmenopausal women. Obstet Gynecol 78:991–995, 1991

Divoll M, Greenblatt DJ, Harmatz JS, et al: Effects of age and gender on temazepam. J Pharm Sci 70:1104–1107, 1981

Dluzen DE, Ramirez VD: Progesterone enhances L-dopa–stimulated dopamine release from the caudate nucleus of freely behaving ovariectomized, estrogen-primed rats. Brain Res 494:122–128, 1989

D'Mello DA, McNeil JA: Sex differences in bipolar affective disorder: neuroleptic dosage variance. Compr Psychiatry 31:80–83, 1990

Domecq C, Naranjo CA, Ruiz I, et al: Sex-related variations in the frequency and characteristics of adverse drug reactions. International Journal of Clinical Pharmacology, Therapy, and Toxicology 18:362–366, 1980

Donaldson GL, Bury RG: Multiple congenital abnormalities in a newborn boy associated with maternal use of fluphenazine enanthate and other drugs during pregnancy. Acta Paediatrica Scandinavica 71:335–338, 1982

Donaldson JO: Control of chorea gravidarum with haloperidol. Obstet Gynecol 59:381–382, 1982

Donnelly EF, Murphy DL, Waldman IN, et al: Prediction of antidepressant responses to imipramine. Neuropsychobiology 5:94–101, 1979

Dorian P, Sellers EM, Reed KL, et al: Amitriptyline and ethanol: pharmacokinetic and pharmacodynamic interaction. Eur J Clin Pharmacol 25:325–331, 1983

Dorus W, Senay EC: Depression, demographic dimensions, and drug abuse. Am J Psychiatry 137:669–704, 1980

Doshi BS, Kulkarni RD, Chauhan BL, et al: Frequency of impaired mephenytoin 4′-hydroxylation in an Indian population (letter). Br J Clin Pharmacol 30:779–780, 1990

Downey G, Coyne JC: Children of depressed parents: an integrative review. Psychol Bull 108:50–76, 1990

Drago F, Scapagnini U: Hormonal modulation of central dopaminergic transmission. J Neural Transm Suppl 22:47–54, 1986

Drago F, Bohus B, Canonico PL, et al: Prolactin induces grooming in the rat: possible involvement of nigrostriatal dopaminergic system. Pharmacol Biochem Behav 15:61–63, 1981

Dresser R: Wanted: single, white male for medical research. Hastings Cent Rep 21:24–29, 1992

Drohse A, Bathum L, Brosen K, et al: Mephenytoin and sparteine oxidation: genetic polymorphism in Denmark. Br J Clin Pharmacol 27:620–625, 1989

Du YL, Lou YQ: Polymorphism of debrisoquine 4-hydroxylation and family studies of poor metabolizers in Chinese population. Acta Pharmacologica Sinica 11:7–10, 1990

Duckert F: Recruitment into treatment and effects of treatment for women problem drinkers. Addict Behav 12:137–150, 1987

Dufour AP, Knight RA, Harria HW: Genetics of isoniazid metabolism in Caucasians, Negroes, and Japanese populations. Science 145:391, 1964

Duke P, Hochman G: A Brilliant Madness: Living With Manic-Depressive Illness. New York, Bantam Books, 1992

Dworkin RH: Patterns of sex differences in negative symptoms and social functioning consistent with separate dimensions of schizophrenic psychopathology. Am J Psychiatry 147:347–349, 1990

Dye L: Measuring the effects of psychotropic drugs during the menstrual cycle: a methodological review, in Human Psychopharmacology: Methods and Measures, Vol 3. Edited by Hindmarch I, Stonier PD. New York, Wiley, 1990, pp 89–110

Eadie MJ, Lander CM Tyrer JH: Plasma drug monitoring in pregnancy. Clin Pharmacokinet 2:427–436, 1977

Eap CB, Baumann P: The genetic polymorphism of human alpha₁-acid glycoprotein: genetics, biochemistry, physiological functions, and pharmacology. Prog Clin Biol Res 300:111–125, 1989

Eap CB, Cuendet C, Baumann P: Binding of d-methadone, 1-methadone, and d-1-methadone to proteins in plasma of healthy volunteers: role of the variants of alpha₁-acid glycoprotein. Clin Pharmacol Ther 47:338–346, 1990

Eaton WW: Marital status and schizophrenia. Acta Psychiatr Scand 52:320–329, 1975

Edelbroek PM, Zitman FG, Schreuder JN, et al: Amitriptyline metabolism in relation to antidepressive effect. Clin Pharmacol Ther 35:467–473, 1984

Edelbroek PM, Linnsen CG, Zitman FG, et al: Analgesic and antidepressive effects of low-dose amitriptyline in relation to its metabolism in patients with chronic pain. Clin Pharmacol Ther 39:156–162, 1986

Editor: Depression and oral contraception. BMJ 4:127–128, 1970

Editor: Drug Facts and Comparisons. St. Louis, MO, Facts and Comparisons, 1993

Edlund MJ, Craig TJ: Antipsychotic drug use and birth defects: an epidemiologic reassessment. Compr Psychiatry 25:32–37, 1984

Edwards G, Brown D, Oppenheimer E, et al: Long-term outcome for patients with drinking problems: the search for predictors. British Journal of Addiction 83:917–927, 1988

Edwards JG, Inman WHW, Pearce GL, et al: Prescription-event monitoring of 10,895 patients treated with alprazolam. Br J Psychiatry 158:387–392, 1991

Edwards RG: Test-tube babies, 1981. Nature 293:253–256, 1981

Edwards RG, Steptoe PC, Purdy JM: Establishing full-term human pregnancies using cleaving embryos grown in vitro. Br J Obstet Gynaecol 87:737–756, 1980a

Edwards RG, Steptoe PC, Fowler RE, et al: Observations on preovulatory human ovarian follicles and their aspirates. Br J Obstet Gynaecol 87:769–779, 1980b

Edwards RG, Anderson G, Pickering J, et al: Rapid assay of urinary LH in women using a simplified method of Hi-Gonavis, in Human Conception In Vitro. Edited by Edwards RG, Purdy JM. New York, Academic Press, 1982, pp 19–49

Eichelbaum M, Bertilsson L, Sawe J, et al: Polymorphic oxidation of sparteine and debrisoquine: related pharmacogenetic entities. Clin Pharmacol Ther 31:184–186, 1982

Eichler A, Parron D: Women's mental health: agenda for research (DHHS Publ No ADM-87-1542). Rockville, MD, National Institute of Mental Health, 1987

Eldred CA, Washington MM: Interpersonal relationships in heroin use by men and women and their role in treatment outcome. Int J Addict 11:117–130, 1976

Elia JE, Katz IR, Simpson GM: Teratogenicity of psychotherapeutic medications. Psychopharmacol Bull 23:531–586, 1987

Elkin I, Shea T, Watkins JT, et al: National Institute of Mental Health Treatment of Depression collaborative research program. Arch Gen Psychiatry 46:971–982, 1989

Elkind-Hirsch K, Goldzieher JW, Gibbons WE, et al: Evaluation of the ovustick urinary luteinizing hormone kit in normal and stimulated menstrual cycles. Obstet Gynecol 67:450–452, 1986

Ellinwood EH, Smith WG, Vaillant GE: Narcotic addictions in males and females: a comparison. Int J Addict 1:33–45, 1966

Ellinwood EH, Easier ME, Linnoila M, et al: Effects of oral contraceptives and diazepam-induced psychomotor impairment. Clin Pharmacol Ther 35:360–366, 1983

Ellinwood EH, Easier ME, Linnoila M, et al: Effects of oral contraceptives and diazepam-induced psychomotor impairment. Clin Pharmacol Ther 35:360–366, 1984

Endicott J, Halbreich U, Schacht S, et al: Premenstrual changes and affective disorders. Psychosom Med 43:519–529, 1981

Endress C, Gray DG, Wollschlaeger G: Bowel ischemia and perforation after cocaine use. American Journal of Roentgenology 159:73–75, 1992

Ereshefsky L, Tran-Johnson T, Davis CM, et al: Pharmacokinetic factors affecting antidepressant drug clearance and clinical effect: evaluation of doxepin and imipramine. Clin Chem 34:863–880, 1988

Ereshefsky L, Saklad SR, Watanabe MD, et al: Thiothixene pharmacokinetic interactions: a study of hepatic enzyme inducers, clearance inhibitors, and demographic variables. J Clin Psychopharmacol 11:296–301, 1991

Erickson J, Fisher A: Myalgia associated with trazodone. Am J Psychiatry 140:1256–1257, 1983

Erickson PG, Murray GF: Sex differences in cocaine use and experiences: a double standard revived? Am J Drug Alcohol Abuse 15:135–152, 1989

Erickson SH, Smith GH, Heidrich F: Tricyclics and breastfeeding. Am J Psychiatry 196:1483, 1979

Eriksson CJP: Ethanol and acetaldehyde metabolism in rat strains genetically selected for their ethanol preference. Biochem Pharmacol 22:2283–2292, 1973

Eriksson E, Sundblad C, Wikander I, et al: The importance of serotonins and androgens for premenstrual dysphoria. CINP XIX Congress, Washington, DC, June 30, 1994

Eriksson K, Malmstrom KK: Sex differences in consumption and elimination of alcohol in albino rats. Ann Med Exp Finn 45:389–392, 1967

Erkkola R, Kanto J: Diazepam and breast-feeding. Lancet 2:1235–1236, 1972

Etchepareborda JJ, Videla L, Bortolussi S, et al: Billings natural FP method: correlation of subjective signs with ovulation and cervical mucus quality, in Research in Family Planning. Edited by Bonnar J, Thompson W, Harrison RF. Boston, MA, MTP Press, 1984, pp 17–20

Ettore E: Women and Substance Use. New Brunswick, NJ, Rutgers University Press, 1992

Evans DA, Mahgoub A, Sloan TP, et al: A family and population study of the genetic polymorphism of debrisoquine oxidation in a white British population. J Med Genet 17:102–105, 1980

Evans J: Fetal crown-rump length values in the first trimester based upon ovulation timing using the luteinizing hormone surge. Br J Obstet Gynaecol 98:48–51, 1991

Everett HC: The use of bethanecol chloride with tricyclic antidepressants. Am J Psychiatry 132:1202–1204, 1975

Facchinetti F, Romano G, Fava M, et al: Lactate infusion induces panic attacks in patients with premenstrual syndrome. Psychosom Med 54:288–296, 1992

Fadel HE, Northrop G, Misenhimer HR, et al: Normal pregnancy: a model of sustained respiratory alkalosis. J Perinat Med 7:195–199, 1979

Fagan TC: Untitled report on sex differences in pharmacology (unpublished manuscript, Department of Internal Medicine, University of Arizona, Tuscon. Presented to the Clinical Pharmacology Panel, Forging a Women's Health Research Agenda Conference, Washington, DC, National Women's Health Resource Center, December 5–6, 1990

Fagan TC: Sex differences in pharmacokinetics and pharmacodynamics: where do they come from? Presentation at the Pharmaceutical Manufacturer's Association Workshop on Special Populations. Washington, DC, May 1992

Fagan TC, Walle T, Walle UK, et al: Ethinyl estradiol alters propranolol metabolism pathway—specifically (abstract). Clin Pharmacol Ther 53:241, 1993

Faiman C, Winter JSD, Reyes FI: Patterns of gonadotrophins and gonadal steroids throughout life. Clinics in Obstetrics and Gynaecology 3:467–484, 1976

Fairman M, Trojan W, Wilkins A, et al: The effect of SSRIs on menstrual cycle length: results of a prospective study of fluoxetine on the treatment of LLPDD. Paper presented at the 23rd annual meeting of the American Society for Psychosomatic Obstetrics and Gynecology, Crystal City, VA, February 24, 1995

Falterman CG, Richardson J: Small left colon syndrome associated with maternal ingestion of psychotropic drugs. J Pediatr 97:308–310, 1980

Faratian B, Gaspar A, O'Brien PMS, et al: Premenstrual syndrome: weight, abdominal swelling, and perceived body image. Am J Obstet Gynecol 150:200–204, 1984

Farina A, Garmezy N, Barry H: Relationship of marital status to incidence and prognosis of schizophrenia. Journal of Abnormal Social Psychology 67:624–630, 1963

Fausto-Sterling A: Myths of Gender: Biological Theories About Women and Men, 2nd Edition. New York, Basic Books, 1992

Fava M, Borofsky GF: Sexual disinhibition during treatment with a benzodiazepine: a case report. Int J Psychiatry Med 21:99–104, 1991

Fazio A: Oral contraceptive drug interactions: important considerations. South Med J 84:997–1002, 1991

Fazleabas AT, Segraves MM, Khan-Dawood FS: Evaluation of salivary and vaginal electrical resistance for determination of the time of ovulation. International Journal of Fertility 35:106–111, 1990

Feder R: Reversal of antidepressant activity of fluoxetine by cyprohep-tadine in three patients. J Clin Psychiatry 52:163–166, 1991

Federman CA, Dumesic DA, Boone WR, et al: Relative efficiency of therapeutic donor insemination using a luteinizing hormone moni-tor. Fertil Steril 54:489–492, 1990

Feksi A, Harris B, Walker RF, et al: Maternity blues and hormone levels in saliva. Journal of Affective Disorders 6:3551–3555, 1984

Ferin J, Thomas K, Johansson EDB: Ovulation detection, in Human Re-production: Conception and Contraception. Edited by Hafez ESE, Evans TN. New York, Harper & Row, 1973, pp 260–283

Fernandez-Ruiz JJ, deMiguel R, Hernandez ML, et al: Time course of the effects of ovarian steroids on the activity of limbic and striatal dopa-minergic neurons in female rats. Pharmacol Biochem Behav 36:603–606, 1990

Fernandez-Ruiz JJ, Hernandez ML, deMiguel R, et al: Nigrostriatal and mesolimbic dopaminergic activities were modified throughout the ovarian cycle of female rats. J Neural Transm Gen Sect 85:223–229, 1991

Ferris RM, Cooper BR, Maxwell RA: Studies of bupropion's mechanism of antidepressant activity. J Clin Psychiatry 44:74–78, 1983

Fesler FA: Valproate in combat-related posttraumatic stress disorder. J Clin Psychiatry 52:361–364, 1991

Fidell LS: Gender and drug use and abuse, in Gender and Psychopathol-ogy. Edited by Al-Issa I. New York, Academic Press, 1982, pp 221–236

Field B, Lu C, Hepner GW: Inhibition of hepatic drug metabolism by norethindrone. Clin Pharmacol Ther 24:196–198, 1979

Field T, Healy B, Goldstein S, et al: Behavior-state matching and syn-chrony in mother-infant interactions of nondepressed vs. depressed dyads. Developmental Psychology 26:7–14, 1990

Fillit H, Weinreb H, Chlost I, et al: Observations in a preliminary open trial of estradiol therapy for senile dementia Alzheimer's type. Psy-choneuroendocrinology 11:337–345, 1986

Fillmore KM, Midanik L: Chronicity of drinking problems among men: a longitudinal study. J Stud Alcohol 45:228–236, 1984

Findlay JWA, Fleet JVW, Smith PG, et al: Pharmacokinetics of bupro-pion, a novel antidepressant agent, following oral administration to healthy subjects. Eur J Pharmacol 21:127–135, 1981

Fink M: Convulsive and drug therapies of depression. Annu Rev Med 32:405–412, 1981

Finney JW, Moos RH: Matching patients with treatments: conceptual and methodological issues. J Stud Alcohol 47:122–134, 1986

Finney JW, Moos RH, Mewborn CR: Posttreatment experiences and treatment outcome of alcoholic patients six months and two years after hospitalization. J Consult Clin Psychol 48:17–29, 1980

Fischer LJ, Thien RL, Charkowski D, et al: Formation and urinary excretion of cyproheptadine in monkeys, chimpanzees and humans. Drug Metab Dispos 8:422–424, 1980

Fiset C, LeBel M: Influence of the menstrual cycle on the absorption and elimination of D-xylose. Clin Pharmacol Ther 48:529–536, 1990

Fisher JB, Edgren BE, Mammel MC, et al: Neonatal apnea associated with maternal clonazepam therapy: a case report. Obstet Gynecol (suppl) 66:34S–35S, 1985

Flaum M, Arndt S, Andreasen NC: The role of gender in studies of ventricle enlargement in schizophrenia: a predominately male effect. Am J Psychiatry 147:1327–1332, 1990

Fleming DE, Anderson RH, Rhees RW, et al: Effects of prenatal stress on sexually dimorphic asymmetries in the cerebral cortex of the male rat. Brain Res Bull 16:395–398, 1986

Floody OR, Pfaff DW: Communication among hamsters by high frequency acoustic signals, III: responses evoked by natural and synthetic ultrasounds. J Comp Psychol 91:820–829, 1977

Fludder MJ, Tonge SR: Variations in concentrations of monoamines in eight regions of rat brain during estrous cycle: a basis for interactions between hormones and psychotropic drugs. Journal of Pharmacy and Pharmacology 27 (suppl):39–42, 1975

Flynn AM, Lynch SS: Cervical mucus and identification of the fertile phase of the menstrual cycle. Br J Obstet Gynaecol 83:656–659, 1976

Flynn AM, Docker M, Morris R, et al: The reliability of women's subjective assessment of the fertile period relative to urinary gonadotrophins and follicular ultrasonic measurements during the menstrual cycle, in Research in Family Planning. Edited by Bonnar J, Thompson W, Harrison RF. Boston, MA, MTP Press, 1984, pp 3–11

Fodor IG: The phobic syndrome in women: implications for treatment, in Women in Therapy: New Psychotherapies for a Changing Society. Edited by Franks V, Buirtle V. New York, Brunner/Mazel, 1974, pp 132–168

Forrest AD, Hay AJ: The influence of sex on schizophrenia. Acta Psychiatr Scand 48:48–58, 1972

Forssman H: Follow-up study of sixteen children whose mothers were given electroconvulsive therapy during gestation. Acta Psychiatrica et Neurologica Scandinavica 30:437–440, 1955

Fortin MT, Evans SB: Correlates of loss of control over drinking in women alcoholics. J Stud Alcohol 44:787–795, 1983

Fotherby K: The progesterone-only pill, in Contraception: Science and Practice. Edited by Filshie M, Guillebaud J. Boston, MA, Butterworths, 1989, pp 94–108

Fowlie S, Burton J: Hyperprolactinemia and nonpuerperal lactation associated with clomipramine (case report). Scott Med J 32:52, 1987

Frank E, Carpenter LL, Kupfer DJ: Sex differences in recurrent depression: are there any that are significant? Am J Psychiatry 145:41–45, 1988

Frank JB, Kosten TR, Giller EL, et al: A randomized clinical trial of phenelzine and imipramine for posttraumatic stress disorder. Am J Psychiatry 145:1289–1291, 1988

Frank R: The hormonal causes of premenstrual tension. Archives of Neurology and Psychiatry 26:1053–1057, 1931

Franks S, Nabarro J, Jacobs H: Prevalence and presentation of hyperprolactinemia in patients with functionless pituitary tumours. Lancet 1:778–780, 1977

Franks S, Van Der Spuy Z, Mason WP, et al: Luteal function after ovulation induction by pulsatile luteinizing hormone releasing hormone, in The Luteal Phase (Current Topics in Reproductive Endocrinology). Edited by Jeffcoate SL. New York, Wiley, 1985, pp 89–100

Fraser AR: Sexual dysfunction following antidepressant drug therapy. J Clin Psychopharmacol 4:62–63, 1984

Fraser I: Systemic hormonal contraception by non-oral routes, in Contraception: Science and Practice. Edited by Filshie M, Guillebaud J. Boston, MA, Butterworths, 1989, pp 109–125

Fraser J: The female alcoholic, in Women and Mental Health. Edited by Howell E, Bayes M. New York, Basic Books, 1981, pp 296–305

Freeman EW, Rickels K: Serotonergic drugs and progesterone in PMS. CINP XIX Congress, Washington, DC, June 30, 1994

Freeman EW, Purdy RH, Coutifaris C, et al: Anxiolytic metabolites of progesterone: correlation with mood and performance on measures following oral progesterone administration to healthy female volunteers. Neuroendocrinology 58:478–484, 1993

Freeman EW, Sondheimer S, Rickels K: Comparisons of the effectiveness of hormonal and CNS medications in PMS treatment. Paper presented at the 23rd annual meeting of the American Society for Psychosomatic Obstetrics and Gynecology, Crystal City, VA, February 23, 1995

French-Mullen JM, Spence KT: Neurosteroids block Ca2+ channel current in freshly isolated hippocampal CA1 neurons. Eur J Pharmacol 202:269–272, 1991

Freud S: Repression (1915), in The Standard Edition of the Complete Psychological Works of Sigmund Freud, Vol 14. Translated and edited by Strachey J. London, Hogarth Press, 1957, pp 141–158

Freud S: Beyond the pleasure principle (1920), in The Standard Edition of the Complete Psychological Works of Sigmund Freud, Vol 18. Translated and edited by Strachey J. London, Hogarth Press, 1955, pp 1–64

Frey B, Schubiger G, Musy JP: Transient cholestatic hepatitis in a neonate associated with carbamazepine exposure during pregnancy and breastfeeding. Eur J Pediatr 150:136–138, 1990

Freyhan F: Loss of ejaculation during mellaril treatment. Am J Psychiatry 118:171–172, 1961

Frezza M, Di Padova C, Pozzato G: High blood alcohol levels in women: the role of decreased gastric alcohol dehydrogenase activity and first-pass metabolism. N Engl J Med 322:95–99, 1990

Froscher W, Stoll K-D, Hildenbrand G, et al: Investigations on the intraindividual constancy of the ratio of carbamazepine to carbamazepine-10, 11-epoxide in man. Arzneimittel-Forschung Drug Research 38 (I-5):724–726, 1988

Fujimoto VY, Clifton DK, Cohen NL, et al: Variability of serum prolactin and progesterone levels in normal women: the relevance of single hormone measurements in the clinical setting. Obstet Gynecol 76:71–78, 1990

Funabashi T, Brooks PJ, Mobbs C, et al: DNA methylation and DNase hypersensitive sites in the 5′ flanking and transcribed regions of the rat preproenkephalin gene: studies of mediobasal hypothalamus. Mol Cell Neurosci 4:499–509, 1993a

Funabashi T, Brooks PJ, Mobbs C, et al: Tissue-specific DNA methylation and DNAse hypersensitive sites in the promoter and transcribed regions of the rat preproenkephalin gene (abstract 112.12). Society for Neuroscience Abstracts 18:240, 1993b

Furlanut M, Montanuri G, Bonin P, et al: Carbamazepine and carbamazepine-10, 11-epoxide serum concentrations in epileptic children. J Pediatr 106:491–495, 1985

Fuxe K, Eneroth P, Gustafson JA, et al: Dopamine in the nucleus accumbens: preferential increase of DA turnover by rat prolactin. Brain Res 122:177–181, 1977

Galeazzi RL: Pharmacodynamics, pharmacokinetics, or both?, in Pharmacokinetics and Pharmacodynamics of Psychoactive Drugs. Edited by Barnett G, Chuiang N. Foster City, CA, Biomedical Publishers, 1985, pp 169–185

Gallant SJ, Popiel DA, Hoffman DM, et al: Using daily ratings to confirm premenstrual syndrome/late luteal phase dysphoric disorder, I: effects of demand characteristics and expectations. Psychosom Med 54:149–166, 1992a

Gallant SJ, Popiel DA, Hoffman DM, et al: Using daily ratings to confirm premenstrual syndrome/late luteal phase dysphoric disorder, II: what makes a real difference? Psychosom Med 54:167–181, 1992b

Gammans RE, Mayol RF, Labudde JA: Metabolism and disposition of buspirone. Am J Med 80:41–51, 1986

Ganrot PO: Variation of the concentrations of some plasma proteins in normal adults, in pregnant women and in newborns. Scand J Clin Lab Invest 29 (suppl 24):83–88, 1972

Garcia JE, Jones GS, Wright GL: Prediction of the time of ovulation. Fertil Steril 36:308–315, 1981

Gardner EA, Johnston JA: Bupropion—an antidepressant without sexual pathophysiological action. J Clin Psychopharmacol 5:24–29, 1985

Gartrell N: Increased libido in women receiving trazodone. Am J Psychiatry 143:781–782, 1986

Garvey MJ, Tollefson GD: Postpartum depression. J Reprod Med 29:113–116, 1984

Garvey MJ, Tuason VB, Lumry AE, et al: Occurrence of depression in the postpartum state. Journal of Affective Disorders 5:97–101, 1983

Gawin FH, Kleber HD: Nueroendocrine findings in chronic cocaine abusers: a preliminary report. Br J Psychiatry 147:569–573, 1985

Gawin FH, Kleber HD, Byck R, et al: Desipramine facilitation of initial cocaine abstinence. Arch Gen Psychiatry 46:117–121, 1989

Gee KW: Steroid modulation of the GABA/benzodiazepine receptor–linked chloride ionophore. Mol Neurobiol 2:291–317, 1988

Gelenberg AJ, Cooper DS, Doller JC, et al: Galactorrhea and hyperprolactinemia associated with amoxapine therapy: report of a case. JAMA 24:1900–1901, 1979

Genazzani AR, Petraglia F, Bergamaschi M: Progesterone and progestins modulate beta-endorphin concentrations in the hypothalamus and in the pituitary of castrated female rats. Gynecol Endocrinol 1:61–69, 1987

Genazzani AR, Petraglia F, Silferi M, et al: Progestins modulate the action of estrogen on gonadrotropin-releasing hormone and prolactin in the rat. Gynecol Obstet Invest 29:197–202, 1990

Gengo F, Fagan SC, Kinkel WR, et al: Serum concentrations of propranolol in migraine prophylaxis. Arch Neurol 41:1306–1308, 1984

Gerner R, Estabrook W, Steuer J, et al: Treatment of geriatric depression with trazodone, imipramine and placebo: a double-blind study. J Clin Psychiatry 41:216–220, 1980

Geschwind N, Galaburda AM: Cerebral lateralization—biological mechanisms, associations, and pathology, I: a hypothesis and program for research. Arch Neurol 42:428–459, 1985a

Geschwind N, Galaburda AM: Cerebral lateralization—biological mechanisms, associations, and pathology, I: a hypothesis and program for research. Arch Neurol 42:634–654, 1985b

Gessa GL, Tagliamonte A: Role of brain monoamines in male sexual behavior. Life Sciences 14:425–436, 1974

Gex-Fabry M, Balant-Georgia A, Balant LP, et al: Clomipramine metabolism: model based analysis of variability factors from drug monitoring data. Clin Pharmacokinet 19:241–255, 1990

Ghadirian AM, Chouinard G, Annable L: Sexual dysfunction and plasma prolactin levels in neuroleptic-treated outpatients. J Nerv Ment Dis 170:463–467, 1982

Ghadirian AM, Annable L, Belanger MC: Lithium, benzodiazepines, and sexual function in bipolar patients. Am J Psychiatry 149:801–805, 1992

Ghose K, Turner P: The menstrual cycle and the tyramine pressor response test. Br J Clin Pharmacol 4:500–502, 1977

Giannini AJ, Martin DM, Turner CE: Beta-endorphin decline in late luteal phase dysphoric disorder. Int J Psychiatry Med 20:279–284, 1990

Giles HG, Sellers EM, Naranjo A, et al: Disposition of intravenous diazepam in young men and women. Eur J Clin Pharmacol 20:207–213, 1981

Gill RC, Murphy PD, Hooper HR, et al: Effect of the menstrual cycle on gastric emptying. Digestion 36:168–174, 1987

Gillberg C: Floppy infant syndrome and maternal diazepam (letter). Lancet 2:244, 1977

Girgis S, Etriby A, El-Hefnawy H, et al: Aspermia: a survey of 40 cases. Fertil Steril 19:580–588, 1968

Gise L (ed): The Premenstrual Syndromes. New York, Churchill Livingston, 1988

Gitlin MJ, Weiss J: Verapamil as maintenance treatment in bipolar illness: a case report. J Clin Psychiatry 4:341–343, 1984

Giudicelli JF, Tillement JP: Influence of sex on drug kinetics in man. Clin Pharmacokinet 2:157–162, 1977

Glassman AH, Perel JM, Shostak et al. 1977: Clinical implications of imipramine plasma levels for depressive illness. Arch Gen Psychiatry 34:197–204, 1977

Gleichauf CN, Roe DA: The menstrual cycle's effect on the reliability of bioimpedance measurements for assessing body composition. Am J Clin Nutr 50:903–907, 1989

Gleichmann W, Bachmann GW, Dengler HJ, et al: Effects of hormonal contraceptives and pregnancy on serum protein pattern. Eur J Clin Pharmacol 5:212–225, 1973

Glick J, Steward D: A new drug treatment for premenstrual exacerbation of schizophrenia. Compr Psychiatry 21:281–287, 1980

Glick SD, Hinds PA, Shapiro RM: Cocaine-induced rotation: sex-dependent differences between left- and right-sided rats. Science 221:775–776, 1983

Goble FC: Sex as a factor in metabolism, toxicity, and efficacy of pharmacodynamic and chemotherapeutic agents, in Advances in Pharmacology and Chemotherapy, Vol 13. Edited by Garattini S, Goldin A, Hawkings F, et al. New York, Academic Press, 1975, pp 173–252

Goethe JW, Szarek BL, Cook WL: A comparison of adequately vs. inadequately treated depressed patients. J Nerv Ment Dis 176:465–470, 1988

Goff DC, Henderson DC, Amico E: Cigarette smoking in schizophrenia: relationship to psychopathology and medication side effects. Am J Psychiatry 149:1189–1194, 1992

Gold BI, Bowers MB Jr, Roth RH, et al: GABA levels of CSF of patients with psychiatric disorders. Am J Psychiatry 137:362–364, 1980

Goldberg HL, Rickels K, Finnerty R: Treatment of neurotic depression with a new antidepressant (abstract). J Clin Psychopharmacol 1 (suppl):35S, 1981

Goldbloom DS, Kennedy SH: Adverse interaction of fluoxetine and cyproheptadine in two patients with bulimia nervosa. J Clin Psychiatry 52:261–262, 1991

Golden RN, DeVane L, Laizure C, et al: Bupropion in depression, II: the role of metabolites in clinical outcome. Arch Gen Psychiatry 45:145–149, 1988

Golden RN, Hsaio J, Lane E, et al: The effects of intravenous clomipramine on neurohormones in normal subjects. J Clin Endocrinol Metab 68:632–637, 1989

Goldstein DB: Pharmacokinetics of alcohol, in Medical Diagnosis and Treatment of Alcoholism. Edited by Mendelson JH, Mello NK. New York, McGraw-Hill, 1992, pp 25–54

Goldstein JM: Gender differences in the course of schizophrenia. Am J Psychiatry 145:684–689, 1988

Goldstein JM, Faraone SV, Chen WJ, et al: Sex differences in the familial transmission of schizophrenia. Br J Psychiatry 156:819–826, 1990

Goldstein MS, Surber M, Wilner DM: Outcome evaluations in substance abuse: a comparison of alcoholism, drug abuse, and other mental health interventions. Int J Addict 19:479–502, 1984

Goldzieher J: Hormonal Contraception: Pills, Injections and Implants, 2nd Edition. Ontario, EMIS-Canada, 1989

Gomberg ESL: Alcoholic women in treatment: the question of stigma and age. Alcohol Alcoholism 23:507–514, 1988

Gomberg ESL: Suicide risk among women with alcohol problems. Am J Public Health 79:1363–1365, 1989

Gomez E: Hypersexuality in men receiving fluphenazine decanoate (letter). Am J Psychiatry 138:1263, 1981

Gonzalez FJ: The molecular biology of cytochrome P450s. Pharmacol Rev 40:243–288, 1988

Gonzalez FJ, Nebert DW: Evolution of the P450 gene superfamily: animal-plant warfare, molecular drive and human genetic differences in drug oxidation. Trends Genetics 6:182–186, 1990

Goodman LS, Gilman A (eds): The Pharmacological Basis of Therapeutics, 5th Edition. New York, Macmillan, 1975

Goodwin DW, Schulsinger F, Hermansen L, et al: Alcohol problems in adoptees raised apart from alcoholic biological parents. Arch Gen Psychiatry 28:238–243, 1973

Goodwin DW, Schulsinger R, Knop J, et al: Alcoholism and depression in adopted-out daughters of alcoholics. Arch Gen Psychiatry 31:164–169, 1977

Gordon CV, Wierenga DE: The Drug Development and Approval Process. Washington, DC, Pharmaceutical Manufacturers Association Office of Research and Development, 1991

Gordon JH: Modulation of apomorphine-induced stereotypy by estrogen: time course and dose response. Brain Res Bull 5:679–682, 1980

Gorelick DA: Alcohol and cocaine: clinical and pharmacological interactions, in Recent Developments in Alcoholism, Vol 10. Edited by Galanter M. New York, Plenum, 1992, pp 37–56

Gorski RA, Harlan, RE, Jacobson CD, et al: Evidence for morphological sex difference within the medial preoptic area of the rat brain. J Comp Neurol 193:529–539, 1980

Gottesman II, Shields J: Schizophrenia: the epigenetic puzzle. Cambridge, UK, Cambridge University Press, 1982

Gouchie C, Kimura D: The relationship between testosterone levels and cognitive ability patterns. Psychoneuroendocrinology 16:323–334, 1991

Gould E, Woolley CS, McEwen BS: The hippocampal formation: morphological changes induced by thyroid, gonadal and adrenal hormones. Psychoneuroendocrinology 16:67–84, 1991

Graeven DB, Schaef RD: Family life and levels of involvement in an adolescent heroin epidemic. Int J Addict 13:747–771, 1978

Gram LF, Christiansen J: First-pass metabolism of imipramine in man. Clin Pharmacol Ther 17:555–563, 1975

Gram LF, Reisby N, Ibsen I, et al: Plasma levels and antidepressive effect of imipramine. Clin Pharmacol Ther 19:318–324, 1976

Gram LF, Sondergaard I, Christiansen J, et al: Steady-state kinetics of imipramine in patients. Psychopharmacology (Berl) 54:255–261, 1977

Gram LF, Bjerre M, Kragh-Sorensen P, et al: Imipramine metabolites in blood of patients during therapy and after overdose. Clin Pharmacol Ther 33:335–342, 1983

Grant DM, Tang BK, Kalow W: Polymorphic N-acetylation of a caffeine metabolite. Clin Pharmacol Ther 33:355–359, 1983

Grant DM, Morike K, Eichelbaum M, et al: Acetylation pharmacogenetics. J Clin Invest 85:968–972, 1990

Gratton L: Neuroleptics, parkinsonisme et schizophrenie. Union Medicale du Canada 89:681–694, 1960

Gray MJ, Strausfeld KS, Watanabe M, et al: Aldosterone secretory rates in the normal menstrual cycle. J Clin Endocrinol Metab 28:1269–1275, 1968

Gray RH, Campbell OM, Apelo R, et al: Risk of ovulation during lactation. Lancet 335:25–29, 1990

Green JG: Recent trends in the treatment of premenstrual syndrome: a critical review, in Behavior and the Menstrual Cycle. Edited by Friedman RC. New York, Marcel Dekker, 1982

Green JG, Cooke DJ: Life stress and symptoms at the climacterium. Br J Psychiatry 136:486–491, 1980

Greenblatt DJ, Shader RI, Franke K, et al: Kinetics of intravenous chlordiazepoxide: sex differences in drug disposition. Clin Pharmacol Ther 22:893–903, 1977

Greenblatt DJ, Divoll M, Harmatz JS, et al: Diazepam disposition determinants. Clin Pharmacol Ther 17:301–312, 1980a

Greenblatt DJ, Allen MD, Harmatz J, et al: Oxazepam kinetics: effects of age and sex. J Pharmacol Exp Ther 215:86–91, 1980b

Greenblatt DJ, Sellers EM, Shader RI: Drug disposition in old age. N Engl J Med 306:1081–1088, 1982

Greenblatt DJ, Abernethy DR, Locniskar A, et al: Age, sex, and nitrazepam kinetics: relation to antipyrine disposition. Clin Pharmacol Ther 38:697–703, 1985

Greenblatt DJ, Friedman H, Burstein ES, et al: Trazodone kinetics: effects of age, gender, and obesity. Clin Pharmacol Ther 42:193–200, 1987

Greenblatt DJ, Divoll MK, Abernethy DR, et al: Age and gender effects on chlordiazepoxide kinetics: relation to antipyrine disposition. Pharmacology 38:327–334, 1989

Greenblatt M, Grosser GH, Wechsler H: Differential response of hospitalized depressed patients to somatic therapy. Am J Psychiatry 120:935–943, 1964

Greene BT, Ryser PE: Impact of sex on length of time spent in treatment and treatment success. Am J Drug Alcohol Abuse 5:97–105, 1978

Greenfield SF, Weiss RD, Mirin SM: Cocaine: a clinical update. Resident and Staff Physician 40:21–24, 1994 [this ref replaces Greenfield, in press and Mirin, in press]

Greenfield SF, Weiss RD, Mirin SM: Psychoactive substance use disorders, in The Practitioner's Guide to Psychoactive Substances. Edited by Gelenberg AJ, Bassuk EL. New York, Plenum (in press)

Griffin J, D'Arcy P: A Manual of Adverse Drug Interactions. Bristol, UK, John Wright, 1975

Griffin ML, Mello NK, Mendelson JH, et al: Alcohol use across the menstrual cycle among marijuana users. Alcohol 4:457–462, 1987

Griffin ML, Weiss RD, Mirin SM, et al: A comparison of male and female cocaine abusers. Arch Gen Psychiatry 46:122–126, 1989

Grimes DA (ed): Drug interactions with OCs. Contraception Report 3:9–12, 1992

Grimes DA (ed): Women's health in the perimenopause. Contraception Report 4:5–10, 1993

Grinsted J, Jacobson JD, Grinsted L, et al: Prediction of ovulation. Fertil Steril 52:388–393, 1989

Gross MD: Reversal by bethanechol of sexual dysfunction caused by anticholinergic antidepressants. Am J Psychiatry 139:1193–1194, 1982

Gross MD: Dr. Gross replies to psychotropic-induced sexual inhibition (letter). Am J Psychiatry 140:515, 1983

Grossman MI, Kirsner JB, Gillespie IA: Basal and histalog-stimulated gastric secretion in control subjects and in patients with peptic ulcer or gastric cancer. Gastroenterol 45:14–26, 1963

Group for the Advancement of Psychiatry: Forced Into Treatment: The Role of Coercion in Clinical Practice. Committee on Government Policy, Group for the Advancement of Psychiatry, Report No. 137. Washington, DC, American Psychiatric Press, 1993

Guelfi JD, Pichot P, Dreyfus JF: Efficacy of tianeptine in anxious-depressed patients: results of a controlled multicenter trial vs. amitriptyline. Neuropsychobiology 22:41–48, 1989

Guengerich FP: Oxidation of 17-alpha-ethinylestradiol by human liver cytochrome P450. Mol Pharmacol 33:500–508, 1988

Guillebaud J: Practical prescribing of the combined oral contraceptive pill, in Contraception: Science and Practice. Edited by Filshie M, Guillebaud J. Boston, MA, Butterworths, 1989, pp 69–93

Guinan ME: Women and crack addiction. J Am Med Wom Assoc 44:129, 1989

Gunne LM, Haggstrom JE, Johansson P, et al: Neurobiochemical changes in tardive dyskinesia. Encephale 14:167–173, 1988

Gur RC, Gur RE, Obrist WD, et al: Sex and handedness differences in cerebral blood flow during rest and cognitive activity. Science 217:659–661, 1982

Gur RC, Mozley LH, Mozley PD, et al: Sex differences in regional cerebral glucose metabolism during a resting state. Science 267:528–531, 1995

Gur RE, Gur RC: Gender difference in regional cerebral blood flow. Schizophr Bull 16:247–254, 1990

Gur RE, Gur RC, Skolnick BE, et al: Brain function in psychiatric disorders, III: regional cerebral blood flow in unmedicated schizophrenics. Arch Gen Psychiatry 42:329–334, 1985

Gureje G: Gender and schizophrenia: age at onset and sociodemographic attributes. Acta Psychiatr Scand 83:402–405, 1991

Haas GL, Sweeney JA: Premorbid and onset features of first-episode schizophrenia. Schizophr Bull 18:373–386, 1992

Haas GL, Hien D, Waked W, et al: Sex differences in schizophrenia (abstract). Schizophr Res 2:11, 1989

Haas GL, Glick ID, Clarkin JF, et al: Gender and schizophrenia outcome: a clinical trial of an inpatient family intervention. Schizophr Bull 16:277–292, 1990

Haastrup S, Jepsen PW: Eleven year follow-up of 300 young opioid addicts. Acta Psychiatr Scand 77:22–26, 1988

Häfner H, Riecher A, Maurer K, et al: How does gender influence age at first hospitalization for schizophrenia? A transnational case register study. Psychol Med 19:903–918, 1989

Häfner H, Behrens S, DeVry J, et al: Oestradiol enhances the vulnerability threshold for schizophrenia in women by an early effect on dopaminergic neurotransmission. Eur Arch Psychiatry Clin Neurosci 241:65–68, 1991

Häfner H, Maurer K, Löffler W, et al: The influence of age and sex on the onset of early course of schizophrenia. Br J Psychiatry 162:80–86, 1993

Hafner RJ: Agoraphobia in men. Aust N Z J Psychiatry 14:243–249, 1981

Hakim C, Pichot D: Le traitement prophylactique de la psychose maniaco-depressive par le carbonate de lithium—Intérêt théorique et pratique de l'étude des variations de la concentration plasmatique. Ann Med Psychol 1:238–246, 1972

Halbreich U (ed): Hormones and Depression. New York, Raven, 1987

Halbreich U, Carson SW: Drug studies in women of child-bearing age: ethical and methodological considerations. J Clin Psychopharmacol 9:328–333, 1989

Halbreich U, Endicott J: A possible involvement of endorphins in premenstrual syndromes and post partum depression. Med Hypotheses 7:1045–1052, 1981

Halbreich U, Endicott J: Methodological issues in studies of premenstrual changes. Psychoneuroendocrinology 10:15–32, 1985a

Halbreich U, Endicott J: The relationship of dysphoric premenstrual changes to depressive disorders. Acta Psychiatr Scand 71:331–338, 1985b

Halbreich U, Tworek H: Altered serotonergic activity in women with dysphoric premenstrual syndrome. Int J Psychiatry Med 23:1–27, 1993

Halbreich U, Ben-David M, Assael M, et al: Serum prolactin in women with premenstrual syndrome. Lancet 2:654–656, 1976

Halbreich U, Asnis G, Ross D, et al: Amphetamine-induced dysphoria in postmenopausal women. Br J Psychiatry 138:470–473, 1981

Halbreich U, Endicott J, Schacht S, et al: The diversity of premenstrual changes as reflected in the Premenstrual Assessment Form. Acta Psychiatr Scand 65:46–65, 1982

Halbreich U, Asnis G, Goldstein S, et al: Sex differences in response to psychological interventions in humans. Schizophr Bull 14:526–530, 1984

Halbreich U, Alt L, Paul L: Premenstrual changes: impaired hormonal homeostasis. Endocrinol Metab Clin North Am 17:173–194, 1988

Halbreich U, Rojansky N, Bakhai Y, et al: Menstrual irregularities associated with bupropion hydrochloride treatment. J Clin Psychiatry 52:15–16, 1991

Halliday A, Bush B: Women and alcohol abuse, in Alcoholism: A Guide for the Primary Care Physician. Edited by Barnes HN, Bronson NM, DelBanco TL. New York, Springer-Verlag, 1987, pp 176–180

Halliday A, Bush B, Cleary P, et al: Alcohol abuse in women seeking gynecologic care. Obstet Gynecol 68:322–326, 1986

Hallonquist JD, Seeman MV, Lang M, et al: Variation in symptom severity over the menstrual cycle of schizophrenics. Biol Psychiatry 33:207–209, 1993

Hällström T, Samuelsson S: Changes in women's sexual desire in middle life: the longitudinal study of women in Gothenberg. Arch Sex Behav 19:259–268, 1990

Hamer DH, Hu S, Magnuson VL, et al: A linkage between DNA markers on the X chromosome and male sexual orientation. Science 261:321–327, 1993

Hamilton J: A rating scale for depression. J Neurol Neurosurg Psychiatry 23:56–62, 1961

Hamilton JA: Avoiding methodological and policy-making biases in gender-related research, in Report of the Public Health Service Task Force on Women's Health Issues, Vol 2. Washington, DC, U.S. Government Printing Office, 1985, pp 54–64

Hamilton JA: An overview of the clinical rationale for advancing gender-related psychopharmacology and drug abuse research, in Women and Drugs: A New Era for Research (NIDA Monograph 65). Edited by Ray BA, Braude MC. Washington, DC, U.S. Government Printing Office, 1986, pp 14–20

Hamilton JA: Clinical pharmacology panel report, in Proceedings, Forging a Women's Health Research Agenda Conference, Washington, DC, December 5–6, 1990. Edited by Blumenthal SJ, Barry B, Hamilton JA, et al. Washington, DC, National Women's Health Resource Center, 1991, pp 1–27

Hamilton JA: Sex and gender as critical variables in psychotropic drug research, in Racism and Sexism and Mental Health. Edited by Brown B, Rieker P, Willie C. Pittsburgh, PA, University of Pittsburgh Press, 1995, pp 297–350

Hamilton JA: Are there sex differences in response to imipramine? Womens Health Forum (in press a)

Hamilton JA: How to include women in clinical trials: debate in the U.S. and international implications, in Gender and Health: An International Perspective. Edited by Sargent C, Bretelle C. Englewood Cliffs, NJ, Simon & Schuster (in press b)

Hamilton JA, Conrad CD: Toward a developmental psychopharmacology: the physiological basis of age, gender, and hormonal effects on drug responsivity, in Basic Handbook of Child Psychiatry, Vol 5. Edited by JD Noshpitz. New York, Basic Books, 1987, pp 6–81

Hamilton JA, Gallant SJ: Premenstrual syndromes: a health psychology critique of biomedically oriented research, in Psychophysiological Disorders (Health Psychology Series). Edited by Gatchel RJ, Blanchard EB. Washington, DC, American Psychological Association, 1993, pp 383–489

Hamilton JA, Grant M: Sex differences in metabolism and pharmacokinetics: effects on agent choice and dosing. Paper presented at the NIMH Conference "Toward a New Psychobiology of Depression in Women: Treatment and Gender," Bethesda, MD, November 4, 1993

Hamilton JA, Halbreich U: Special aspects of neuropsychiatric illness in women: with a focus on depression. Annu Rev Med 44:355–364, 1993

Hamilton JA, Jensvold MF: Pharmacotherapy for complicated depressions in women. Psychiatric Times 8:1, 47–49, 51–54, 1991

Hamilton JA, Jensvold MF: Personality, psychopathology and depression in women, in Personality and Psychopathology: Feminist Reappraisals. Edited by Brown LS, Ballou M. New York, Guilford, 1992, pp 116–143

Hamilton JA, Parry BL: Sex-related differences in clinical drug response: implications for women's health. J Am Med Wom Assoc 38:126–132, 1983

Hamilton JA, Lloyd C, Alagna SW, et al: Gender, depressive subtypes, and gender-age effects on antidepressant response: hormonal hypotheses. Psychopharmacol Bull 20:475–480, 1984a

Hamilton JA, Parry BL, Alagna SW, et al: Premenstrual mood changes: a guide to evaluation and treatment. Psychiatric Annals 14:426–435, 1984b

Hamilton JA, Parry BL, Blumenthal SJ: The menstrual cycle in context, I: affective syndromes associated with reproductive hormonal changes. J Clin Psychiatry 49:474–480, 1988

Hamilton JA, Jensvold MF, Rothblum E, et al. (eds): Psychopharmacology From a Feminist Perspective (special issue of Women and Therapy). New York, Haworth, 1995

Hammar M, Berg G, Fahraeus L, et al: Climacteric symptoms in an unselected sample of Swedish women. Maturitas 6:345–350, 1984

Hammarback S, Bäckström T: Induced anovulation as treatment of premenstrual tension syndrome. Acta Obstet Gynecol Scand 67:159–166, 1988

Hammond JE, Toseland PA: Placental transfer of chlorpromazine. Arch Dis Child 45:139–140, 1970

Hanley SP: Asthma variation with menstruation. British Journal of Diseases of the Chest 75:306–308, 1981

Hansten P: Drug Interactions, 3rd Edition. Philadelphia, PA, Lea & Febiger, 1976

Harada S: Genetic polymorphism of aldehyde dehydrogenase and its physiological significance to alcohol metabolism. Prog Clin Biol Res 344:289–291, 1990

Haring C, Meise U, Humpel C, et al: Dose-related plasma levels of clozapine: influence of smoking, behavior, sex and age. Psychopharmacology (Berl) 99:538–540, 1989

Harlan RE, Shivers BD, Romano GJ, et al: Localization of preproenkephalin mRNA in the rat brain and spinal cord by in situ hybridization. J Comp Neurol 258:159–184, 1987

Harris RB, Laws A, Reddy VM, et al: Are women using postmenopausal estrogens? a community survey. Am J Public Health 80:1266–1268, 1990

Harrison WM, Stewart J, Ehrhardt AA, et al: A controlled study of the effects of antidepressant medication on sexual function. Psychopharmacol Bull 21:85–88, 1985

Harrison WM, Rabkin JG, Ehrhardt AA, et al: Effects of antidepressant medication on sexual function: a controlled study. J Clin Psychopharmacol 6:144–149, 1986

Harrison WM, Sandberg D, Gorman J, et al: Provocation of panic with carbon dioxide inhalation in patients with premenstrual dysphoria. Psychiatry Res 27:183–192, 1989

Harrison WM, Endocott J, Nee J: Treatment of premenstrual dysphoria with alprazolam: a controlled study. Arch Gen Psychiatry 47:270–275, 1990

Hartley LR, Ungapen S, Davie I: The effect of beta adrenergic blocking drugs on speaker's performance and memory. Br J Psychiatry 142:512–517, 1983

Hartz SC, Heinonen OP, Shapiro S, et al: Antenatal exposure to meprobamate and chlordiazepoxide in relation to malformations, mental development and childhood mortality. N Engl J Med 292:726–728, 1975

Harvey AM, Malvin RL, Vander AJ: Comparison of creatinine secretion in men and women. Nephron 3:201–205, 1966

Hashimoto S, Miwa M, Akasofu K, et al: Changes in 40 serum proteins of post-menopausal women. Maturitas 13:23–33, 1991

Hassler M: Testosterone and artistic talents. Int J Neurosci 56:25–38, 1991

Hatazawa J, Masatoshi I, Harutsugu Y, et al: Sex difference in brain atrophy during aging: a quantitative study with computer tomography. J Am Geriatr Soc 30:235–239, 1982

Hatcher R, Stewart F, Trussel J, et al: Contraceptive Technology: 1990–1992, 15th Revised Edition. New York, Irvington, 1990

Hatotani N, Kitayama I, Inoue K, et al: Psychoneuroendocrine studies of recurrent psychoses, in Neurobiology of Periodic Psychoses. Edited by Hatotani N, Nomura J. Tokyo, Japan, Igaku-Shoin, 1983, pp 77–92

Haukkamaa M: Contraception by Norplant subdermal capsules is not reliable in epileptic patients on anticonvulsant treatment. Contraception 33:559–565, 1986

Hauser PI, Dauphinais D, Berrettini W, et al: Corpus callosum dimensions measured by magnetic resonance imaging in bipolar affective disorder and schizophrenia. Biol Psychiatry 26:659–668, 1989

Haver B: Female alcoholics, IV: the relationship between family violence and outcome 3–10 years after treatment. Acta Psychiatr Scand 75:445–449, 1987

Hay WM, Nathan PE, Heermans HW, et al: Menstrual cycle, tolerance and blood alcohol level discrimination ability. Addict Behav 9:67–77, 1984

Heinonen OP, Slone D, Shapiro S: Birth Defects in Pregnancy. Littleton, MA, Publishing Sciences Group, 1977

Hekimian L, Friedhoff A, Deever E: A comparison of the onset of action and therapeutic efficacy of amoxapine and amitriptyline. J Clin Psychiatry 39:633–637, 1978

Helzer JE, Robins LN, McEvoy L: Post traumatic stress disorder in the general population. N Engl J Med 317:1630–1634, 1987

Helzer JE, Burnam A, McEvoy LT: Alcohol abuse and dependence, in Psychiatric Disorders in America. Edited by Robins LN, Regier DA. New York, Free Press, 1991, pp 81–115

Herman JL, Perry JC, van der Kolk BA: Childhood trauma in borderline personality disorder. Am J Psychiatry 146:490–495, 1989

Herr BM, Pettinati HM: Long term outcome in working and homemaking alcoholic women. Alcohol Clin Exp Res 8:576–579, 1984

Herrick A, McColl K, Wallace A, et al: LHRH analogue treatment for the prevention of premenstrual attacks of acute porphyria. Quarterly Journal of Medicine 75:355–363, 1990

Hesselbrock MN, Meyer RE, Keener JJ: Psychopathology in hospitalized alcoholics. Arch Gen Psychiatry 42:1050–1055, 1985

Hesselbrock VM, Stabenau JR, Hesselbrock MN, et al: The nature of alcoholism in patients with different family histories for alcoholism. Prog Neuropsychopharmacol Biol Psychiatry 6:607–614, 1982

Hesselbrock VM, Hesselbrock MN, Workman-Daniels KL: Effect of major depression and antisocial personality on alcoholism: course and motivational patterns. J Stud Alcohol 47:207–212, 1986

Hier DB: Sex differences in hemispheric specialization: hypothesis for the excess of dyslexia in boys. Bulletin of the Orton Society 29:74–83, 1979

Higgins ST, Delaney DD, Budney AJ, et al: A behavioral approach to achieving initial cocaine abstinence. Am J Psychiatry 148:1218–1224, 1991

Hillesmaa VK, Bardy AH, Granstrom ML, et al: Valproic acid during pregnancy (letter). Lancet 1:883, 1980

Hillesmaa VK, Teramo K, Granstrom ML, et al: Fetal heat growth retardation associated with maternal antiepileptic drugs. Lancet 2:165–167, 1981

Hobbes J, Boutagy J, Shenfield GM: Interactions between ethanol and oral contraceptive steroids. Clin Pharmacol Ther 38:371–380, 1985

Hoff JD, Quigley ME, Yen SSC: Hormonal dynamics at midcycle: a reevaluation. J Clin Endocrinol Metab 57:792–796, 1983

Hohmann AA: Gender bias in psychotropic drug prescribing in primary care. Med Care 27:478–490, 1989

Hollander E, McCarley A: Yohimbine treatment of sexual side effects induced by serotonin reuptake blockers. J Clin Psychiatry 53:207–209, 1992

Hollister LE: Treatment of depression with drugs. Ann Intern Med 89:78–84, 1978

Holst J, Bäckström T, Hammerbäck S, et al: Progestin addition during oestrogen replacement therapy—effects on vasomotor symptoms and mood. Maturitas 11:13–20, 1989

Holt JP, Wright ER, Hecker AO: Comparative clinical experience with five antidepressants. Am J Psychiatry 117:533–538, 1960

Homeida M, Halliwell M, Branch RA: Effects of an oral contraceptive on hepatic size and antipyrine metabolism in premenopausal women. Clin Pharmacol Ther 24:228–232, 1978

Honjo H, Ogins Y, Natitoh K, et al: In vivo effects by estrone sulphate on the central nervous system—on senile dementia (Alzheimer's type). Journal of Steroid Biochemistry 34:521–525, 1989

Hooper WD, Quing MS: The influence of age and gender on stereoselective metabolism and pharmacokinetics of mephobarbital in humans. Clin Pharmacol Ther 48:633–640, 1990

Hooshmand H, Sepdham T, Vries JK: Klüver-Bucy syndrome: successful treatment with carbamazepine (case report). JAMA 229:1782, 1974

Hopkins HS: Antidotes for antidepressant-induced sexual dysfunction. Biological Therapies in Psychiatry Newsletter 15:33–36, 1992

Horai Y, Nakano M, Ishizaki T, et al: Metoprolol and mephenytoin oxidation polymorphisms in far eastern oriental subjects: Japanese versus mainland Chinese. Clin Pharmacol Ther 6:198–207, 1989

Horai Y, Taga J, Ishizaki T, et al: Correlations among the metabolic ratios of three test probes (metoprolol, debrisoquine, sparteine) for genetically determined oxidation polymorphism in a Japanese population. Br J Clin Pharmacol 29:111–115, 1990

Horowitz M, Maddern GJ, Chatterton BE, et al: Changes in gastric emptying rates with age. Clin Sci 67:213–218, 1984

Horowitz M, Maddern GJ, Chatterton BE, et al: The normal menstrual cycle has no effect on gastric emptying. Br J Obstet Gynaecol 92:743–746, 1985

Horvath TL, Naftolin F, Leranth C: Luteinizing hormone–releasing hormone and gamma-aminobutyric acid neurons in the medial preoptic area are synaptic targets of dopamine axons originating in anterior periventricular areas. J Neuroendocrinol 5:71–79, 1993

Howland RH: Pharmacotherapy of dysthymia: a review. J Clin Psychopharmacol 11:83–91, 1991

Hruska RE, Ludmer LM, Silbergold EK: Hypophysectomy prevents the striatal dopamine receptor supersensitivity produced by chronic haloperidol treatment. Eur J Pharamol 65:445–456, 1980

Hruska RE, Ludmer LM, Pitman KT, et al: Effects of estrogen on striatal dopamine receptor function in male and female rats. Pharmacol Biochem Behav 16:285–291, 1982

Hser Y, Anglin MD, McGlothin W: Sex differences in addict careers, I: initiation of use. Am J Drug Alcohol Abuse 13:33–57, 1987

Hsu JJ, Kim CH, O'Connor MK, et al: Effect of menstrual cycle on esophageal emptying of liquid and solid boluses. Mayo Clin Proc 68:753–756, 1993

Hsu LC, Tani K, Fujiyoshi T, et al: Cloning of cDNAs for human aldehyde dehydrogenase 1 and 2. Proc Natl Acad Sci U S A 82:3771–3775, 1985

Hunt CM, Westerkam WR, Stave GM: Effect of age and gender on the activity of human hepatic CYP3A. Biochem Pharmacol 44:275–283, 1992

Hunter MS, Whitehead MJ: Psychological experience of the climacteric and postmenopause, in Menopause: Evaluation, Treatment and Health Concerns. Edited by Hammond CB, Haseltine FP. New York, Alan R Liss, 1989, pp 211–224

Hurley DL: Women, alcohol and incest: an analytical review. J Stud Alcohol 52:253–268, 1991

Hurwitz N: Predisposing factors in adverse reactions to drugs. BMJ 1:536–539, 1969

Hutson WR, Roehrkasse RL, Wald A: Influence of gender and menopause on gastric emptying and motility. Gastroenterol 96:11–17, 1989

Huybrechts I: The pharmacology of alprazolam: a review. Clin Ther 13:100–117, 1991

Hyman MM: Alcoholics fifteen years later. Ann N Y Acad Sci 273:613–623, 1976

Iacono WG, Beiser M: Where are the women in first-episode studies of schizophrenia? Schizophr Bull 18:471–480, 1992

Impastato DJ, Gabriel AR, Lardaro HH: Electric and insulin shock therapy during pregnancy. Diseases of the Nervous System 25:542–546, 1964

Inaba T, Arias TD: On phenotyping with isoniazid: the use of urinary acetylation ratio and the uniqueness of antimodes—study of two Amerindian populations. Clin Pharmacol Ther 42:493–497, 1987

Inaba T, Otton SV, Kalow W: Debrisoquine hydroxylation capacity: problems of assessment in two populations. Clin Pharmacol Ther 29:218–223, 1981

Inaba T, Vinks A, Otton SV, et al: Comparative pharmacogenetics of sparteine and debrisoquine. Clin Pharmacol Ther 33:394–399, 1983

Inaba T, Jurima M, Nakano M, et al: Mephenytoin and sparteine pharmacogenetics in Canadian-Caucasians. Clin Pharmacol Ther 36:670–676, 1984

Inaba T, Jorge LF, Arias TD: Mephenytoin hydroxylation in the Cuna Amerindians of Panama. Br J Clin Pharmacol 25:75–79, 1988

Insel TR: New pharmacologic approaches to obsessive compulsive disorder. J Clin Psychiatry 51 (suppl 20):47–51, 1990

Insel TR, Zohar J: Psychopharmacologic approaches to obsessive-compulsive disorder, in Psychopharmacology: The Third Generation of Progress, Vol 1. Edited by Meltzer HY. New York, Raven, 1987, pp 1205–1210

Insel TR, Murphy DL, Cohen RM, et al: Obsessive-compulsive disorder: a double-blind trial of clomipramine and clorgyline. Arch Gen Psychiatry 40:605–612, 1983

Isaksson A, Larkander O, Morsing C, et al: A controlled comparison between imipramine and protriptyline. Acta Psychiatr Scand Suppl 203:239, 1968

Iselius L, Evans DAP: Formal genetics of isoniazid metabolism in man. Clin Pharmacokinet 8:541–544, 1983

Ishizaki T, Eichelbaum M, Horai Y, et al: Evidence for polymorphic oxidation of sparteine in Japanese subjects. Br J Clin Pharmacol 23:482–485, 1987

Islam SI, Idle JR, Smith RL: The polymorphic 4-hydroxylation of debrisoquine in a Saudi Arab population. Xenobiotica 10:819–825, 1980

Istvan J: Stress anxiety, and birth outcomes: a critical review of the evidence. Psychol Bull 100:331–348, 1986

Iyun AO, Lennard MS, Tucker GT, et al: Metoprolol and debrisoquin metabolism in Nigerians: lack of evidence for polymorphic oxidation. Clin Pharmacol Ther 40:387–394, 1986

Jack DB, Quarterman CP, Zaman R, et al: Variability of beta-blocker pharmacokinetics in young volunteers. Eur J Clin Pharmacol 23:37–42, 1982

Jackson D: Memorandum: guidelines on bias for the Publication Manual. Washington, DC, American Psychological Association, November 3, 1993

Jacobsen FM: Fluoxetine-induced sexual dysfunction and an open trial of yohimbine. J Clin Psychiatry 53:119–122, 1992

Jacobsen SJ, Jones K, Johnson K, et al: Prospective multicenter study of pregnancy outcome after lithium exposure during first trimester. Lancet 339:530–533, 1992

Jacobson JN: Anorgasmia caused by an MAOI (letter). Am J Psychiatry 144:527, 1987

Jacqz E, Dulac H, Mathieu H: Phenotyping polymorphic drug metabolism in the French Caucasian Population. Eur J Clin Pharmacol 35:167–171, 1988

Jagiello G, Karnicki J, Ryan R: Superovulation with pituitary gonadotrophins: method for obtaining meiotic metaphase figures in human ova. Lancet 1:178–180. January 27, 1968

Jamison KR, Gerner RH, Goodwin FK: Patient and physician attitudes toward lithium: relationship to compliance. Arch Gen Psychiatry 36 (8 spec no):866–869, 1979

Jani NN, Wise TN: Antidepressants and inhibited female orgasm. J Sex Marital Ther 14:179–184, 1988

Jani NN, Wise TN, Kass E, et al: Trazodone and anorgasmia (letter). Am J Psychiatry 145:896, 1988

Janowsky DS, Rausch J: Biochemical hypotheses of premenstrual tension syndrome. Psychol Med 15:3–8, 1985

Janowsky DS, Fann WE, Davis JM: Monoamines and ovarian hormone–linked sexual and emotional changes. Arch Sex Behav 1:205–218, 1971

Janowsky DS, El-Yousef MK, David JM, et al: A cholinergic-adrenergic hypothesis of mania and depression. Lancet 2:632–635, 1972

Janowsky DS, Berens SC, Davis JM: Correlations between mood, weight, and electrolytes during the menstrual cycle: a renin-angiotensin-aldosterone hypothesis of premenstrual tension. Psychosom Med 35:143–152, 1973

Jansson JO, Ekberg S, Isaksson O, et al: Imprinting of growth hormone secretion, body growth, and hepatic steroid metabolism by neonatal testosterone. Endocrinology 117:1881–1889, 1985

Jeavons PM: Sodium valproate and neural tube defects. Lancet 2:1282–1283, 1982

Jellinek EM: Immanuel Kant on drinking. Quarterly Journal of Studies on Alcohol 1:777–778, 1941

Jensen J, Christiansen C, Rodbro P: Cigarette smoking, serum estrogens, and bone loss during hormone-replacement therapy early after menopause. N Engl J Med 313:973–975, 1985

Jensen J, Christiansen C, Rodbro P: Oestrogen-progestogen replacement therapy changes body composition in early postmenopausal women. Maturitas 8:209–216, 1986

Jensvold MF: Psychiatric aspects of the menstrual cycle, in Psychological Aspects of Women's Health Care: The Interface Between Psychiatry and Obstetrics and Gynecology. Edited by Stewart D, Stotland N. Washington, DC, American Psychiatric Press, 1993a, pp 165–192

Jensvold MF: Workplace sexual harassment: the use, misuse and abuse of psychiatry. Psychiatric Annals 23:438–445, 1993b

Jensvold MF: The female brain: the intersection of traumatic experience and hormonal events in the lives of women. Trauma, Loss, and Dissociation: The Foundations of 21st-Century Traumatology, First Annual Conference, Alexandria, VA, February 20, 1995

Jensvold MF: Menopause and psychopharmacology, in A Clinician's Guide to Menopause. Edited by Stewart DE, Robinson G. Washington, DC, American Psychiatric Press (in press)

Jensvold MF, Hamilton JA: Sex and gender effects in psychopharmacology: contributory factors and implications for pharmacotherapy, in Psychiatric Issues in Women (Clinical Psychiatry Series). Edited by Halbreich U. London, England, Bailliere's (in press)

Jensvold MF, Putnam F: Post abuse syndromes in premenstrual syndrome patients and controls. Paper presented at the annual meeting of the Association for Women in Psychology, Tempe, AZ, March 9, 1990

Jensvold MF, Grover G, Muller K, et al: Effects of clonidine and placebo infusions upon premenstrual syndrome patients and controls. Biol Psychiatry 27 (suppl):85A, 1990a

Jensvold MF, Grover G, Muller K, et al: Growth hormone, cortisol and prolactin responses to intravenous clonidine in PMS patients and controls. Paper presented at the XXI International Congress of the International Society of Psychoneuroendocrinology, Buffalo, NY, August 1990b

Jensvold MF, Rehm D, Temple R: Is there gender bias in drug testing? FDA Consumer 25(3):8–13, 1991

Jensvold MF, Reed K, Jarrett DB, et al: Menstrual cycle–related depressive symptoms treated with variable antidepressant dosage. Journal of Women's Health 1:109–115, 1992

Jochemsen R, van der Graaff M, Boeijinga JK, et al: Influence of sex, menstrual cycle and oral contraception on the disposition of nitrazepam. Br J Clin Pharmacol 13:319–324, 1982

John VA, Luscombe DK, Kemp H: Effects of age, cigarette smoking and the oral contraceptive on the pharmacokinetics of clomipramine and its desmethyl metabolite during chronic dosing. J Int Med Res 8:88–95, 1980

Johnson TL, Fee E: Women's participation in clinical research: from protectionism to access. Paper presented at Workshop, Committee on the Legal and Ethical Issues Relating to the Inclusion of Women in Clinical Studies, Institute of Medicine, National Academy of Sciences, Washington, DC, March 1993

Jonderko K: Effect of the menstrual cycle on gastric emptying. Acta Physiologia Polonica 40:504–510, 1989

Jones BM, Jones MK: Male and female intoxication levels for three alcohol doses or do women really get higher than men? Alc Tech Rep 5:11–14, 1976

Jones KL, Lacro RV, Johnson KA, et al: Pattern of malformations in the children of women treated with carbamazepine during pregnancy. N Engl J Med 320:1661–1666, 1989

Jones MK, Jones BM: Ethanol metabolism in women taking oral contraceptives. Alcoholism (NY) 8:24–28, 1984

Jones SB, Bylund DB, Rieser CA, et al: Alpha2-adrenergic receptor binding in human platelets: alterations during the menstrual cycle. Clin Pharmacol Ther 34:90–96, 1983

Jones SD: Ejaculatory inhibition with trazodone. J Clin Psychopharmacol 4:279–281, 1984

Jorge LF, Arias TD, Inaba T, et al: Unimodal distribution of the metabolic ratio for debrisoquine in Cuna Amerindians of Panama. Br J Clin Pharmacol 30:281–285, 1990

Josiassen RC, Roemer RA, Johnson MM, et al: Are gender differences in schizophrenia reflected in brain event–related potentials? Schizophr Bull 16:229–246, 1990

Juchau MR, Fouts JR: Effects of norethynodrel and progesterone on hepatic microsomal drug-metabolizing enzyme systems. Biochem Pharmacol 15:891–898, 1966

Juraska JM: Sex differences in cognitive regions of the brain. Psychoneuroendocrinology 16:105–119, 1991

Jurima M, Inaba T, Kodar D, et al: Genetic polymorphism of mephenytoin p(4') hydroxylation: difference between Orientals and Caucasians. Br J Clin Pharmacol 19:43–47, 1985

Jussofie A: Brain region–specific effects of neuroactive steroids on the affinity and density of the GABA-binding site. Biol Chem Hoppe Seyler 374:265–270, 1993

Kafka MP: Successful antidepressant treatment of nonparaphilic sexual addictions and paraphilias in men. J Clin Psychiatry 52:60–65, 1991

Kahn DA: Possible toxic interaction between cyproheptadine and phenelzine (letter). Am J Psychiatry 144:1242–1243, 1987

Kalkhoff RK: Metabolic effects of progesterone. Am J Obstet Gynecol 142:735–738, 1982

Kallen B: Comments on teratogen update: lithium. Teratology 38:597, 1988

Kallen B, Tandberg A: Lithium and pregnancy: a cohort study on manic-depressive women. Acta Psychiatr Scand 68:134–139, 1983

Kalow W: Ethnic differences in drug metabolism. Clin Pharmacokinet 7:373–400, 1982

Kalow W: Interethnic variation of drug metabolism. Trends Pharmacol Sci 12:102–107, 1991

Kalow W, Otton SV, Kadar D, et al: Ethnic difference in drug metabolism: debrisoquine 4-hydroxylation in Caucasians and Orientals. Can J Physiol Pharmacol 58:1142–1144, 1980

Kalra SP, Gallo RV: Effects of intraventricular administration of cat-echolamines on luteinizing hormone release in morphine-treated rats. Endocrinology 113:23–28, 1983

Kalra SP, Kalra PS: Opioid-adrenergic-steroid connection in neural regulation of luteinizing hormone secretion in the rat. Endocr Rev 4:311–351, 1983

Kampen DL, Sherwin BB: Estrogen use and verbal memory in healthy postmenopausal women. Obstet Gynecol 83:979–983, 1994

Kane FJ, Treadway CR, Ewing JA: Emotional changes associated with oral contraceptives in female psychiatric patients. Compr Psychiatry 10:16–30, 1969

Kane JM, Smith JM: Tardive dyskinesia: prevalence and risk factors, 1959–1979. Arch Gen Psychiatry 39:473–481, 1982

Kanto JH: Use of benzodiazepines during pregnancy, labour and lacta-tion, with particular reference to pharmacokinetic considerations. Drugs 23:354–380, 1982

Kaplan HS: The New Sex Therapy: Active Treatment of Sexual Dysfunc-tion. New York, Brunner/Mazel, 1974

Kaplan HS: The Evolution of Sexual Disorders. New York, Brunner/Ma-zel, 1983

Kaplitt MG, Pfaus JG, Kleopoulos SP, et al: Expression of a functional foreign gene in adult mammalian brain following in vivo transfer via a herpes simplex virus type 1 defective viral vector. Mol Cell Neurosci 2:320–330, 1991

Kaplitt MG, Rabkin S, Pfaff DW: Molecular alterations in nerve cells: direct manipulation and physiological mediation, in Current Topics in Neuroendocrinology, Vol 11. Edited by Imura M. Berlin, Springer-Verlag, 1993, pp 169–191

Kaplitt MG, Kwong AD, Kleopoulos SP, et al: Preproenkephalin pro-moter yields region-specific and long-term expression in adult brain after direct in vivo gene transfer via a defective herpes simplex viral vector. Proc Natl Acad Sci U S A 91:8979–8983, 1994

Kargas GA, Kargas SA, Bruyere HJ Jr, et al: Perinatal mortality due to interaction of dephenhydramine and temazepam (letter). N Engl J Med 313:14–17, 1985

Kashiwagi T, McClure J, Wetzel RD: Premenstrual affective syndrome and psychiatric disorder. Diseases of the Nervous System 37:116–119, 1976

Kasvikis JG, Tsakiris F, Marks IM: Women with obsessive-compulsive disorder frequently report a past history of anorexia nervosa. Int J Eat Disord 5:1069–1075, 1986

Kato R: Sex-related differences in drug metabolism. Drug Metab Rev 3:32–40, 1974

Kato R, Yamazoe Y, Shimada M, et al: Effect of growth hormone and ectopic transplantation of pituitary gland on sex-specific forms of cytochrome P450 and testosterone and drug oxidations in rat liver. J Biochem 100:895–902, 1986

Katz FH, Romf HP: Plasma aldosterone and renin activity during the menstrual cycle. J Clin Endocrinol Metab 34:819–823, 1972

Kay CR: Progestogens and arterial disease—evidence from the Royal College of General Practitioners' Study. Am J Obstet Gynecol 142:762–765, 1982

Kay CR: The Royal College of General Practitioners' Oral Contraception Study: some recent observations. Clin Obstet Gynecol 11:759–786, 1984

Keats JS, Fitzgerald DE: Limb volume and blood flow changes during the menstrual cycle, in Sportsmedicine. Edited by Williams JGP, Sperry CPN. Baltimore, MD, Williams & Wilkins, 1976, pp 210–225

Keck PE, McElroy SL, Friedman LM: Valproate and carbamazepine in the treatment of panic and posttraumatic stress disorders, withdrawal states, and behavioral dyscontrol syndromes. J Clin Psychopharmacol 12 (suppl 1):36S–41S, 1992

Keepers GA, Casey DE: Prediction of neuroleptic-induced dystonia. J Clin Psychopharmacol 7:342–345, 1987

Keller MB, Lavori PW: Commentary: the adequacy of treating depression. J Nerv Ment Dis 176:471–474, 1988

Keller MB, Lavori PW, Mueller TI, et al: Time to recovery, chronicity and levels of psychopathology in major depression. Arch Gen Psychiatry 49:809–816, 1992

Kellner R, Buckman MT, Fava M, et al: Prolactin, aggression and hostility: a discussion of recent studies. Psychiatric Developments 2:131–138, 1984

Kemali D, Pacini A, Vacca L, et al: Sull'attività timolettica di un nuovo farmaco antidepressivo: il benzocazone (FI 6654). Prime osservazioni clinico-terapeutiche. Acta Neurol (Napoli) 27:57–67, 1972

Kemp J, Ilett KF, Booth J, et al: Excretion of doxepin and *N*-desmethyl-doxepin in human milk. Br J Clin Pharmacol 20:497–499, 1985

Kendall D, Stancel G, Enna S: The influence of sex hormones on anti-depressant-induced alteration in neurotransmitter receptor binding. J Neurosci 2:354–360, 1982

Kendall MJ, Quarterman CP, Jack DB, et al: Metoprolol pharmacokinetics and the oral contraceptive pill. Br J Clin Pharmacol 14:120–122, 1984

Kendell RE, McGuire RJ, Connor Y: Mood changes in the first three weeks after childbirth. Journal of Affective Disorders 3:317–326, 1981

Kendell RE, Chalmers JC, Platz C: Epidemiology of puerperal psychoses. Br J Psychiatry 150:662–673, 1987

Kendler KS, Heath AC, Neale MC, et al: A population-based twin study of alcoholism in women. JAMA 268:1877–1882, 1992

Kerin JF, Warnes GM, Crocker J, et al: Three-hour urinary radioimmunoassay for luteinizing hormone to detect onset of preovulatory LH surge. Lancet 2:430–431, 1980

Kerin JF, Edmonds DK, Warnes GM, et al: Morphological and functional relations of graafian follicle growth to ovulation in women using ultrasonic, laparoscopic and biochemical measurements. Br J Obstet Gynaecol 88:81–90, 1981

Kernberg OF: Aggression in Personality Disorders and Perversions. New Haven, CT, Yale University Press, 1992

Kessler RC, McLeod JD: Sex differences in vulnerability to undesirable life events. Sociological Review 49:620–631, 1984

Khalsa H, Paredes A, Anglin MD: The role of alcohol in cocaine dependence, in Recent Developments in Alcoholism, Vol 10. Edited by Galanter M. New York, Plenum, 1992, pp 7–35

Khandelwal SK: Complete loss of libido with short-term use of lorazepam. Am J Psychiatry 145:1313–1314, 1988

Kilbey MM, Sobeck JP: Epidemiology of alcoholism, in Women and Health Psychology. Edited by Travis CB. Hillsdale, NJ, Lawrence Erlbaum, 1988, pp 92–107

Kimmel S, Gonsalves L, Youngs D, et al: Fluctuating levels of antidepressants premenstrually. J Psychosom Obstet Gynecol 13:277–280, 1992

Kinney EL, Trautman J, Gold JA, et al: Underrepresentation of women in new drug trials. Ann Intern Med 95:495–499, 1981

Kinzie JD, Leung P: Clonidine in Cambodian patients with posttraumatic stress disorder. J Nerv Ment Dis 177:546–550, 1989

Kirkwood C, Moore A, Hayes P, et al: Influence of the menstrual cycle on alprazolam pharmacokinetics. Clin Pharmacol Ther 50:404–409, 1991

Klaiber EL, Kobayahi Y, Broverman DM, et al: Plasma monoamine oxidase activity in regularly menstruating women and in amenorrheic women receiving cyclic treatment with estrogens and a progestin. J Clin Endocrinol Metab 33:630–638, 1971

Klaiber EL, Broverman DM, Vogel W, et al: Effects of estrogen therapy on plasma MAO activity and EEG driving responses of depressed women. Am J Psychiatry 128:1492–1498, 1972

Klaiber EL, Broverman DM, Vogel W, et al: Estrogen therapy for severe persistent depression in women. Arch Gen Psychiatry 36:550–554, 1979

Klein DF: Delineation of two drug-responsive anxiety syndromes. Psychopharmacologia (Berl) 5:397–408, 1964

Klein DF: False suffocation alarms, spontaneous panics, and related conditions: an integrative hypothesis. Arch Gen Psychiatry 50:306–317, 1993

Klein DF, Fink M: Psychiatric reactions to imipramine. Am J Psychiatry 119:432–438, 1962

Klein DF, Gorman JM: A model of panic and agoraphobic development. Acta Psychiatr Scand 76 (suppl):87–95, 1987

Klein U, Klein M, Sturm H, et al: The frequency of adverse drug reactions as dependent upon age, sex, and duration of hospitalization. International Journal of Clinical Pharmacology and Biopharmacy 13:187–195, 1976

Kline MD: Fluoxetine and anorgasmia. Am J Psychiatry 146:804–805, 1989

Kocsis JH, Hanin I, Bowden C, et al: Imipramine and amitriptyline plasma concentrations and clinical response in major depression. Br J Psychiatry 148:52–57, 1986

Kocsis JH, Frances, AJ, Voss C, et al: Imipramine treatment for chronic depression. Arch Gen Psychiatry 45:253–257, 1988

Kocsis JH, Mason BJ, Frances AJ, et al: Prediction of response of chronic depression to imipramine. Journal of Affective Disorders 17:255–260, 1989

Kok EC, Wilson BJ, Potgieter B: Influence of estrogen levels on anticholinergic activity of tricyclic antidepressants. Prog Neuropsychopharmacol Biol Psychiatry 10:49–55, 1986

Kolb LS, Burris B, Griffiths S: Propranolol and clonidine in treatment of the chronic post-traumatic stress disorders of war, in Post-Traumatic Stress Disorder: Psychological and Biological Sequelae. Edited by van der Kolk B. Washington, DC, American Psychiatric Press, 1984, pp 97–105

Koninckx PR, Heyns WJ, Corvelyn PA, et al: Delayed onset of luteinization as a cause of infertility. Fertil Steril 29:266–269, 1978

Konradi C, Kornhuber J, Sofic E, et al: Variations of monoamines and their metabolites in the human brain putamen. Brain Res 579:285–290, 1992

Kook KA, Stimmel GL, Wilkins JN, et al: Accuracy and safety of a priori lithium loading. J Clin Psychiatry 46:49–51, 1985

Koopman P, Gubbay J, Vivian N, et al: Male development of chromosomally female mice transgenic for Sry. Nature 351:117–121, 1991

Kopala L, Clark C: Implications of olfactory agnosia for understanding sex differences in schizophrenia. Schizophr Bull 16:255–261, 1990

Kopala L, Clark C, Hurwitz T: Sex differences in olfactory function in schizophrenia. Am J Psychiatry 146:1320–1322, 1989

Koren G, Graham K: Cocaine in pregnancy: analysis of fetal risk. Vet Hum Toxicol 34:263–264, 1992

Kornguth ML, Hutchins LG, Eichelman BS: Binding of psychotropic drugs to isolated alpha$_1$-acid glycoprotein. Biochem Pharmacol 30:2435–2441, 1981

Kossoy LR, Hill GA, Herbert CM, et al: Therapeutic donor insemination: the impact of insemination timing with the aid of a urinary luteinizing hormone immunoassay. Fertil Steril 49:1026–1029, 1988

Kosten T, Gawin FH, Kosten TR, et al: Gender difference in cocaine use and treatment response. J Subst Abuse Treat 10:63–66, 1993

Kosten TR, Rounsaville BJ: Psychopathology in opioid addicts. Psychiatr Clin North Am 9:515–532, 1986

Kosten TR, Rounsaville BJ, Kleber HD: Parental alcoholism in opioid addicts. J Nerv Ment Dis 173:461–469, 1985

Kotin J, Wilbert D, Verburg D, et al: Thioridazine and sexual dysfunction. Am J Psychiatry 133:82–85, 1976

Kovach JA: Incest as a treatment issue for alcoholic women. Alcoholism Treatment Quarterly 3:1–15, 1986

Kowalski A, Stanley RO, Dennerstein L, et al: The sexual side effects of antidepressant medication: a double-blind comparison of two anti-depressants in a non-psychiatric population. Br J Psychiatry 147:413–418, 1985

Kragh-Hansen U: Molecular aspects of ligand binding to serum albumin. Pharmacol Rev 33:17–53, 1981

Kramer PD: Listening to Prozac. New York, Viking, 1993

Kräupl Taylor F: Loss of libido in depression (letter). BMJ 1:305, 1972

Kremer JM, Witting J, Janssen LH: Drug binding to human alpha$_1$-acid glycoprotein in health and disease. Pharmacol Rev 40:1–47, 1988

Krey LC, Luine VN: Effect of progesterone on monoamine turnover in the brain of the estrogen-primed rat. Brain Res Bull 19:195–202, 1987

Kris EB: Children born to mothers maintained on pharmacotherapy during pregnancy and postpartum. Recent Advances in Biological Psychiatry 4:180–187, 1961

Krishnan KR, France RD, Ellinwood EH: Tricyclic-induced akathisia in patients taking conjugated estrogens. Am J Psychiatry 141:696–697, 1984

Kristansson F, Thorsteinsson SB: Disposition of alprazolam in human volunteers: differences between genders. Acta Pharmaceutica Nordica 3:249–250, 1991

Kristensen CB: Imipramine serum protein binding in healthy subjects. Clin Pharmacol Ther 34:689–694, 1983

Kristensen E, Jorgensen P: Sexual function in lithium treated manic-depressive patients. Pharmacopsychiatry 20:165–167, 1987

Kroboth PD, Smith RB, Sorkin MI, et al:. Triazolam protein binding and correlation with α_1-acid glycoprotein concentration. Clin Pharmacol Ther 36:379–383, 1984

Kroboth PD, Smith RB, Stoehr GP, et al: Pharmacodynamic evaluation of the benzodiazepine–oral contraceptive interaction. Clin Pharmacol Ther 38:525–532, 1985

Kubacki A: Sexual disinhibition on clonazepam. Can J Psychiatry 32:643–645, 1987

Kuenssberg EV, Knox JDE: Imipramine in pregnancy (letter). BMJ 2:292, 1972

Kuevi V, Causon R, Dixson AF, et al: Plasma amine and hormone changes in post-partum blues. Clin Endocrinol (Oxford) 19:39–46, 1983

Kukopulos A, Reginaldi D: Variations of serum lithium concentrations correlated with the phases of manic-depressive psychosis. Agressologie 19D:219–222, 1978

Kukopulos A, Minnai G, Muller-Oerlinghausen B: The influence of mania and depression on the pharmacokinetics of lithium. Journal of Affective Disorders 8:159–166, 1985

Kulik FA, Wilbur R: Case report of painful ejaculation as a side effect of amoxapine. Am J Psychiatry 4:28–40, 1982

Kumar N, Behari M, Ahyja GK, et al: Phenytoin levels in catamenial epilepsy. Epilepsia 29:155–158, 1988

Kupfer A, Preisig R: Pharmacogenetics of mephenytoin: a new drug hydroxylation polymorphism in man. Eur J Clin Pharmacol 26:753–759, 1984

Laatikainen TJ: Corticotropin-releasing hormone and opioid peptides in reproduction and stress. Ann Med 23:489–496, 1991

Labbate L, Pollack MH: Treatment of fluoxetine-induced sexual dysfunction with bupropion: a case report. Ann Clin Psychiatry 6:13–15, 1994

Ladwig GB, Andersen MD: Substance abuse in women: relationship between chemical dependency of women and past reports of physical and/or sexual abuse. Int J Addict 24:739–754, 1989

Laegreid L, Olegard R, Conradi N, et al: Congenital malformations and maternal consumption of benzodiazepines: a case-control study. Dev Med Child Neurol 32:432–441, 1990

Lake CR, Chernow B, Zaloga G, et al: The effects of phenylpropanolamine on human sympathetic nervous system function. Neuropsychopharmacology 1:163–167, 1988

Lake CR, Gallant SJ, Masson E, et al: Adverse drug effects attributed to phenylpropanololamine: a review of 142 case reports. Am J Med 89:195–208, 1990

Lam YWF, Casto DT, Dunn JF: Drug metabolizing capacity in Mexican Americans (abstract). Clin Pharmacol Ther 49:159, 1991

Landau RL, Lugibihl K: Metabolic and natriuretic effects of progesterone in man. Recent Prog Horm Res 17:249–292, 1961

Landgren BM, Aedo AR, Diczfalusy E: Hormonal changes associated with ovulation and luteal function, in The Gonadotropins: Basic Science and Clinical Aspects in Females (Proceedings of the Serono Symposia, Vol 42). Edited by Flamigni C, Givens JR. New York, Academic Press, 1982, pp 187–201

Lane EA, Guthrie S, Linnoila M: Effects of ethanol on drug and metabolite pharmacokinetics. Clin Pharmacokinet 10:228–247, 1985

Lasagna L: Phenylpropanololamine—A Review. New York, Wiley, 1988

Lauber AH, Romano GJ, Mobbs CV, et al: Estradiol induction of preproenkephalin messenger RNA in hypothalamus: dose-response and relation to reproductive behavior in the female rat. Molecular Brain Research 8:47–54, 1990a

Lauber AH, Romano GJ, Mobbs CV, et al: Estradiol regulation of estrogen receptor messenger ribonucleic acid in rat mediobasal hypothalamus: an in situ hybridization study. J Neuroendocrinol 2:605–611, 1990b

Lauber AH, Romano GJ, Pfaff DW: Sex differences in estradiol regulation of progestin receptor mRNA in rat mediobasal hypothalamus as demonstrated by in situ hybridization. Neuroendocrinology 53:608–613, 1991

Laughren T, Brown W, Petrucci J: Effect of thioridazine on serum testosterone. Am J Psychiatry 135:982–984, 1978

Laurell C, Kullander S, Thorell J: Plasma protein changes induced by sequential type of contraceptive steroid pills. Clin Chim Acta 25:294–296, 1969

Leclercq V, Desager JP, van Nieuwenhuyze Y, et al: Prevalence of drug hydroxylator phenotypes in Belgium. Eur J Clin Pharmacol 33:439–440, 1987

Lee EJ, Nam YP, Hee GN: Oxidation phenotyping in Chinese and Malay populations. Clin Exp Pharmacol Physiol 15:889–891, 1988

Leetz K, Rodenhauser P, Wheelock J: Medroxyprogesterone in the treatment of periodic menstrual psychosis. J Clin Psychiatry 49:372–373, 1988

Leland J: Gender, drinking, and alcohol abuse, in Gender and Psychopathology. Edited by Al-Issa I. New York, Academic Press, 1982, pp 201–220

Lemay A, Bastide A, Lambert R, et al: Prediction of human ovulation by rapid luteinizing hormone (LH) radioimmunoassay and ovarian ultrasonography. Fertil Steril 38:194–201, 1982

Lenton EA, Weston GA, Cooke ID: Problems in using basal body temperature recordings in an infertility clinic. BMJ 1:803–805, 1977

Leranth C, Shanabrough M, Naftolin F: Estrogen induces ultrastructural changes in progesterone receptor–containing GABA neurons of the primate hypothalamus. Neuroendocrinology 54:571–579, 1991

Lerer B: Alternative therapies for bipolar disorder. J Clin Psychiatry 46:309–316, 1985

Lesar TS, Tollefson G, Koch M: Relationship between patient variables and lithium dosage requirements. J Clin Psychiatry 46:133–136, 1985

Lesko LM, Stotland NL, Segraves RT: Three cases of female anorgasmia associated with MAOIs. Am J Psychiatry 139:1353–1354, 1982

Lester BM, Cucca J, Andreozzi L, et al: Possible association between fluoxetine hydrochloride and colic in an infant. J Am Acad Child Adolesc Psychiatry 32:1253–1255, 1993

LeVay S: A difference in hypothalamic structure between heterosexual and homosexual men. Science 253:1034–1037, 1991

LeVay S: The Sexual Brain. Cambridge, MA, MIT Press, 1993

Levy RH, Moreland TA: Rationale for monitoring free drug levels. Clin Pharmacokinet 9 (suppl 1):1–9, 1984

Levy SJ, Doyle KM: Attitudes to women in a drug treatment program. Journal of Drug Issues 4:423–434, 1974

Lewine RRJ: Gender and Schizophrenia, in Handbook of Schizophrenia, Vol 3: Nosology, Epidemiology and Genetics. Edited by Tsuang M, Simpson J. Amsterdam, Elsevier Science, 1988, pp 379–397

Lewine RRJ, Burbach D, Meltzer HY: Effect of diagnostic criteria on ratio of male to female schizophrenic patients. Am J Psychiatry 141:84–87, 1984

Lewine RRJ, Gulley LR, Risch CR, et al: Sexual dimorphism, brain morphology and schizophrenia. Schizophr Bull 16:195–203, 1990

Lex BW: Gender differences and substance abuse, in Advances in Substance Abuse: Behavioral and Biological Research, Vol 4. Edited by Mello NK. London, Jessica Kingsley, 1991, pp 225–296

Lex BW: Alcohol problems in special populations, in Medical Diagnosis and Treatment of Alcoholism. Edited by Mendelson JH, Mello NK. New York, McGraw-Hill, 1992, pp 71–154

Lex BW, Griffin ML, Mello NK, et al: Alcohol, marijuana, and mood states in young women. Int J Addictions 24:405–424, 1989

Liebenluft E: Do gonadal steroids regulate circadian rhythms in humans? J Affective Disorders 29:175–181, 1993

Lieberman JA, Alvir JM: A report of clozapine-induced agranulocytosis in the United States. Drug Saf 7 (suppl 1):1–2, 1992

Liebowitz MR, Gorman JM, Fyer AJ, et al: Social phobia: review of a neglected anxiety disorder. Arch Gen Psychiatry 42:729–736, 1985

Liebowitz MR, Fyer AJ, Gorman JM, et al: Tricyclic therapy of the DSM-III anxiety disorders: a review with implications for further research. J Psychiatr Res 22 (suppl 1):7–31, 1988

Liebowitz MR, Schneier F, Campeas R, et al: Phenelzine vs atenolol in social phobia: a placebo-controlled comparison. Arch Gen Psychiatry 49:290–300, 1992

Lin KM, Poland RE, Nuccio I, et al: Longitudinal assessment of haloperidol doses and serum concentrations in Asian and Caucasian schizophrenic patients. Am J Psychiatry 146:1307–1311, 1989

Lin KM, Poland RE, Smith MW, et al: Pharmacokinetic and other related factors affecting psychotropic responses in Asians. Psychopharmacol Bull 27:427–439, 1991

Lin KM, Poland RE, Nakasaki G: Psychopharmacology and Psychobiology of Ethnicity. Washington, DC, American Psychiatric Press, 1993

Lindberg S, Agren G: Mortality among male and female hospitalized alcoholics in Stockholm 1962–1983. British Journal of Addiction 83:1193–1200, 1988

Lipper S, Davidson JR, Grady TA, et al: Preliminary study of carbamazepine in post-traumatic stress disorder. Psychosomatics 27:849–854, 1986

Lipsett MB: Steroid hormones, in Reproductive Endocrinology, Physiology, Pathophysiology and Clinical Management. Edited by Yen SSC, Jaffe RB. Philadelphia, PA, WB Saunders, 1986

Litt MD, Babor TF, Delboca FK, et al: Types of alcoholics, II: application of an empirically derived typology to treatment matching. Arch Gen Psychiatry 49:609–614, 1992

Lloyd KG, Zivkovic B, Scatton B, et al: The GABA-ergic hypothesis of depression. Prog Neuropsychopharmacol Biol Psychiatry 13:341–351, 1989

Lloyd R, Coulam CB: The accuracy of urinary luteinizing hormone testing in predicting ovulation. Am J Obstet Gynecol 160:1370–1375, 1989

Lo WH, Lo T: A ten-year follow-up study of Chinese schizophrenics in Hong Kong. Br J Psychiatry 131:63–66, 1977

Lobo RA: Hormones, hormone replacement therapy, and heart disease, in Cardiovascular Health and Disease in Women. Edited by Douglas PS. Philadelphia, PA, WB Saunders, 1993, pp 153–173

Loebel AD, Lieberman JA, Alvir JM, et al: Duration of psychosis and outcome in first-episode schizophrenia. Am J Psychiatry 149:1183–1188, 1992

Longcope C: Metabolic clearance and blood production rates in postmenopausal women. Am J Obstet Gynecol 111:779–785, 1981

Longcope C: Adrenal and gonadal steroid secretion in normal females. Clinics in Endocrinology and Metabolism 15:213–228, 1986

Loriaux DL: Hormonal contraceptives: mechanisms of action, in Preventing Unwanted Pregnancies: The Role of Hormonal Contraceptives. Bethesda, MD, National Institute of Child Health and Human Development and Association of Reproductive Health Professionals, April 27, 1993, pp 53–54

Loscher W, Wahnschaffe U, Rundfeldt C, et al: Regional alterations in brain amino acids during the estrous cycle of the rat. Neurochem Res 17:973–977, 1992

Lou Y, Ying L, Bertilsson L, et al: Low frequency of slow debrisoquine hydroxylation in a native Chinese population (letter). Lancet 2:852–853, 1987

Loyd DW, Simpson JC, Tsuang MT: A family study of sex differences in the diagnosis of atypical schizophrenia. Am J Psychiatry 142:1366–1368, 1985

Luciano AA, Peluso J, Koch EI, et al: Temporal relationship and reliability of the clinical, hormonal, and ultrasonographic indices of ovulation in infertile women. Obstet Gynecol 75:412–416, 1990

Luine VN: Estradiol increases choline acetyltransferase activity in specific basal forebrain nuclei and projection areas of female rats. Exp Neurol 89:489–490, 1985

Luine VN, Hearns M: Spatial memory deficits in aged rats: contributions of the cholinergic system assessed by ChAT. Brain Res 523:321–324, 1990

Luine VN, Rhodes JC: Gonadal hormone regulation of MAO and other enzymes in hypothalamic areas. Neuroendocrinology 36:235–241, 1983

Luine VN, Khylchevskaya RJ, McEwen BS: Effect of gonadal steroids on activities of monoamine oxidase and choline acetylase in rat brain. Brain Res 86:293–306, 1975

Lunde PKM, Frislid K, Hansteen V: Disease and acetylation polymorphism. Clin Pharmacokinet 2:182–196, 1977

Lusseveld EM, Peters ET, Deurenberg P: Multifrequency bioelectrical impedance as a measure of differences in body water distribution. Ann Nutr Metab 37:44–51, 1993

Lux-Lantos V, Rey E, Libertun C: Activation of GABA-B receptors in the anterior pituitary inhibits prolactin and luteinizing hormone secretion. Neuroendocrinology 56:687–693, 1992

Lydiard RB: Tricyclic-resistant depression: treatment resistance or inadequate treatment? J Clin Psychiatry 46:412–417, 1985

Lydiard RB, Gelenberg AJ: Amoxapine antidepressant with some neuroleptic properties? A review of its chemistry and animal pharmacology, and toxicity, human pharmacology and clinical efficacy. Pharmacotherapy 1:163–178, 1981

Lydiard RB, Howell EF, Laraia MT, et al: Sexual side effects of alprazolam. Am J Psychiatry 144:254–255, 1987

Lydiard RB, Lesser IM, Ballenger JC, et al: A fixed-dose study of alprazolam 2mg, 6mg and placebo in panic disorder. J Clin Psychopharmacol 12:96–103, 1992

Maas JW: Biogenic amines and depression: biochemical and pharmacological separation of two types of depression. Arch Gen Psychiatry 32:1357–1361, 1975

MacDonald I: Gastric activity during the menstrual cycle. Gastroenterol 30:602–607, 1956

MacDonald PC, Dombrowski RA, Casey ML: Recurrent secretion of progesterone in large amounts: an endocrine/metabolic disorder unique to young women? Endocrine Review 12:372–401, 1991

MacKinnon M, Sutherlan E, Simon FR: Effects of ethinyl estradiol on hepatic microsomal proteins and turnover of cytochrome P450. J Lab Clin Med 90:1096–1106, 1977

MacLeod SM, Giles HG, Bengert B, et al: Age- and gender-related differences in diazepam pharmacokinetics. J Clin Pharmacol 19:15–19, 1979

Maddux JF, Desmond DP: Family and environment in the choice of opioid dependence or alcoholism. Am J Drug Alcohol Abuse 15:117–134, 1989

Madeira MD, Lieberman AR: Sexual dimorphism in the mammalian limbic system. Prog Neurobiol 45:275–333, 1995

Maggi A, Perez J: Estrogen-induced up-regulation of gamma-aminobutyric acid receptors in the CNS of rodents. J Neurochem 47:1793–1797, 1986

Mahgoub A, Idle JR, Dring LG, et al: Polymorphic hydroxylation of debrisoquine in man. Lancet 2:584–586, 1977

Mahgoub A, Idle JR, Smith RL: A population and familial study of the defective alicyclic hydroxylation of debrisoquine among Egyptians. Xenobiotica 9:51–56, 1979

Maier W, Lichtermann D, Minges J, et al: The impact of gender and age at onset on the familial aggregration of schizophrenia. Eur Arch Psychiatry Clin Neurosci 242:279–285, 1993

Majewska MD: Neurosteroids: endogenous modulators of the GABA-A receptor: mechanism of action and physiological significance. Prog Neurobiol 38:379–395, 1992

Majewska MD: Dehydroepiandrosterone (DHEA) and aging. Ann N Y Acad Sci 774:111–120, 1995

Majewska MD, Schwartz RD: Pregnenolone-sulfate: an endogenous antagonist of the γ-aminobutyric acid receptor complex in brain? Brain Res 404:355–360, 1987

Majewska MD, Harrison NL, Schwartz RD, et al: Metabolites of steroid hormones are barbiturate-like modulators of the aminobutyric acid receptors. Science 232:1004–1007, 1986

Majewska MD, Ford-Rice F, Falkay G: Pregnancy-induced alterations of GABA$_A$ receptor sensitivity in maternal brain: an antecedent of postpartum blues? Brain Res 482:397–401, 1989

Majewska MD, Demirgoren S, Spivak CH, et al: Neurosteroid dehydroepiandrosterone sulfate is an allosteric antagonist of the GABA$_A$ receptor. Brain Res 526:143–146, 1990

Maneshka S, Harry TA: Lorazepam in sexual disorders. Br J Clin Pract 29:175–176, 1975

Mannisto PT, Laakso ML, Jarvinen A, et al: Effects of central and peripheral type benzodiazepine ligands on growth hormone and gonadotropin secretion in male rats. Pharmacol Toxicol 71:75–80, 1992

Mansky T, Mestres-Ventura P, Wuttke W: Involvement of GABA in the feedback action of estradiol on gonadotropin and prolactin release: hypothalamic GABA and catecholamine turnover rates. Brain Res 231:353–364, 1982

Marks IM: Fears, Phobias, and Rituals. New York, Oxford University Press, 1987

Marsh KL, Simpson DD: Sex differences in opioid addiction careers. Am J Drug Alcohol Abuse 12:309–329, 1986

Marshall AW, Kingstone D, Boss M, et al: Ethanol elimination in males and females: relationship to menstrual cycle and body composition. Hepatology 3:701–706, 1983

Marshall J: Regulation of gonadotropin secretion, in Endocrinology. Edited by DeGroot L, Besser G, Marshall J, et al. Philadelphia, PA, WB Saunders, 1989, pp 1903–1914

Marshall J, Odell W: The menstrual cycle—hormonal regulation, mechanisms of anovulation, and responses of the reproductive tract to steroid hormones, in Endocrinology. Edited by DeGroot L, Besser G, Marshall J, et al. Philadelphia, PA, WB Saunders, 1989, pp 1940–1949

Martin E: Drug Interactions Index 1978/1979. Philadelphia, PA, JB Lippincott, 1978

Martin E: The Woman in the Body: A Cultural Analysis of Reproduction. Boston, MA, Beacon Press, 1992

Masters WH, Johnson VE: Human Sexual Inadequacy. Boston, MA, Little, Brown, 1970

Mastroianni L, Donaldson PJ, Kante TT (eds): Developing New Contraceptives: Obstacles and Opportunities. Washington, DC, National Research Council and Institute of Medicine, National Academy Press, 1990

Matheson I, Pande H, Alertsen AR: Respiratory depression caused by N-desmethyldoxepin in breast milk (letter). Lancet 2:1124, 1985

Matsuda T, Nakano Y, Kanda T, et al: Gonadal hormones affect the hypothermia induced by serotonin$_{1A}$ (5-HT$_{1A}$) receptor activation. Life Sciences 48:1627–1632, 1991

Matthews CD, Broom TJ, Black T, et al: Optimal features of basal body temperature recordings associated with conceptional cycles. International Journal of Fertility 2:319–320, 1980

Mattson R, Cramer J, Darney P, et al: Use of oral contraceptives by women with epilepsy. JAMA 256:238–240, 1986

May PR, Tuma AH, Dixon WJ: Schizophrenia: a follow-up study of the results of five forms of treatment. Arch Gen Psychiatry 38:776–784, 1981

Mayer GA: Blood viscosity in healthy subjects and patients with coronary heart disease. Can Med Assoc J 91:951–954, 1964

Mayersohn M: Drug disposition, in Drug Therapy for the Elderly. Edited by Conrad KA, Bressler R. St. Louis, MO, CV Mosby, 1982, pp 31–63

Mayeux R, Denaro J, Hemenegildo N, et al: A population-based investigation of the Parkinson's disease with and without dementia: relationship to age and gender. Arch Neurol 49:492–497, 1992

Mbanefo C, Bababunmi EA, Mahgoub A, et al: A study of the debrisoquine hydroxylation polymorphism in a Nigerian population. Xenobiotica 10:811–818, 1980

McCabe MS: Demographic differences in functional psychoses. Br J Psychiatry 127:320–323, 1975

McClintock MK: A functional approach to behavioral endocrinology of rodents, in Psychobiology of Reproduction. Edited by Crews D. New York, Prentice Hall, 1987, pp 176–203

McEwen BS: Binding and metabolism of sex steroids by the hypothalamic-pituitary unit: physiological implications. Annu Rev Physiol 42:97–110, 1980

McEwen BS: Non-genomic and genomic effects of steroids on neural activity. Trends Pharmacol Sci 12:141–147, 1991

McEwen BS: Effects of the steroid/thyroid hormone family on neural and behavioral plasticity, in Neuroendocrinology. Edited by Nemeroff CB. Boca Raton, FL, CRC Press, 1992, pp 333–351

McEwen BS, Parsons B: Gonadal steroid action on the brain: neurochemistry and neuropharmacology. Ann Rev Pharmacol Toxicol 22:555–598, 1982

McEwen BS, Jones KJ, Pfaff DW: Hormonal control of sexual behavior in the female rat: Molecular, cellular and neurochemical studies. Biol Reprod 36:37–45, 1987

McGrath E, Keita GP, Strickland BR, et al. (eds): Women and Depression: Risk Factors and Treatment Issues. Washington, DC, American Psychological Association, 1990

McKinlay SM, Jeffreys M: The menopausal syndrome. Br J Prev Soc Med 28:108–115, 1974

McMillan M, Pihl R: Premenstrual depression: a distinct entity. Journal of Abnormal Psychology 96:149–154, 1987

Meade T, Greenberg G, Thompson S: Progestogens and cardiovascular reactions associated with oral contraceptives and a comparison of safety of 50- and 30-µg estrogen preparations. BMJ 1:1157–1161, 1980

Mello NK: Some behavioral and biological aspects of alcohol problems in women, in Alcohol and Drug Problems in Women, Vol 5: Research Advances in Alcoholism and Drug Problems. Edited by Kalant OJ. New York, Plenum, 1980, pp 263–298

Mello NK, Mendelson JH: Operant acquisition of marijuana in women. Pharmacol Exp Ther 235:162–171, 1985

Mello NK, Mendelson JH, Lex BW: Alcohol use and premenstrual symptoms in social drinkers. Psychopharmacology (Berl) 101:448–455, 1990

Mellstrom B, Bertilsson L, Lou YC, et al: Amitriptyline metabolism: relationship to polymorphic debrisoquine hydroxylation. Clin Pharmacol Ther 34:516–520, 1983

Meltzer HY, Fang VS, Tricou BJ, et al: Effect of antidepressants on neuroendocrine axis in humans, in Typical and Atypical Antidepressants: Clinical Practice. Edited by Costa E, Racagui G. New York, Raven, 1982, pp 303–16

Meltzer HY, Busch D, Fang V: Serum neuroleptic and prolactin levels in schizophrenic patients and clinical response. Psychiatry Res 9:271–283, 1983

Mendelson JH, Teoh SK, Lange U, et al: Anterior pituitary, adrenal, and gonadal hormones during cocaine withdrawal. Am J Psychiatry 145:1094–1098, 1988

Mendelson SD, Gorzalka BB: Effects of 5-HT$_{1A}$ selective anxiolytics on lordosis behavior: interactions with progesterone. Eur J Pharmacol 132:323–326, 1986

Mendoza R, Smith MW, Poland RE, et al: Ethnic psychopharmacology: the Hispanic and Native American perspective. Psychopharmacol Bull 27:449–461, 1991

Menzies KD, Drysdale DB, Waite PME: Effects of prenatal progesterone on development of pyramidal cells in rat cerebral cortex. Exp Neurol 77:654–667, 1982

Mercke C, Lundh B: Erythrocyte filterability and heme catabolism during the menstrual cycle. Ann Intern Med 85:322–324, 1976

Merkatz RB, Temple R, Sobel S, et al: Inclusion of women in clinical trials—Policies for population subgroups. N Engl J Med 329:288–291, 1993a

Merkatz RB, Temple R, Sobel S, et al: Women in clinical trials of new drugs: a change in Food and Drug Administration policy. N Engl J Med 329:292–296, 1993b

Merlob P, Mor N, Litwin A: Transient hepatic dysfunction in an infant of an epileptic mother treated with carbamazepine during pregnancy and breastfeeding. Ann Pharmacother 26:1563–1565, 1992

Merryman W, Boiman R, Barnes L, et al: Progesterone anesthesia in human subjects. Journal of Clinical Endocrinology 14:1567–1569, 1954

Meston CM, Gorzalka BB: Psychoactive drugs and human sexual behavior: the role of serotonergic activity. J Psychoactive Drugs 24:1–40, 1992

Metz AM, Stump G, Cowen PJ, et al: Changes in platelet alpha$_2$-adrenoreceptor binding post-partum: possible relation to maternity blues. Lancet 1:495–498, 1983

Metz AM, Sichel DA, Goff DC: Postpartum panic disorder. J Clin Psychiatry 49:278–279, 1988

Meyer DC, McRee C, Jacobs M: Role of 5-hydroxytryptamine receptors on luteinizing-hormone–releasing hormone release in the ovariectomized, estradiol-treated rat. Brain Res Bull 28:853–860, 1992

Meyer G, Ferres-Torres R, Mas M: The effects of puberty and castration on hippocampal dendritic spines of mice: a Golgi study. Brain Res 155:108–112, 1978

Meyer UA, Zanger UM, Grant D, et al: Genetic polymorphisms of drug metabolism. Advances in Drug Research 19:198–242, 1990

Middlefell R, Frost L, Eagan GP, et al: A report on the effects of phenelzine (Nardil), a monoamine oxidase inhibitor, in depressed patients. J Nerv Ment Dis 106:1533–1538, 1960

Milkovich L, van den Berg BJ: Effects of prenatal meprobamate and chlordiazepoxide hydrochloride on human embryonic and fetal development. N Engl J Med 291:1268–1271, 1974

Miller BA, Downs WR, Gondoli DM, et al: The role of childhood sexual abuse in the development of alcoholism in women. Violence Vict 2:157–172, 1987

Miller JB: Toward a New Psychology of Women. Boston, MA, Beacon Press, 1976

Miller JB, Stiver I: A relational approach to understanding women's lives and problems. Psychiatric Annals 23:424–431, 1993

Miller JC: Sex differences in dopaminergic and cholinergic activity and function in nigro-striatal system of the rat. Psychoneuroendocrinology 8:225–236, 1983

Miller LG: Cigarettes and drug therapy: pharmacokinetic and pharmacodynamic considerations. Clinical Psychiatry 9:125–135, 1990

Miller LJ: Clinical strategies for the use of psychotropic drugs during pregnancy. Psychiatric Medicine 9:275–298, 1991

Miller NS, Gold MS, Belkin BM, et al: Family history and diagnosis of alcohol dependence in cocaine dependence. Psychiatry Res 29:113–121, 1989

Mindham RHS, Howland C, Sheperd M: An evaluation of continuation therapy with antidepressants in depressive illness. Psychol Med 3:5–17, 1973

Miners JO, Atwood J, Birkett DJ: Influence of sex and oral contraceptive steroids on paracetamol metabolism. Br J Clin Pharmacol 16:503–509, 1983

Mishell DR: Contraception. N Engl J Med 320:777–787, 1989

Mitchell JE, Popkin MK: Antipsychotic drug therapy and sexual dysfunction in men. Am J Psychiatry 139:633–637, 1982

Mitchell JE, Popkin MK: Antidepressant drug therapy and sexual dysfunction in men: a review. J Clin Psychopharmacol 3:76–79, 1983

Mitchell MC, Hanew T, Meredith CG, et al: Effects of oral contraceptive steroids on acetaminophen metabolism and elimination. Clin Pharmacol Ther 34:48–55, 1983

Mitchell MD, Haynes P, Anderson A, et al: Plasma oxytocin concentrations during the menstrual cycle. Eur J Obstet Gynecol Reprod Biol 12:195–200, 1981

Mizoi Y, Ijiri I, Tatsuno Y, et al: Relationship between facial flushing and blood acetaldehyde levels after alcohol intake. Pharmacol Biochem Behav 10:301–311, 1979

Mode A, Norstedt G, Simic B, et al: Continuous infusion of growth hormone feminizes hepatic steroid metabolism in the rat. Endocrinology 108:2163–2168, 1981

Modell JG: Repeated observations of yawning, clitoral engorgement, and orgasm associated with fluoxetine administration. J Clin Psychopharmacol 9:63–65, 1989

Moghissi KS: Accuracy of basal body temperature for ovulation detection. Fertil Steril 27:1415–1421, 1976

Moghissi KS, Syner FN, Evans TN: A composite picture of the menstrual cycle. Am J Obstet Gynecol 114:405–418, 1972

Mogul KM: Psychological considerations in the use of psychotropic drugs with women patients. Hosp Community Psychiatry 36:1080–1085, 1985

Monteiro WO, Noshirvani HF, Marks IM, et al: Anorgasmia from clomipramine in obsessive-compulsive disorder: a controlled trial. Br J Psychiatry 151:107–112, 1987

Montiel MD, Carracedo A, Blazquez-Caeiro JL, et al: Orosomucoid (ORM1 and ORM2) types in the Spanish Basque country, Galicia, and Northern Portugal. Hum Hered 40:330–334, 1990

Moody JP, Tait AC, Todrick A: Plasma levels of imipramine and desmethylimipramine during therapy. Br J Psychiatry 113:183–193, 1967

Morgan ET, MacGeoch C, Gustafsson JA: Hormonal and developmental regulation of expression of the hepatic microsomal steroid 16-alpha-hydroxylase cytochrome P450 apoprotein in the rat. J Biol Chem 260:11895–11898, 1985

Morgan ET, MacGeoch C, Gustafsson JA: Sexual differentiation of cytochrome P450 in rat liver: evidence for a constitutive isoenzyme as the male specific 16-alpha-hydroxylase. Mol Pharmacol 27:471–479, 1986

Morgan MY, Sherlock S: Sex-related differences among 100 patients with alcoholic liver disease. BMJ 1:939–941, 1977

Morgan WW, Herbert DC: Elevation of serum prolactin levels after inhibition of serotonin uptake. Endocrinology 103:1016–1022, 1978

Morishita H, Hashimoto T, Mitani H, et al: Cervical mucus and prediction of the time of ovulation. Gynecol Obstet Invest 10:157–162, 1979

Morley K, Parke A, Hughes G: Systemic lupus erythematosis: two patients treated with danazol. BMJ 284:1431–1432, 1982

Morris JB, Beck AT: The efficacy of antidepressant drugs: a review of research. Arch Gen Psychiatry 30:667–674, 1974

Morris NM, Underwood LE, Easterling WJ: Temporal relationship between basal body temperature nadir and luteinizing hormone surge in normal women. Fertil Steril 27:780–783, 1976

Mortola JF: The use of psychotropic agents in pregnancy and lactation. Psychiatr Clin North Am 12:69–87, 1989

Mosher W: Contraceptive practice in the United States, 1982–1988. Fam Plann Perspect 22:198–205, 1990

Moss HB: More cases of anorgasmia after MAOI treatment (letter). Am J Psychiatry 140:266, 1983

Moyer TP, Boeckx RL (eds): Applied Therapeutic Drug Monitoring, Vol 1: Fundamentals. Washington, DC, American Association for Clinical Chemistry, 1982

Mumme D: Aftercare: its role in primary and secondary recovery of women from alcohol and other drug dependence. Int J Addict 26:549–564, 1991

Munemura M, Agui T, Sibley DR: Chronic estrogen treatment promotes a functional uncoupling of the D_2 dopamine receptor in rat anterior pituitary gland. Endocrinology 124:346–355, 1989

Munoz RF, Hollon SD, McGrath E, et al: On the AHCPR depression in primary care guidelines: further considerations for practitioners (Agency for Health Care Policy and Research). Am Psychol 49:42–61, 1994

Murphy DL, Pato MT, Pigott TA: Obsessive-compulsive disorder: treatment with serotonin-selective uptake inhibitors, azapirones, and other agents. J Clin Psychopharmacol 10 (suppl):91–100, 1990

Murphy M: Down regulation of post-synaptic serotonin receptors as a mechanism for clomipramine-induced anorgasmia (letter). Br J Psychiatry 151:704, 1987

Murray R: The neurodevelopmental basis of sex differences in schizophrenia. Psychol Med 21:565–575, 1991

Muscettola G, Goodwin FK, Potter WZ, et al: Imipramine and desipramine in plasma and spinal fluid: relationship to clinical response and serotonin metabolism. Arch Gen Psychiatry 35:621–625, 1978

Musher JS: Anorgasmia with the use of fluoxetine (letter). Am J Psychiatry 147:948, 1990

Myers LS, Morokoff PJ: Physiological and subjective sexual arousal in pre- and postmenopausal women taking replacement therapy. Psychophysiology 23:283–290, 1986

Nafziger AN, Schwartzman MS, Bertino JS Jr: Absence of tobramycin pharmacokinetic and creatinine clearance variation during the menstrual cycle: implied absence of variation in glomerular filtration rate. J Clin Pharmacol 29:757–763, 1989

Nagy A, Johansson R: The demethylation of imipramine and clomipramine as apparent from their plasma kinetics. Psychopharmacology (Berl) 54:125–131, 1977

Nakamura K, Goto F, Ray WA, et al: Interethnic differences in genetic polymorphism of debrisoquine and mephenytoin hydroxylation between Japanese and Caucasian populations. Clin Pharmacol Ther 38:402–408, 1985

Nakane Y, Okuma T, Takahashi, et al: Multi-institutional study on the teratogenicity and fetal toxicity of antiepileptic drugs: a report of a collaborative study group in Japan. Epilepsia 21:663–680, 1980

Narbone MC, Ruello C, Oliva A, et al: Hormonal dysregulation and catemenial epilepsy. Funct Neurol 5:49–53, 1990

Nasrallah HA, Andreasen NC, Coffman JA, et al: A controlled magnetic resonance imaging study of corpus callosum thickness in schizophrenia. Biol Psychiatry 21:274–282, 1986

Nasrallah HA, Schwarzkopf SB, Olson SC, et al: Gender differences in schizophrenia on MRI brain scans. Schizophr Bull 16:205–210, 1990

National Institute on Drug Abuse: Drug use among American high school seniors, college students and young adults, 1975–1990, Vol 2 (DHHS Publ No ADM-91-1835). Washington, DC, U.S. Government Printing Office, 1991a

National Institute on Drug Abuse: National Household Survey on Drug Abuse: population estimates—1990 (DHHS Publ No ADM-91-1732). Washington, DC, U.S. Government Printing Office, 1991b

Nau H, Rating D, Koch S, et al: Valproic acid and its metabolites: placental transfer, neonatal pharmacokinetics, transfer via mother's milk and clinical status in neonates of epileptic mothers. J Pharmacol Exp Ther 219:768–777, 1981

Nausieda PA, Koller WC, Weiner WJ, et al: Modification of postsynaptic dopaminergic sensitivity by female sex hormones. Life Sciences 25:521–530, 1979

Nebert DW, Weber WW: Pharmacogenetics, in Principles of Drug Action. Edited by Pratt WB, Taylor P. New York, Churchill Livingston, 1990

Nelson RP: Nonoperative management of impotence. J Urol 139:2–5, 1988

Nestoros JN, Lehmann HE, Ban TA: Neuroleptic drugs and sexual function in schizophrenics. Modern Problems in Pharmacopsychiatry 15:111–130, 1980

Nestoros JN, Lehmann HE, Ban TA: Sexual behavior of the male schizophrenic: the impact of illness and medications. Arch Sex Behav 10:421–442, 1981

Nielsen HK, Brixen K, Bouillon R, et al: Changes in biochemical markers of osteoblastic activity during the menstrual cycle. J Clin Endocrinol Metab 70:1431–1437, 1990

Noel B, Watterson K: You Must Be Dreaming. New York, Poseidon, 1992

Nolen-Hoeksema S: Sex Differences in Depression. Stanford, CA, Stanford University Press, 1990

Nordin BE, Need AG, Morris HA, et al: Evidence for a renal calcium leak in postmenopausal women. J Clin Endocrinol Metab 72:401–407, 1991

Noshirvani HF, Kasvikis Y, Marks IM, et al: Gender-divergent aetiological factors in obsessive-compulsive disorder. Br J Psychiatry 158:260–263, 1991

Notivol R, Carrio I, Cano L, et al: Gastric emptying of solid and liquid meals in healthy young subjects. Scand J Gastroenterol 19:1107–1113, 1984

Nott PN, Franklin M, Armitage C, et al: Hormonal changes in mood in the puerperium. Br J Psychiatry 128:379–383, 1976

Nowaczynski W, Koiw E, Biron P, et al: Effects of angiotensin infusions on urinary excretion of compound III and substances other than aldosterone. Canadian Journal of Biochemistry and Physiology 40:727–738, 1962

Noyes R, Garvey MJ, Cook BL, et al: Problems with tricyclic antidepressant use in patients with panic disorder or agoraphobia: results of a naturalistic follow-up study. J Clin Psychiatry 50:163–169, 1989

Nulsen J, Wheeler C, Ausmanas M, et al: Cervical mucus changes in relationship to urinary luteinizing hormone. Fertil Steril 48:783–786, 1987

Nurco DN, Wegner N, Stephenson F: Female narcotic addicts: changing profiles. Journal on Addiction and Health 3:62–105, 1982

Nurnberg HG, Levine PE: Spontaneous remission of MAOI-induced anorgasmia. Am J Psychiatry 144:805–807, 1987

Nutt D, Hackman A, Hawton K: Increased sexual function in benzodiazepine withdrawal (letter). Lancet 2:1101–1102, 1986

O'Brien PMS, Craven D, Selby C, et al: Treatment of premenstrual syndrome by spironolactone. Br J Obstet Gynaecol 86:142–147, 1979

Ochs HR, Greenblatt DJ, Divoll M, et al: Diazepam kinetics in relation to age and sex. Pharmacol 23:24–30, 1981

O'Connor LH, Nock B, McEwen BS: Regional specificity of gamma-aminobutyric acid receptor regulation by estradiol. Neuroendocrinology 47:473–481, 1988

Odejide AO: Prevalence of persistent abnormal involuntary movements among patients in a Nigerian long-stay psychiatric unit. International Pharmacopsychiatry 15:292–300, 1980

Odlind V, Olsson SE: Enhanced metabolism of levonorgestrel during phenytoin treatment in a woman with Norplant implants. Contraception 33:257–261, 1986

Ogawa S, Olazabal UE, Parhar IS, et al: Effects of intrahypothalamic administration of antisense DNA for progesterone receptor mRNA on reproductive behavior and progesterone receptor immunoreactivity in female rat. J Neurosci 14:1766–1774, 1994

O'Keane V, Dinan TG: Sex steroid priming effects on growth hormone response to pyridostigmine throughout the menstrual cycle. J Clin Endocrinol Metab 75:11–14, 1992

Olson S, Schwarzkopf S, Coffman J, et al: Anterior coronal brain and ventricular measures in male schizophrenics using MRI. Schizophr Res 2:126–131, 1989

Olster DH, Blaustein JD: Immunocytochemical colocalization of progestin receptors and beta-endorphin or enkephalin in the hypothalamus of female guinea pigs. J Neurobiol 21:768–780, 1990

O'Malley BW, Means AR: Female steroid hormone and target cell nuclei. Science 183:610–620, 1993

O'Malley K, Crooks J, Duke E, et al: Effects of age and sex on human drug metabolism. BMJ 3:607–704, 1971

Omtzigt JG, Nau H, Los FJ, et al: The disposition of valproate and its metabolites in the late first trimester and early second trimester of pregnancy in maternal serum, urine, and amniotic fluid: effect of dose, co-medication, and the presence of spinal bifida. Eur J Clin Pharmacol 43:381–388, 1992a

Omtzigt JG, Los FJ, Hagenaars AM, et al: Prenatal diagnosis of spina bifida aperta after first-trimester valproate exposure. Prenatal Diagnosis 12:893–897, 1992b

Oppenheim G: Estrogen in the treatment of depression: neuropharmacological mechanisms. Arch Gen Psychiatry 43:569–573, 1986

Orford J, Keddie A: Gender differences in the functions and effects of moderate and excessive drinking. Br J Clin Psychol 24:265–279, 1985

Ostheimer G, Warren TM: Obstetric analgesia and anesthesia, in Drug Use in Pregnancy. Edited by Stern L. Sydney, Australia, Adis Health Science Press, 1984, pp 216–269

Ostrow DC, Trevisan M, Okonek A, et al: Sodium dependent membrane processes in major affective disorders, in Biological Markers in Psychiatry and Neurology. Edited by Usdin E, Handin I. New York, Pergamon, 1982, pp 153–167

Othmar E, Othmar S: Effect of buspirone on sexual dysfunction in patients with generalized anxiety disorder. J Clin Psychiatry 48:201–203, 1987

O'Toole ML: Exercise and physical activity, in Cardiovascular Health and Disease in Women. Edited by Douglas PS. Philadelphia, PA, WB Saunders, 1993, pp 253–257

Otton SV, Inaba T, Kalow W: Inhibition of sparteine oxidation in human liver by tricyclic antidepressants and other drugs. Life Sciences 32:795–800, 1983

Ouslander JG: Drug therapy in the elderly. Ann Intern Med 95:711–722, 1981

Owens WD, Zeitlin GL: Hypoventilation in a newborn following administration of succinylcholine to the mother. Anesth Analg 54:38–39, 1975

Paaby P, Moller-Petersen J, Larsen CE, et al: Endogenous overnight creatinine clearance, serum B_2-microglobulin and serum water during the menstrual cycle. Acta Medica Scandinavica 221:191–197, 1987

Pache TD, Wladimiroff JW, De Jong FH, et al: Growth patterns of nondominant ovarian follicles during the normal menstrual cycle. Fertil Steril 54:638–642, 1990

Palermo-Neto J, Dorce VA: Influence of estrogen and/or progesterone on some dopamine related behavior in rats. Gen Pharmacol 21:83–87, 1990

Palinkas LA, Barrett-Connor E: Estrogen use and depressive symptoms in postmenopausal women. Obstet Gynecol 80:30–36, 1992

Parella DP, Filstead WJ: Definition of onset in the development of onset-based alcoholism typologies. J Stud Alcohol 49:85–92, 1988

Parish RC, Spivey C: Influence of menstrual cycle phase on serum concentration of α_1-acid glycoprotein. Br J Clin Pharmacol 31:197–199, 1991

Pastuszak A, Schick-Boschetto B, Zuber C, et al: Pregnancy outcome following first-trimester exposure to fluoxetine (Prozac). JAMA 269:2246–2248, 1993

Patterson JF: Treatment of chorea gravidarum with haloperidol. South Med J 72:1220–1221, 1979

Patwardhan RV, Mitchell MC, Johnson RF, et al: Induction of glucuronidation by oral contraceptive steroids (OCs). Clin Res 29:861A, 1981

Patwardhan RV, Mitchell MC, Johnson RF, et al: Differential effects of oral contraceptive steroids on the metabolism of benzodiazepines. Hepatology 3:248–253, 1983

Pauerstein CJ, Eddy CA, Croxatto HD, et al: Temporal relationship of estrogen, progesterone, and luteinizing hormone levels to ovulation in women and infrahuman primates. Am J Obstet Gynecol 130:876–886, 1978

Paul SM, Axelrod J, Saavedra JM, et al: Estrogen-induced efflux of endogenous catecholamines from the hypothalamus in vitro. Brain Res 178:479–505, 1979

Paul SM, Rehavi M, Skolnick P, et al: High affinity binding of antidepressants to biogenic amine transport sites in human brain and platelet: studies in depression, in Neurobiology of Mood Disorders. Edited by Post RM, Ballenger JC. Baltimore, MD, Williams & Wilkins, 1984, pp 846–853

Paulson JD, Speck G, Albarelli JN: The use of ultrasonography to detect ovulation, in Ovulation and Its Disorders (Studies in Fertility and Sterility). Edited by Thompson W, Harrison RF, Bonnar J. Boston, MA, MTP Press, 1984, pp 7–12

Paykel ES, Hollyman JA, Freeling P, et al: Predictors of therapeutic benefit from amitriptyline in mild depression: a general practice placebo-controlled trial. Journal of Affective Disorders 14:83–95, 1988

Paz G, Yogev L, Gottreich A, et al: Determination of urinary luteinizing hormone for prediction of ovulation. Gynecol Obstet Invest 29:207–210, 1990

Peart GF, Boutagy J, Shenfield GM: Debrisoquine oxidation in an Australian population. Br J Clin Pharmacol 21:465–471, 1986

Peck C: FDC Reports, Inc. Pink Sheet, July 26, 1993

Penniman LJ, Agnew J: Women, work, and alcohol: occupational medicine, in Alcoholism and Chemical Dependency in the Workplace. Edited by Wright C. Philadelphia, PA, Hanley & Belfus, 1989, pp 264–273

Perel JM, Shostak M, Gann E, et al: Pharmacodynamics of imipramine and clinical outcome in depressed patients, in Pharmacokinetics, Psychoactive Drug Blood Levels and Clinical Outcome. Edited by Gottschalk L, Merlis S. New York, Wiley, 1975a, pp 229–241

Perel JM, Hurwic MJ, Kanzler MB: Pharmacodynamics of imipramine in depressed patients. Psychopharmacol Bull 11:16, 1975b

Perez OE, Henriquez N: Galactorrhea associated with maprotiline HCl. Am J Psychiatry 140:641–642, 1983

Perier M, Eslami H: Evaluation clinique des effets anti-depresseurs de la doxepine [Clinical evaluation of the antidepressive effects of doxepine]. Annales Medico-Psychologiques (Paris) 1:581–587, 1971

Perper JA, Van Thiel DH: Respiratory complications of cocaine abuse. Recent Dev Alcohol 10:363–377, 1992

Perrini M, Piliego N: The increase of aldosterone in the premenstrual syndrome. Minerva Med 50:2897–2899, 1959

Perse TL, Greist JH, Jefferson JW, et al: Fluvoxamine treatment of OCD. Am J Psychiatry 144:1543–1548, 1988

Persky H: Reproductive hormones, moods, and the menstrual cycle, in Sex Differences in Behavior. Edited by Friedman R. New York, Wiley, 1974, pp 455–466

Perucca E, Crema A: Plasma protein binding of drugs in pregnancy. Clin Pharmacokinet 7:336–356, 1982

Peselow ED, Felippi AM, Goodnick R, et al: The short- and long-term efficacy of paroxetine HCl, A: data from a 6-week double-blind parallel design trial vs. imipramine and placebo. Psychopharmacol Bull 25:267–271, 1989

Petersen WF, Milles G: Relation of menstruation to permeability of capillaries and autonomic tonus of skin vessels. Arch Int Med 38:730–735, 1926

Petring OU, Flachs H: Inter- and intrasubject variability of gastric emptying in healthy volunteers measured by scintigraphy and paracetamol absorption. Br J Clin Pharmacol 29:703–708, 1990

Pettinati HM, Sugerman AA, Maurer HS: Four-year MMPI changes in abstinent and drinking alcoholics. Alcohol Clin Exp Res 6:487–494, 1982

Pettinati HM, Cabezas RA, Jensen J, et al: Incidence of personality disorders in cocaine vs. alcohol-dependent females. NIDA Research Monographs 105:369–370, 1991

Pfaff DW: Estrogens and Brain Function: Neural Analysis of a Hormone-Controlled Mammalian Reproductive Behavior. New York, Springer-Verlag, 1980

Pfaff DW (ed): The Physiological Mechanisms of Motivation. Heidelberg, Germany, Springer-Verlag, 1982

Pfaff DW, Schwartz-Giblin S, McCarthy MM, et al: Cellular and molecular mechanisms of female reproductive behaviors, in The Physiology of Reproduction, 2nd Edition. Edited by Knobil E, Neill JD. New York, Raven, 1994, pp 107–220

Pfaus JG, Gorzalka BB: Opioids and sexual behavior. Neuroscience Biobehavioral Review 11:1–34, 1987a

Pfaus JG, Gorzalka BB: Selective activation of opioid receptors differentially affects lordosis behavior in female rats. Peptides 8:309–317, 1987b

Pfaus JG, Pfaff DW: Mu, delta, and kappa opioid receptor agonists selectively modulate sexual behaviors in the female rat: differential dependence on progesterone. Horm Behav 26:457–473, 1992

Pfeiffer E, Davis GC: Determinants of sexual behavior in middle and old age. J Am Geriatr Soc 4:151–160, 1972

Pharmaceutical Manufacturers Association: Guidelines for the Assessment of Drug and Medical Device Safety in Animals. Washington, DC, Pharmaceutical Manufacturers Association, February 1977

Phillips SM, Sherwin BB: Effects of estrogen on memory function in surgically menopausal women. Psychoneuroendocrinology 17:485–495, 1992

Physicians' Desk Reference, 47th Edition. Montvale, NJ, Medical Economics Data, 1993

Piafsky KM, Borga O, Odar-Cedarlof E, et al: Increased binding of propranolol and chlorpromazine in disease. N Engl J Med 299:1435–1439, 1978

Piazza NJ, Vrbka JF, Yeager RD: Telescoping of alcoholism in women alcoholics. Int J Addict 24:19–28, 1989

Piscotta V: Drug-induced agranulocytosis. Drugs 15:132–143, 1978

Pohl R, Yeragani V, Balon R, et al: The jitteriness syndrome in panic disorder patients treated with antidepressants. J Clin Psychiatry 49:100–104, 1988

Poirier MF, Loo H, Scatton B, et al: Platelet monoamine oxidase activity and dihydroxyphenyl glycol during the menstrual cycle. Neuropsychobiology 14:165–169, 1985

Poirier MF, Benkelfat C, Galzin AM, et al: Platelet ^{3}H-imipramine binding and steroid hormones serum concentrations during the menstrual cycle. Psychopharmacology (Berl) 88:86–89, 1986

Polefrone JM, Manuck SB: Gender differences in cardiovascular and neuroendocrine reponse to stressors, in Gender and Stress. Edited by Barnett RC, Biener L, Baruch GK. New York, Free Press, 1987, pp 13–38

Polich JM, Armor DJ, Braiker HB: The course of alcoholism: four years after treatment (National Institute on Alcohol Abuse and Alcoholism Publ No R-2433-NIAAA). Washington, DC, Rand Corporation, 1981

Pollack MH, Rosenbaum JF: Management of antidepressant-induced side effects: a practical guide for the clinician. J Clin Psychiatry 48:3–8, 1987

Pollack MH, Tesar GE, Rosenbaum JF, et al: Clonazepam in the treatment of panic disorder and agoraphobia: a one-year follow-up. J Clin Psychopharmacol 6:302–304, 1982

Pollack MH, Reiter S, Hammerness P: Genitourinary and sexual adverse effects of psychotropic medication. Int J Psychiatry Med 22:305–327, 1992

Pollock BG, Perel JM, Kirshner M, et al: S-mephenytoin 4-hydroxylation in older Americans. Eur J Clin Pharmacol 40:609–611, 1991

Pontius EB: An anticholinergic crisis associated with cyproheptadine treatment of desipramine-induced anorgasmia. J Clin Psychopharmacol 8:230–231, 1988

Poortman J, Andriesse R, Agema A, et al: Adrenal androgen secretion and metabolism in postmenopausal women, in Adrenal Androgens. Edited by Gemazzini AR, Thyssen JHH, Suteri PK. New York, Raven, 1980, 219–240

Popkin CL, Rudisill LC, Waller PF, et al: Female drinking and driving: recent trends in North Carolina. Accid Anal Prev 20:219–255, 1988

Popour J: Planning women's alcohol and drug services in Michigan. Lansing, MI, Michigan Department of Public Health, Office of Substance Abuse Services, 1983

Post RM: Effectiveness of carbamazepine in the treatment of bipolar affective disorder, in Use of Anticonvulsants in Psychiatry: Recent Advances. Edited by McElroy SL, Pope HGJ. Clifton, NJ, Oxford Health Care, 1988, pp 1–24

Post RM: Non-lithium treatment for bipolar disorder. J Clin Psychiatry 51 (suppl):9–16, 1990

Potter WZ: Pharmacokinetics in special populations. Conference presentation in Pharmacokinetics and Psychiatric Drugs symposium, American Psychiatric Association Annual Meeting, San Francisco, CA, May 25, 1993

Prange AJ, Wilson IC, Rabon AM, et al: Clinical and theoretical implications of the enhancement of imipramine by tri-iodothyronine in the full spectrum of depressive illnesses, in Recent Advances in the Psychobiology of Depressive Illness. Edited by Williams T, Katz M, Shield JA. Washington, DC, U.S. Government Printing Office, 1972, pp 249–255

Preedy J, Aitken E: The effect of estrogen on water and electrolyte metabolism: the normal. J Clin Invest 35:423–429, 1956

Prendiville W, Baker TS: The relationship between the ratio of El-3-G/Pd-3-G and the fertile period, in Research in Family Planning (Studies in Fertility and Sterility). Edited by Bonnar J, Thompson W, Harrison RF. Boston, MA, MTP Press, 1984, pp 53–54

Preskorn SH, Mac DS: Plasma levels of amitriptyline: effects of age and sex. J Clin Psychopharmacol 46:276–277, 1985

Price J, Grunhaus LJ: Treatment of clomipramine-induced anorgasmia with yohimbine: a case report. J Clin Psychiatry 51:31–32, 1990

Pulver AE, Brown CH, Wolniec P, et al: Schizophrenia: age at onset, gender and familial risk. Acta Psychiatr Scand 82:344–351, 1990

Putnam FW, Gurroff JJ, Silberman EK, et al: The clinical phenomenology of multiple personality disorder: review of 100 recent cases. J Clin Psychiatry 51:470–472, 1986

Quagliarello J, Arny M: Inaccuracy of basal body temperature charts in predicting urinary luteinizing hormone surges. Fertil Steril 45:334–337, 1986

Quigley M, Yen S: The role of endogenous opiates on LH secretion during the menstrual cycle. J Clin Endocrinol Metab 51:179–181, 1980

Quirk KC, Einarson TR: Sexual dysfunction and clomipramine. Can J Psychiatry 27:228–231, 1982

Quitkin FM, Stewart JW, McGrath PJ, et al: Phenelzine versus imipramine in the treatment of probable atypical depression. Am J Psychiatry 145:306–311, 1988

Quitkin FM, McGrath PJ, Stewart JW, et al:. Phenelzine and imipramine in mood-reactive depressives: further delineation of the syndrome of atypical depression. Arch Gen Psychiatry 46:787–793, 1989

Rabkin J, Quitkin F, Harrison W, et al: Adverse reactions to monoamine oxidase inhibitors, II: treatment correlates and clinical management. J Clin Psychopharmacol 5:2–9, 1985

Rachamin G, MacDonald JA, Wahid S, et al: Modulation of alcohol dehydrogenase and ethanol metabolism by sex hormones in the spontaneously hypertensive rat. Biochem J 186:483–490, 1980

Rainbow TC, DeGroff V, Luine VN, et al: Estradiol 17-beta increases the number of muscarinic receptors in hypothalamic nuclei. Brain Res 198:239–243, 1980

Rao SSC, Read NW, Brown C, et al: Studies on the mechanism of bowel disturbance in ulcerative colitis. Gastroenterol 93:934–940, 1987

Rapkin AJ, Edelmuth E, Chang L, et al: Whole-blood serotonin in premenstrual syndrome. Obstet Gynecol 70:533–537, 1987

Rapkin AJ, Buckman TD, Sutphin MS, et al: Platelet monoamine oxidase B activity in women with premenstrual syndrome. Am J Obstet Gynecol 159:1536–1540, 1988

Raskin A: Age-sex differences in response to antidepressant drugs. J Nerv Ment Dis 159:120–130, 1974

Rasmussen SA, Tsuang MT: The epidemiology of obsessive compulsive disorder. J Clin Psychiatry 45:450–457, 1984

Rausch JL, Parry BL: Treatment of premenstrual mood symptoms. Psychiatr Clin North Am 16:829–839, 1993

Rausch JL, Janowsky DS, Risch SC, et al: Hormonal and neurotransmitter hypotheses of premenstrual tension. Psychopharmacol Bull 18:26–34, 1982

Rawson RA, Obert JL, McCann MJ, et al: Cocaine treatment outcome: cocaine use following inpatient, outpatient, and no treatment, in Problems of Drug Dependence, 1985. Proceedings of the 47th Annual Scientific Meeting, The Committee on Problems of Drug Dependence (NIDA Research Monograph 67; DHHS Publ No ADM-86-1448). Edited by Harris LA. Washington, DC, U.S. Department of Health and Human Services, 1986, pp 111–120

Raymond V, Beaulieu M, Labrie F, et al: Potent antidopaminergic activity of estradiol at the pituitary level on prolactin release. Science 200:1173–1175, 1978

Reame N, Sauder S, Kelch R, et al: Pulsatile gonadotropin secretion during the human menstrual cycle: evidence for altered frequency of gonadotropin-releasing hormone secretion. J Clin Endocrinol Metab 59:328–337, 1984

Reddi K, Wickings EJ, McNeilly AS, et al: Circulating bioactive follicle stimulating hormone and immunoreactive inhibin levels during the normal human menstrual cycle. Clin Endocrinol (Oxford) 33:547–557, 1990

Rees WDW, Rhodes J: Altered bowel habit and menstruation (letter). Lancet 2:475, 1976

Regier DA, Farmer ME, Rae DS, et al: Comorbidity of mental disorders with alcohol and other drug abuse: results from the Epidemiologic Catchment Area (ECA) Study. JAMA 264:2511–2518, 1990

Rehavi M, Sepcuti H, Weizman A: Upregulation of imipramine binding and serotonin uptake by estradiol in female rat brain. Brain Res 410:135–139, 1987

Reich M: The variations in urinary aldosterone levels of normal females during their menstrual cycle. Australasian Annals of Medicine (Sydney) 11:41–49, 1962

Reich T, Cloninger R, Eerdewegh PV, et al: Secular trends in familial transmission of alcoholism. Alcohol Clin Exp Res 12:458–464, 1988

Reid RL, Yen SS: Premenstrual syndrome. Am J Obstet Gynecol 139:85–104, 1981

Reisby N, Gram LF, Bech P, et al: Imipramine: clinical effects and pharmacokinetic variability. Psychopharmacology 54:263–272, 1977

Relling MV, Cherrie J, Schell MJ, et al: Lower prevalence of the debrisoquin oxidative poor metabolizer phenotype in American black versus white subjects. Clin Pharmacol Ther 50:308–313, 1991

Rementeria JL, Bhatt K: Withdrawal symptoms in neonates from intrauterine exposure to diazepam. J Pediatr 90:123–126, 1977

Remick RA, Maurice WL: ECT in pregnancy. Am J Psychiatry 135:761–762, 1978

Repke JT, Berger NG: Electroconvulsive therapy in pregnancy. Obstet Gynecol 63 (suppl):39–41, 1984

Reubens JR: The physiology of normal sexual response in females. J Psychoactive Drugs 14:45–46, 1982

Ribeiro WO, Mishell DR, Thorneycroft IH: Comparison of the patterns of androstenedione, progesterone, and estradiol during the human menstrual cycle. Am J Obstet Gynecol 119:1026–1032, 1974

Richardson CJ, Blocka KLN, Ross SG, et al: Effects of age and sex on piroxicam disposition. Clin Pharmacol Ther 37:13–18, 1985

Richardson CJ, Blocka KLN, Ross SG, et al: The menstrual cycle, cognition, and paramenstrual symptomatology, in Cognition and the Menstrual Cycle. Edited by Richardson JTE. New York, Springer-Verlag, 1992, pp 1–38

Rickels K, Schweizer E: The clinical course and long-term management of generalized anxiety disorder. J Clin Psychopharmacol 10 (suppl 3):101S–110S, 1990

Rickels K, Raab E, DeSilverio R, et al: Drug treatment in depression: antidepressant or tranquilizer. JAMA 201:105–111, 1967

Rickels K, Norstad N, Singer M, et al: Buspirone and diazepam in the treatment of anxiety: a controlled study. J Clin Psychiatry 43:81–86, 1982a

Rickels K, Case WG, Downing RW: Issues in long-term treatment with diazepam. Psychopharmacol Bull 18:38–41, 1982b

Rickels K, Freeman E, Sondheimer S: Buspirone in treatment of premenstrual syndrome (letter). Lancet 1:177, 1989

Rickels K, Schweizer E, Clary C, et al: Nefazodone and imipramine in major depression: a placebo-controlled trial. Br J Psychiatry 164:802–805, 1994

Rieder MJ, Shear NH, Kanee A, et al: Prominence of slow acetylator phenotype among patients with sulfonamide hypersensitivity reactions. Clin Pharmacol Ther 49:13–17, 1991

Riester EF, Pantuck EJ, Pantuck CB, et al: Antipyrine metabolism and the menstrual cycle. Clin Pharmacol Ther 28:384–391, 1980

Rietveld EC, Broekman MM, Houben JJ, et al: Rapid onset of an increase in caffeine residence time in young women due to oral contraceptive steroids. Eur J Clin Pharmacol 26:371–373, 1984

Riley AJ, Riley EJ: Cyproheptadine and antidepressant-induced anorgasmia. Br J Psychiatry 148:217–218, 1986

Ring N, Tantam D, Montague L, et al: Gender differences in the incidence of definite schizophrenia and atypical psychosis—focus on negative symptoms of schizophrenia. Acta Psychiatr Scand 84:489–496, 1991

Rizack M, Hillman C: The Medical Letter Handbook of Adverse Drug Interactions. New Rochelle, NY, The Medical Letter, 1991

Robert E, Guibaud P: Maternal valproic acid and congenital neural tube defects. Lancet 2:937, 1982

Roberts RK, Desmond PV, Wilkinson GR, et al: Disposition of chlordiazepoxide: sex differences and effects of oral contraceptives. Clin Pharmacol Ther 25:826–858, 1979

Robins LN, Regier DA (eds): Psychiatric Disorders in America. New York, Free Press, 1991

Robins LN, Helzer JE, Weissman MM, et al: Lifetime prevalence of specific psychiatric disorders in three sites. Arch Gen Psychiatry 41:949–958, 1984

Robinson TE, Becker JB, Ramirez VD: Sex differences in amphetamine-elicited rotational behavior and lateralization of striatal dopamine in rats. Brain Res Bull 5:539–545, 1980

Robinson TE, Becker JB, Presty SK: Long term facilitation of amphetamine-induced rotational behavior and striatal dopamine release produced by a single exposure to amphetamine: sex differences. Brain Res 253:231–241, 1982

Rogers SM, Back DJ, Stevenson PJ, et al: Paracetamol interaction with oral contraceptive steroids: increased plasma concentrations of ethinyloestradiol. Br J Clin Pharmacol 23:721–725, 1987

Rojansky N, Halbreich U, Zander K, et al: Imipramine receptor binding and serotonin uptake in platelets of women with premenstrual changes. Gynecol Obstet Invest 31:146–152, 1991

Rojansky N, Wang K, Halbreich U: Reproductive and sexual adverse effects of psychotropic drugs, in Adverse Effects of Psychotropic Drugs. Edited by Lieberman J, Kane J. New York, Guilford, 1992, pp 356–375

Romano GJ, Shivers BD, Harlan RE, et al: Haloperidol increases preproenkephalin mRNA levels in the caudate-putamen of the rat: a quantitative study at the cellular level using in situ hybridization. Molecular Brain Research 2:23–41, 1987

Romano GJ, Harlan RE, Shivers BD, et al: Estrogen increases preproenkephalin messenger ribonucleic acid levels in the ventromedial hypothalamus of the rat. Mol Endocrinol 2:1320–1328, 1988

Romano GJ, Mobbs CV, Howells RD, et al: Estrogen regulation of preproenkephalin gene expression in the ventromedial hypothalamus of the rat: temporal qualities and synergism with progesterone. Molecular Brain Research 5:51–58, 1989

Romano GJ, Mobbs CV, Lauber A, et al: Differential regulation of proenkephalin gene expression by estrogen in the ventromedial hypothalamus of male and female rats. Brain Res 536:63–68, 1990

Roof RL, Duvdevani R, Stein DG: Progesterone treatment attenuates brain edema following contusion injury in male and female rats. Restorative Neurology and Neuroscience 4:425–427, 1992

Roof RL, Duvdevani R, Stein DG: Gender influences outcome of brain injury: progesterone plays a protective role. Brain Res 607:333–336, 1993

Root MP: Treatment failures: the role of sexual victimization in women's addictive behavior. Am J Orthopsychiatry 59:542–549, 1989

Roper WL, Winkenwerder W, Hackbarin GM, et al: Effectiveness in health care: an initiative to evaluate and improve medical practice. N Engl J Med 319:1197–1202, 1988

Rosa FW: Spina bifida in infants of women treated with carbamazepine during pregnancy. N Engl J Med 324:674–677, 1991

Rosciszewska D, Buntner B, Guz I, et al: Ovarian hormones, anticonvulsant drugs and seizures during the menstrual cycle in women with epilepsy. J Neurol Neurosurg Psychiatry 49:47–51, 1986

Rose D, Adams P: Oral contraceptives and tryptophan metabolism: effects of oestrogen in low dose combined with a progestagen and of a low-dose progestagen (megestrol acetate) given alone. J Clin Pathol 25:252–258, 1972

Rosenbaum M: Becoming addicted: the woman addict. Contemporary Drug Problems 8:141–167, 1979

Rosenbaum M: Women on Heroin. New Brunswick, Rutgers University Press, 1981

Rosenberg L, Mitchell AA, Parsells JL, et al: Lack of relation of oral clefts to diazepam use during pregnancy. N Engl J Med 309:1282–1285, 1983

Rosenthal BJ, Savoy MJ, Greene BT, et al: Drug treatment outcomes: is sex a factor? Int J Addict 14:45–62, 1979

Rosenthal J, Hemlock C, Hellerstein DJ, et al: A preliminary study of serotonergic antidepressants in treatment of dysthymia. Prog Neuropsychopharmacol Biol Psychiatry 16:933–941, 1992

Rosenthal R: Meta-analysis: a review. Psychosom Med 53:247–271, 1991

Rosenthal R, Rubin DB: A simple, general purpose display of magnitude of experimental effect. Journal of Educational Psychology 74:166–169, 1982

Roskos LK, Boudinot FD: Effects of dose and sex on the pharmacokinetics of piroxicam in the rat. Biopharm Drug Dispos 11:215–225, 1990

Ross HE, Glaser FB, Stiasny S: Sex differences in the prevalence of psychiatric disorders in patients with alcohol and drug problems. British Journal of Addiction 83:1179–1192, 1988

Rothschild AJ: Selective serotonin reuptake inhibitor-induced sexual dysfunction: efficacy of a drug holiday. Am J Psychiatry 152:1514–1516, 1995

Rounsaville BJ, Kleber HD: Untreated opiate addicts: how do they differ from those seeking treatment? Arch Gen Psychiatry 42:1072–1077, 1985

Rounsaville BJ, Weissman MM, Kleber H, et al: Heterogeneity of psychiatric diagnosis in treated opiate addicts. Arch Gen Psychiatry 39:161–166, 1982a

Rounsaville BJ, Weissman MM, Wilber CH, et al: Pathways to opiate addiction: an evaluation of differing antecedents. Br J Psychiatry 141:437–446, 1982b

Rounsaville BJ, Dolinsky ZS, Babor TF, et al: Psychopathology as a predictor of treatment outcome in alcoholics. 6:607–614, 1987

Rounsaville BJ, Anton SF, Carroll K, et al: Psychiatric diagnoses of treatment seeking cocaine abusers. Arch Gen Psychiatry 48:43–51, 1991

Routledge PA: The plasma protein binding of basic drugs. Br J Clin Pharmacol 22:499–506, 1986

Routledge PA, Shand DG, Barchowsky A, et al: Relationship between alpha$_1$-acid glycoprotein and lidocaine disposition in myocardial infarction. Clin Pharmacol Ther 30:154–157, 1981

Rowan PK, Paykel ES, Parker RR: Phenelzine and amitriptyline: effects on symptoms of neurotic depression. Br J Psychiatry 140:475–483, 1982

Rowe I: Prescriptions of psychotropic drugs by general practioners: antidepressants. Med J Aust 1:642–644, 1973

Roy EJ, Buyer DR, Licari VA: Estradiol in the striatum: effects on behavior and dopamine receptors but no evidence for membrane steroid receptors. Brain Res Bull 25:221–227, 1990

Roy-Byrne P, Rubinow D, Gold P, et al: Possible antidepressant effect of oral contraceptives: case report. J Clin Psychiatry 45:350–352, 1984

Rutter M, Quinton D: Parental psychiatric disorder: effects on children. Psychol Med 14:853–880, 1984

Ryan V, Popour J: Five-year women's plan (IV:4c, 12c). Capitol Area Substance Abuse Commission, for the Office of Substance Abuse, Michigan Department of Health, Lansing, MI, 1983

Safra JM, Oakley GP: Association between cleft lip with or without cleft palate and prenatal exposure to diazepam. Lancet 2:476–480, 1980

St. Clair SM, Schirmer RG: First-trimester exposure to alprazolam. Obstet Gynecol 80:843–846, 1992

Sakaguchi T, Yamazaki M, Itoh S, et al: Gastric acid secretion controlled by oestrogen in women. J Int Med Res 19:384–388, 1991

Sallee FR, Pollock BG: Clinical pharmacokinetics of imipramine and desipramine. Clin Pharmacokinet 18:346–364, 1990

Salokangas RKR: Prognostic implications of the sex of schizophrenic patients. Br J Psychiatry 142:145–151, 1983

Sameroff AT, Seifer R, Zax M: Early development of children at risk for emotional disorder. Monogr Soc Res Child Dev 47, serial no 199, 1982

Sanders SA, Reinish JM: Behavioral effects on humans of progesterone related compounds during development and in the adult, in Actions of Progesterone on the Brain. Edited by Ganten D, Pfaff D. Berlin, Springer, 1985, pp 175–206

Sandison RA, Whitelaw E, Currie JD: Clinical trials with melleril [sic] (TP21) in the treatment of schizophrenia: a two-year study. J Ment Sci 106:732–741, 1960

Sandmeier M: The Invisible Alcoholics: Women and Alcohol Abuse in America. New York, McGraw-Hill, 1980

Sangal R: Inhibited female orgasm as a side effect of alprazolam. Am J Psychiatry 142:1223–1224, 1985

Sanz EJ, Villen T, Alm C, et al: S-mephenytoin hydroxylation phenotypes in a Swedish population determined after coadministration with debrisoquine. Clin Pharmacol Ther 45:495–499, 1989

Saunders EA, Arnold F: Borderline personality disorder and childhood abuse: revisions in clinical thinking and treatment approach (Work in Process 59). Wellesley, MA, Stone Center, 1991

Scambler G, Scambler A: Minor psychiatric morbidity and menstruation. Int J Soc Psychiatry 32:9–14, 1986

Scanlon FJ: Use of antidepressant drugs during the first trimester (letter). Med J Aust 2:1077, 1969

Schank J, McClintock MK: A coupled-oscillator model of ovarian cycle synchrony among female rats. J Theor Biol 157:317–362, 1992

Schatzberg AF, Cole JO: Manual of Clinical Psychopharmacology, 2nd Edition. Washington, DC, American Psychiatric Press, 1992

Scheibe G, Albus M: Age at onset, precipitating events, sex distribution, and co-occurrence of anxiety disorders. Psychopathology 25:11–18, 1992

Scher M, Kreiger JN, Juergens S: Trazodone and priapism. Am J Psychiatry 140:1362–1363, 1983

Schiebel AB, Kovelman JA: Disorientation of hippocampal pyramidal cell and its processes in the schizophrenic patient. Biol Psychiatry 16:101–102, 1981

Schimmell MS, Katz EZ, Shaag Y, et al: Toxic neonatal effects following maternal clomipramine therapy. Clinical Toxicology 29:479–484, 1991

Schmid B, Bircher J, Preisig R, et al: Polymorphic dextromethorphan metabolism: co-segregation of oxidative O-demethylation with debrisoquin hydroxylation. Clin Pharmacol Ther 38:618–624, 1985

Schmidt LG, Grohmann R, Muller-Oerlinghausen B, et al: Adverse drug reactions to first- and second-generation antidepressants: a critical evaluation of drug surveillance data. Br J Psychiatry 148:38–43, 1986

Schmidt PJ, Rubinow DR: Menopause-related affective disorders: a justification for further study. Am J Psychiatry 148:844–852, 1991

Schmidt PJ, Nieman LK, Grover GN, et al: Lack of effect of induced menses on symptoms in women with premenstrual syndrome. N Engl J Med 324:1174–1179, 1991

Schmidt PJ, Grover GN, Rubinow DR: Alprazolam in the treatment of premenstrual syndrome: a double-blind, placebo-controlled trial. Arch Gen Psychiatry 50:467–473, 1993

Schmidt PJ, Purdy RH, Moore PH, et al: Circulating levels of anxiolytic steroids in the luteal phase in women with premenstrual syndrome and in control subjects. J Clin Endocrinol Metab 79:1256–1260, 1994

Schneider LS, Cooper TB, Severson JA, et al: Electrocardiographic changes with nortriptyline and 10-hydroxynortriptyline in elderly depressed outpatients. J Clin Psychopharmacol 8:402–408, 1988

Schneider MA, Brotherton PL, Hailes J: The effect of exogenous oestrogens on depression in menopausal women. Med J Aust 2:162–165, 1977

Schneider RJ, Khantzian EJ: Psychotherapy and patient needs in treatment of alcohol and cocaine abuse. Recent Dev Alcohol 10:179–191, 1992

Schneier FR, Liebowitz MR, Davies SO, et al: Fluoxetine in panic disorder. J Clin Psychopharmacol 10:119–121, 1990

Schneier FR, Johnson J, Hornig CD, et al: Social phobia: comorbidity and morbidity in an epidemiologic sample. Arch Gen Psychiatry 49:282–288, 1992

Schooler N: Affliation among schizophrenics: preferred characteristics of the other. J Nerv Ment Dis 137:438–446, 1963

Schou M: What happened later to the lithium babies? A follow-up study of children born without malformations. Acta Psychiatr Scand 54:193–197, 1976

Schou M, Amdisen A: Lithium and pregnancy, III: lithium ingestion by children breast-fed by women on lithium treatment. BMJ 2:138, 1973

Schou M, Amdisen A, Streenstrup OR: Lithium and pregnancy, II: hazards to women given lithium during pregnancy and delivery. BMJ 2:137–138, 1973

Schou M, Thomsen K, Vestergaard P: The renal lithium clearance and its correlations with other biological variables: observations in a large group of physically healthy persons. Clin Nephrol 25:207–211, 1986

Schubert DSP: Reversal of doxepin-induced hypoactive sexual desire by substitution of nortriptyline. Journal of Sex Education and Therapy 18:42–44, 1992

Schuckit MA, Daly V, Herrman G, et al: Premenstrual symptoms and depression in a university population. Diseases of the Nervous System 36:516–517, 1975

Schuckit MA, Irwin M, Brown SA: The history of anxiety symptoms among 171 primary alcoholics. J Stud Alcohol 51:34–41, 1990

Schuckit MA, Smith TL, Anthenelli R, et al: Clinical course of alcoholism in 636 male inpatients. Am J Psychiatry 150:786–792, 1993

Schulterbrandt JG, Raskin A, Reatig N: True and apparent side effects in a controlled trial of chlorpromazine and imipramine in depression. Psychopharmacologia (Berl) 38:303–317, 1974

Schumacher M, Coirini H, Frankfurt M, et al: Localized actions of progesterone in hypothalamus involve oxytocin. Proc Natl Acad Sci U S A 86:6798–6801, 1989a

Schumacher M, Coirini H, McEwen BS: Regulation of high-affinity $GABA_A$ receptors in specific brain regions by ovarian hormones. Neuroendocrinology 50:315–320, 1989b

Schurz B, Wimmer-Greinecker G, Metka M, et al: Beta-endorphin levels during the climacteric period. Maturitas 10:45–50, 1988

Schwallie P, Assenzo J: Contraceptive use-efficacy study utilizing Depo-Provera administered as an injection once every six months. Contraception 6:315–322, 1972

Scokel PW III, Jones WN: Infant jaundice after phenothiazine drugs for labor: an enigma. Obstet Gynecol 20:124–127, 1962

Scolnik MB, Nulman I, Rovet J, et al: Neurodevelopment of children exposed in utero to phenytoin and carbamazepine monotherapy. JAMA 271:767–770, 1994

Scutchfield F, Long W, Correy B, et al: Medroxyprogesterone acetate as an injectable female contraceptive. Contraception 3:21–32, 1971

Seeman MV: Gender differences in schizophrenia. Can J Psychiatry 27:108–111, 1982

Seeman MV: Interactions of sex, age, and neuroleptic dose. Compr Psychiatry 24:125–128, 1983

Seeman MV: Current outcome in schizophrenia: women vs men. Acta Psychiatr Scand 73:609–617, 1986

Seeman MV: Neuroleptic prescriptions for men and women. Social Pharmacology 3:219–236, 1989

Seeman MV, Lang M: The role of estrogens in schizophrenic gender differences. Schizophr Bull 16:185–194, 1990

Segarra AC, Luine VN, Strand FL: Sexual behavior of male rats is differentially affected by timing of perinatal ACTH administration. Physiol Behav 50:689–697, 1991

Segraves RT: Reversal by bethanechol of imipramine-induced ejaculatory dysfunction. Am J Psychiatry 144:1243–1244, 1987a

Segraves RT: Treatment of premature ejaculation with lorazepam (letter). Am J Psychiatry 144:1240, 1987b

Segraves RT: Psychiatric drugs and inhibited female orgasm. J Sex Marital Ther 14:202–207, 1988

Segraves RT: Overview of sexual dysfunction complicating the treatment of depression. J Clin Psychiatry Monograph 10:4–10, 1992

Seibel MM, Shine W, Smith DM, et al: Biological rhythm of the luteinizing hormone surge in women. Fertil Steril 37:709–711, 1982a

Seibel MM, Smith DM, Levesque L, et al: The temporal relationship between the luteinizing hormone surge and human oocyte maturation. Am J Obstet Gynecol 142:568–572, 1982b

Seidl LG, Thornton GF, Smith JW, et al: Studies on the epidemiology of adverse drug reactions, III: reactions in patients on a general medical service. Bulletin of the Johns Hopkins Hospital 119:299–315, 1966

Sell MB: Sensitization to thioridazine through sexual intercourse. Am J Psychiatry 142:271–272, 1985

Sellers EM: Drug interactions, in Principles of Medical Pharmacology, 4th Edition. Edited by Kalant H, Roschlau WHE, Sellers EM. New York, Oxford University Press, 1985, pp 129–140

Sellers EM, Holloway MR: Drug kinetics and alcohol ingestion, in Handbook of Clinical Pharmacokinetics. Edited by Gibaldi M, Prescott L. Balgowlah, Australia, ADIS Health Science Press, 1983, pp 267–281

Semmens JP, Wagner G: Estrogen deprivation and vaginal function in postmenopausal women. JAMA 248:445–448, 1982

Severino S, Moline M: Premenstrual Syndrome: A Clinician's Guide. New York, Guilford, 1989

Shaarawy M, Fayad M, Nagui AR, et al: Serotonin metabolism and depression in oral contraceptive users. Contraception 26:193–204, 1985

Shader RI, Harmatz JS: Premenstrual tension in biochemical and psychotropic drug assessment. Psychopharmacol Bull 18:113–123, 1982

Shaheen O, Biollaz J, Koshakji RP, et al: Influence of debrisoquine phenotype on the inducibility of propranolol metabolism. Clin Pharmacol Ther 45:439–443, 1989

Shapira B, Oppenheim G, Zohar J, et al: Lack of efficacy of estrogen supplementation to imipramine in resistant female depressives. Biol Psychiatry 20:576–578, 1985

Sharpey-Shafer EP, Shrire I: Effect of oestrogens on urinary volume. Lancet 2:973–974, 1939

Shavit G, Lerman P, Korczyn S, et al: Phenytoin pharmacokinetics in catamenial epilepsy. Neurology 34:959–961, 1984

Shaw T, Meyer JS, Mortel K, et al: Effects of normal aging, sex and risk factors for stroke on regional cerebral blood flow (rCBF) in normal volunteers. Acta Neurol Scand 72 (suppl):462–463, 1979

Shay S, Eggli D, McDonald C, et al: Gastric emptying of solid food in patients with gastroesophageal reflux. Gastroenterology 92:459–465, 1987

Shaywitz B, Shaywitz SG, Pugh KR, et al: Sex differences in the functional organization of the brain for language. Nature 373:607–609, 1995

Sheehan DV: Current perspectives in the treatment of panic and phobic disorders. Drug Therapeutics 9:179–193, 1982

Sheehan DV, Ballenger J, Jacobsen G: Treatment of endogenous anxiety with phobic, hysterical, and hypochondriacal symptoms. Arch Gen Psychiatry 37:51–59, 1980

Sheftell F, Silberstein S, Rapoport A, et al: Migraine and women: diagnosis, pathophysiology and treatment. Journal of Women's Health 1:5–19, 1992

Shen WW: Female orgasmic inhibition by amoxapine. Am J Psychiatry 139:1220–1221, 1982

Shen WW, Lin KM: Cytochrome P450 monooxygenases and interactions of psychotropic drugs. Int J Psychiatry Med 21:21–30, 1990

Shen WW, Park S: Thioridazine-induced inhibition of female orgasm. Psychiatric Journal of the University of Ottawa 7:249–250, 1982

Shen WW, Lindbergh S, Hofstatter L: Thioridazine and understanding sexual phases in both sexes. Psychiatric Journal of the University of Ottawa 9:187–190, 1984

Sherwin BB: Affective changes with estrogen and androgen replacement therapy in surgically menopausal women. Journal of Affective Disorders 14:177–187, 1988a

Sherwin BB: Estrogen and/or androgen replacement therapy and cognitive functioning in surgically menopausal women. Psychoneuroendocrinology 13:345–357, 1988b

Sherwin BB: The psychoendocrinology of aging and female sexuality. Annual Review of Sex Research 2:181–198, 1991

Sherwin BB: Estrogenic effect on memory in women. Ann N Y Acad Sci 743:213–231, 1994

Sherwin BB, Gelfand MM: The role of androgen in the maintenance of sexual functioning in oophorectomized women. Psychosom Med 49:397–409, 1987

Sherwin BB, Phillips S: Estrogen and cognitive functioning in surgically menopausal women. Ann N Y Acad Sci 592:474–476, 1990

Sherwin BB, Suranyi-Cadotte BE: Up-regulatory effect of estrogen on platelet 3H-imipramine binding sites in surgically menopausal women. Biol Psychiatry 28:339–348, 1990

Sherwin BB, Gelfand MM, Brender W: Androgen enhances sexual motivation in females: a prospective, crossover study of sex steroid administration in the surgical menopause. Psychosom Med 47:339–351, 1985

Shibuya A, Yoshida A: Frequency of the atypical aldehyde dehydrogenase-2 gene (ALDH2) in Japanese and Caucasians. Am J Hum Genet 43:744–748, 1988

Sholomskas DE, Wickamaratne PJ, Dogolo L, et al: Postpartum onset of panic disorder: a coincidental event? J Clin Psychiatry 54:476–480, 1993

Shores MM, Glubin T, Cowley DS, et al: The relationship between anxiety and depression: a clinical comparison of generalized anxiety disorder, dysthymic disorder, panic disorder, and major depressive disorder. Compr Psychiatry 33:237–244, 1992

Shtasel DL, Gur RE, Gallacher F, et al: Gender differences in the clinical expression of schizophrenia. Schizophr Res 7:225–231, 1992

Silberstein SD, Merriam GR: Sex hormones and headache. J Pain Symptom Manage 8:98–114, 1993

Simpson GM, Blair JH, Amuso D: Effects of antidepressants on genitourinary function. Diseases of the Nervous System 26:787–789, 1965

Simpson GM, Varga E, Lee JH, et al: Tardive dyskinesia and psychoactive drug history. Psychopharmacology (Berl) 58:117–124, 1978

Simpson GM, Yadalam KG, Levinson DF, et al: Single-dose pharmacokinetics of fluphenazine after fluphenazine decanoate administration. J Clin Psychopharmacol 10:417–421, 1990

Simpson JM, Bateman DN, Rawlins MD: Using the adverse reactions register to study the effects of age and sex on adverse drug reactions. Stat Med 6:863–867, 1987

Singh M, Saxena BB, Rathnam P: Clinical validation of enzyme immunoassay of human luteinizing hormone (hLH) in the detection of the preovulatory luteinizing hormone (LH) surge in urine. Fertil Steril 41:210–217, 1984

Skett P, Mode A, Rafter J, et al: The effects of gonadectomy and hypophysectomy on the metabolism of imipramine and lidocaine by the liver of male and female rats. Biochem Pharmacol 29:2759–2762, 1980

Skjelbo E, Brosen K, Hallas J, et al: The mephenytoin oxidation polymorphism is partially responsible for the *N*-demethylation of imipramine. Clin Pharmacol Ther 49:18–23, 1991

Slap GB: Oral contraceptives and depression: impact, prevalence and cause. Journal of Adolescent Health Care 2:53–64, 1981

Slone D, Siskind V, Heinonen OP: Antenatal exposure to the phenothiazines in relation to congenital malformations, perinatal mortality rate, birth weight, and intelligence quotient score. Am J Obstet Gynecol 128:486–488, 1977

Slutsker L: Risks associated with cocaine use during pregnancy. Obstet Gynecol 79 (5, pt 1):778–789, 1992

Smith JM, Oswald WT, Kucharski T, et al: Tardive dyskinesia: age and sex differences in hospitalized schizophrenics. Psychopharmacology (Berl) 58:207–211, 1978

Smith RB, Divoll M, Gillespie WR, et al: Effects of subject age and gender on pharmacokinetics of oral triazolam and temazepam. J Clin Psychopharmacol 3:172–176, 1983

Smith SS: Estrogen administration increases neuronal responses to excitatory amino acids as a long-term effect. Brain Res 503:354–357, 1989

Smith SS: Progesterone administration attenuates excitatory amino acid responses of cerebellar Purkinje cells. Neuroscience 42:309–320, 1991

Smith TJ, Talbert RL: Sexual dysfunction with antihypertensive and antipsychotic agents. Clinical Pharmacy 5:373–384, 1986

Snyder SH, Yamamura HI: Antidepressant in the muscarinic acetylcholine receptor. Arch Gen Psychiatry 34:236–239, 1977

Sobel DE: Fetal damage due to ECT insulin coma, chlorpromazine and reserpine. Arch Gen Psychiatry 2:603–611, 1960

Society for Menstrual Cycle Research (SMCR) Newsletter. Winter 1986a, Vol 2(3) [as cited in Dye 1990]

Society for Menstrual Cycle Research (SMCR) Newsletter. Summer 1986b, Vol 3(1) [as cited in Dye 1990]

Soloff PH, Millward JW: Developmental histories of borderline patients. Compr Psychiatry 24:574–578, 1983

Solomon SD, Gerrity ET, Muff AM: Efficacy of treatments for posttraumatic stress disorder. JAMA 268:633–638, 1992

Solyom L, Solyom C, Ledwidge B: The fluoxetine treatment of low-weight chronic bulimia nervosa. J Clin Psychopharmacol 10:421–425, 1990

Someya T, Sibasaki M, Noguchi T, et al: Haloperidol metabolism in psychiatric patients: importance of glucuronidation and carbonyl reduction. J Clin Psychopharmacol 12:169–174, 1992

Sommers DK, Moncrieff J, Avenant J: Polymorphism of the 4-hydroxylation of debrisoquine in the San Bushmen of southern Africa. Human Toxicology 7:273–276, 1988

Sommers DK, Moncrieff J, Avenant J: Non-correlation between debrisoquine and metoprolol polymorphisms in the Venda. Human Toxicology 8:365–368, 1989

Sommers DK, Moncrieff J, Avenant JC: Absence of polymorphism of sparteine oxidation in the South African Venda. Hum Exp Toxicol 10:175–178, 1991

Song CS, Merkatz IR, Rifkind AB, et al: The influence of pregnancy and oral contraceptive steroids on the concentration of plasma proteins. Am J Obstet Gynecol 108:277–231, 1970

Sorscher SM, Dilsaver SC: Antidepressant-induced sexual dysfunction in men: Due to cholinergic blockade? (letter). J Clin Psychopharmacol 6:53–55, 1986

Sorvino AR: Painful postcoital testicular retraction linked with desipramine. Am J Psychiatry 143:682–683, 1986

Sotsky SM, Shea MT, Pilkonis PA, et al: Patient predictors of response to psychotherapy and pharmacotherapy: findings in the NIMH Treatment of Depression Collaborative Research Program. Am J Psychiatry 148:997–1008, 1991

Southam A, Gonzaga F: Systemic changes during the menstrual cycle. Am J Obstet Gynecol 91:142–165, 1965

Sovner R: Anorgasmia associated with imipramine but not desipramine: case report. J Clin Psychiatry 44:345–346, 1983

Sovner R: Treatment of tricyclic antidepressant–induced orgasmic inhibition with cyproheptadine (letter). J Clin Psychopharmacol 4:169, 1984

Squire L: Memory and the hippocampus: a synthesis from findings with rats, monkeys and humans. Psychol Rev 99:195–231, 1992

Stancer HC, Reed KL: Desipramine and 2-hydroxydesipramine in human breast milk and the nursing infant's serum. Am J Psychiatry 143:1595–1600, 1986

Steele TE, Howell EF: Cyproheptadine for imipramine-induced anorgasmia. J Clin Psychopharmacol 6:326–327, 1986

Stein MB, Schmidt PJ, Rubinow DR, et al: Panic disorder and the menstrual cycle: panic disorder patients, healthy control subjects, and patients with premenstrual syndrome. Am J Psychiatry 146:1299–1303, 1989

Steiner E, Bertilsson L, Sawe J, et al: Polymorphic debrisoquin hydroxylation in 757 Swedish subjects. Clin Pharmacol Ther 44:431–435, 1988

Steiner M, Wheadon DE, Kreider MS, et al: Antidepressant response to paroxetine by gender (NR462). Program and Abstracts on New Research, 146th Annual Meeting, American Psychiatric Association, San Francisco, CA, May 26, 1993, p 176

Stevens JR: An anatomy of schizophrenia? Arch Gen Psychiatry 29:177–189, 1973

Steward J, Kolb B: The effects of neonatal gonadectomy and prenatal stress on cortical thickness and asymmetry in rats. Behavioral and Neural Biology 49:344–360, 1988

Stewart DE, Klompenhouwer JL, Kondell RE, et al: Prophylactic lithium in puerperal psychosis: the experience of three centres. Br J Psychiatry 158:393–397, 1991

Stewart DE, Fairman M, Barbadoro S, et al: Follicular and late luteal phase serum fluoxetine levels in women suffering from late luteal phase dysphoric disorder. Biol Psychiatry 36:201–202, 1994

Stewart JT: Carbamazepine treatment of a patient with Klüver-Bucy syndrome. J Clin Psychiatry 46:496–497, 1985

Stewart JW, Quitkin FM, Liebowitz MR, et al: Efficacy of desipramine in depressed outpatients: response according to RDC diagnoses and severity of illness. Arch Gen Psychiatry 40:202–207, 1983

Stewart JW, McGrath PJ, Quitkin FM, et al: Relevance of DSM-III depressive subtype and chronicity of antidepressant efficacy in atypical depression. Arch Gen Psychiatry 46:1080–1087, 1989

Stoehr GP, Kroboth PD, Juhl RP, et al: Effect of oral contraceptives on triazolam, temazepam, alprazolam and lorazepam kinetics. Clin Pharmacol Ther 36:683–690, 1984

Stone AB, Pearlstein T, Brown WA: Fluoxetine in the treatment of premenstrual syndrome. Psychopharmacol Bull 26:331–335, 1990

Stone E: The personality pill. Mirabella, June 1993, pp 60–64

Stover E, Nightingale EO (eds): The Breaking of Bodies and Minds: Torture, Psychiatric Abuse, and the Health Professions (American Association for the Advancement of Science). New York, WH Freeman, 1985

Stowell LI, McIntosh CJ, Cooke R, et al: Adrenoceptor and imipramine receptor binding during the menstrual cycle. Acta Psychiatr Scand 78:366–368, 1988

Strain SL: Fluoxetine-initiated ovulatory cycles in two clomiphene-resistant women (letter). Am J Psychiatry 151:620, 1994

Sullivan G: Increased libido in three men treated with trazodone. J Clin Psychiatry 49:202–203, 1988

Sullivan G, Lukoff D: Sexual side effects of antipsychotic medication: evaluation and interventions. Hosp Community Psychiatry 41:1238–1241, 1990

Summers B, Summers RS: Carbamazepine clearance in paediatric epilepsy patients: influence of body mass, dose, sex and co-medication. Clin Pharmacokinet 17:208–216, 1989

Sundsfjord JA, Aakvaag A: Variations in plasma aldosterone and plasma renin activity throughout the menstrual cycle. Acta Endocrinol (Copenhagen) 73:499–508, 1973

Sussman N: The uses of buspirone in psychiatry. J Clin Psychopharmacol 12:3–19, 1994

Sutfin TA, Perini GI, Molnar G, et al: Multiple-dose pharmacokinetics of imipramine and its major active and conjugated metabolites in depressed patients. J Clin Psychopharmacol 8:48–53, 1988

Sutker PB, Goist KC, King A: Acute alcohol intoxication in women: relationship to dose and menstrual cycle phase. Alcohol Clin Exp Res 11:74–79, 1987a

Sutker PB, Goist KC, Allain AN, et al: Acute alcohol intoxication: sex comparisons on pharmacokinetic and mood measures. Alcohol Clin Exp Res 11:507–512, 1987b

Svanum S, McAdoo G: Parental alcoholism: an examination of male and female alcoholics in treatment. J Stud Alcohol 52:127–132, 1991

Swayze VW, Andreasen NC, Ehrhardt JC, et al: Developmental abnormalities of the corpus callosum in schizophrenia. Biol Psychiatry 47:805–808, 1990

Sykes PA, Quarrie J, Alexander FW: Lithium carbonate and breast-feeding (case report). BMJ 2:1299, 1976

Syvalahti EK, Lindberg R, Kallio J, et al: Inhibitory effects of neuroleptics on debrisoquine oxidation in man. Br J Clin Pharmacol 22:89–92, 1986

Szorady I, Santa A: Drug hydroxylator phenotype in Hungary (letter). Eur J Clin Pharmacol 32:325, 1987

Szymanski S, Masiar S, Mayerhoff D, et al: Clozapine response in treatment-refractory first-episode schizophrenia. Biol Psychiatry 35:278–280, 1994

Szymanski S, Lieberman JA, Alvir JM, et al: Gender differences in onset of illness, treatment response, course, and biologic indexes in first-episode schizophrenic patients. Am J Psychiatry 152:698–703, 1995

Takahashi R, Inabi Y, Inanaga K, et al: CT scanning and the investigation of schizophrenia. Biol Psychiatry 9:259–268, 1981

Tallal P: Hormonal influences in developmental learning disabilities. Psychoendocrinology 16:203–211, 1991

Tanaka E, Baba N, Toshida K, et al: Evidence for 5-HT$_2$ receptor involvement in the stimulation of preovulatory LH and prolactin release and ovulation in normal cycling rats. Life Sciences 52:669–676, 1993

Taymor ML, Seibel MM, Smith D, et al: Ovulation timing by luteinizing hormone assay and follicle puncture. Obstet Gynecol 62:191–195, 1983

Teichmann AT: Influence of oral contraceptives on drug therapy. Am J Obstet Gynecol 163:2208–2213, 1990

Temple R: Speaking at Food and Drug Law Institute Meeting, Women in Clinical Trials of FDA-Regulated Products, Washington, DC, October 1992

Templeton AA, Penney GC, Lees MM: Relation between the luteinizing hormone peak, the nadir of the basal body temperature and the cervical mucus score. Br J Obstet Gynaecol 89:985–988, 1982

Tepper SJ, Haas JR: Prevalence of tardive dyskinesia. J Clin Psychiatry 40:508–516, 1979

Testart J, Frydman R: Minimum time lapse between luteinizing hormone surge or human chorionic gonadotropin administration and follicular rupture. Fertil Steril 37:50–53, 1982

Testart J, Frydman R, Feinstein MC, et al: Interpretation of plasma luteinizing hormone assay for the collection of mature oocytes from women: definition of a luteinizing hormone surge–initiating rise. Fertil Steril 36:50–54, 1981

Testart J, Frydman R, Roger M: Seasonal influence of diurnal rhythms in the onset of the plasma luteinizing hormone surge in women. J Clin Endocrinol Metab 55:374–377, 1982

Thom B: Sex differences in help-seeking for alcohol problems, I: the barriers to help-seeking. British Journal of Addiction 81:777–788, 1986

Thomasson HR, Edenberg HJ, Crabb DW, et al: Alcohol and aldehyde dehydrogenase genotypes and alcoholism in Chinese men. Am J Hum Genet 48:677–681, 1991

Thompson B, Hart SA, Durno D: Menopausal age and symptomatology in a general practice. J Biosoc Sci 5:71–82, 1973

Thompson JW, Ware MR, Blashfield RK: Psychotropic medication and priapism: a comprehensive review. J Clin Psychiatry 51:430–433, 1990

Thorén P, Åsberg M, Cronholm B, et al: Clomipramine treatment of obsessive-compulsive disorder, I: a controlled clinical trial. Arch Gen Psychiatry 37:1281–1289, 1980

Thorn GW, Nelson KR, Thorn DW: A study of mechanism of edema associated with menstruation. Endocrinology 22:155–163, 1938

Thorner M, Besser B: Bromocriptine treatment for hyperprolactinemic hypogonadism. Acta Endocrinologica 88 (suppl 216):131–146, 1978

Thorneycroft IH, Sribyatta B, Tom WK, et al: Measurement of serum LH, FSH, progesterone, 17-hydroxyprogesterone and estradiol-17b levels at 4-hour intervals during the periovulatory phase of the menstrual cycle. J Clin Endocrinol Metab 39:754–758, 1974

Tillet Y, Batailler M, Thibault J: Neuronal projections to the medial preoptic area of the sheep, with special reference to monoaminergic afferents: immunohistochemical and retrograde tract tracing studies. J Comp Neurol 330:195–220, 1993

Tinguely D, Bauman P, Conti M, et al: Interindividual differences in the binding of antidepressants to plasma proteins: the role of variants of alpha₁-acid glycoprotein. Eur J Clin Pharmacol 27:661–666, 1985

Tollan A, Oian P: Changes in transcapillary fluid dynamics—a possible explanation of the fluid retention in the premenstrual phase? in Hormones and Behaviour. Edited by Dennerstein L, Fraser I. New York, Elsevier Science, 1986, pp 143–146

Toone BK, Wheeler M, Nanjee M, et al: Sex hormones, sexual activity and plasma anticonvulsant levels in male epileptics. J Neurol Neurosurg Psychiatry 46:824–826, 1983

Tredway DR, Chan P, Henig I, et al: Effectiveness of stimulated menstrual cycles and Percoll sperm penetration in intrauterine insemination. J Reprod Med 35:103–108, 1990

Treloar A, Boynton R, Behn B, et al: Variation of the human menstrual cycle through reproductive life. International Journal of Infertility 12:77–126, 1967

Trimble MR: Worldwide use of clomipramine. J Clin Psychiatry 51:51–54, 1990

Trinkoff AM, Anthony JC: Gender differences in initiation of psychotherapeutic medicine use. Acta Psychiatr Scand 81:32–38, 1990

Tunnessen WW Jr, Hertz CG: Toxic effects of lithium in newborn infants: a commentary. J Pediatr 81:804–807, 1972

Udry JR, Morris NM: The distribution of events in the human menstrual cycle. J Reprod Fertil 51:419–425, 1977

Uhde TW, Tancer ME, Shea CA: Sexual dysfunction related to alprazolam treatment of social phobia. Am J Psychiatry 145:531–532, 1988

Uhde TW, Tancer ME, Black B: Phenomenology and neurobiology of social phobia: comparison with panic disorder. J Clin Psychiatry 52 (suppl):31–40, 1991

Underhill BL: Issues relevant to aftercare programs for women. Alcohol Health and Research World 11:46–48, 1994

U.S. Food and Drug Administration: Guidelines for preclinical toxicity testing of investigational drugs for human use. Washington, DC, U.S. Department of Health and Human Services (DHHS), U.S. Government Printing Office, 1966

U.S. Food and Drug Administration: General considerations for the clinical evaluation of drugs. Washington, DC, U.S. Department of Health and Human Services (DHHS), U.S. Government Printing Office, 1979

U.S. Food and Drug Administration: Guideline for the format and content of the clinical and statistical sections of new drug applications. Rockville, MD, U.S. Department of Health and Human Services, Public Health Service, July 1988

U.S. Food and Drug Administration: Guideline for the study of drugs likely to be used in the elderly. Rockville, MD, U.S. Department of Health and Human Services, Public Health Service, November 1989

U.S. Food and Drug Administration: Geriatric uses labeling. Federal Register (55 FR 46134), November 1, 1990

U.S. Food and Drug Administration: Labeling: inclusion of information on the use of drugs in children. Federal Register (57 FR 47423), October 16, 1992

U.S. Food and Drug Administration: Guideline for the study and evaluation of gender differences in the clinical evaluation of drugs. Notice, Federal Register, July 22, 1993

U.S. Food and Drug Administration: Guideline for the study and evaluation of gender differences in the clinical evaluation of drugs (U.S. Food and Drug Administration Docket No. 93D-0236). Rockville, MD, 1993, pp 1–53

U.S. General Accounting Office: National Institutes of Health: Problems in implementing policy on women in study populations (GAO/T-HRD-90-38). Washington, DC, U.S. Superintendent of Documents, June 18, 1990

U.S. General Accounting Office: Women's health: FDA needs to ensure more study of gender differences in prescription drug testing (GAO/HRD-93-17). Washington, DC, U.S. Superintendent of Documents, October 1992

Vaillant G: Alcoholism. Cambridge, MA, Harvard University Press, 1983

Valera S, Ballivet M, Bertrand D: Progesterone modulates a neuronal nicotinic acetylcholine receptor. Proc Natl Acad Sci U S A 89:9949–9953, 1992

Vallejo J, Gasto C, Catalan R, et al: Double-blind study of imipramine versus phenelzine in melancholias and dysthymic disorders. Br J Psychiatry 151:639–642, 1987

Van Cauter E, Aschoff J: Endocrine and other biological rhythms, in Endocrinology. Edited by DeGroot L, Besser G, Marshall J, et al. Philadelphia, PA, WB Saunders, 1989, pp 2658–2705

van der Kolk BA (ed): Psychological Trauma. Washington, DC, American Psychiatric Press, 1987

van Harten J: Clinical pharmacokinetics of selective serotonin reuptake inhibitors. Clin Pharmacokinet 24:203–220, 1993

van Waes A, van de Velde E: Safety evaluation of haloperidol in the treatment of hyperemesis gravidarum. J Clin Pharmacol 9:224–227, 1969

Vance M, Thorner M: Prolactin: hyperprolactinemic syndromes and management, in Endocrinology. Edited by DeGroot L, Besser G, Marshall J, et al. Philadelphia, PA, WB Saunders, 1989, pp 408–409

Vanhulle G, Demol P: A double-blind study into the influence of estriol on a number of psychological tests in post-menopausal women, in Consensus on Menopause Research: Monograph, First International Congress on the Menopause, La Grande Motte, France, June 1976. Edited by Keep PAV, Greenblatt RB, Albeaux-Fernet M, et al. Baltimore, MD, University Park Press, 1976, pp 84–93

Varan LR, Gillieson MS, Skene DS, et al: ECT in an acutely psychotic pregnant woman with actively aggressive (homicidal) impulses. Can J Psychiatry 30:363–376, 1985

Vazquez Rodriquez AM, Arranz Pena MI, Lopez Ibor JJ, et al: Clomipramine test: serum level determination in three groups of psychiatric patients. J Pharm Biomed Analysis 9:949–952, 1991

Veldhuis JD, Evans WS, Rogol AD, et al: Intensified rates of venous sampling unmask the presence of spontaneous high frequency pulsations of luteinizing hormones in man. J Clin Endocrinol Metab 59:96–102, 1984

Vener AM, Krupka LR: Over-the-counter anorexiants: use and perceptions among young adults, in Phenylpropranolamine: Risks, Benefits and Controversies. Edited by Morgan JP, Kagan DJ, Brody JS. New York, Praeger, 1985, pp 132–149

Vermesh M, Kletzky OA, Davajan V, et al: Monitoring techniques to predict and detect ovulation. Fertil Steril 47:259–264, 1987

Vermeulen A, Verdonck L: Plasma androgen levels during the menstrual cycle. Am J Obstet Gynecol 125:491–494, 1976

Veronese ME, McLean S: Debrisoquine oxidation polymorphism in a Tasmanian population. Eur J Clin Pharmacol 40:529–532, 1991

Vessman J, Alexanderson B, Sjoqvist F, et al: Comparative pharmacokinetics of oxazepam and nortriptyline after single oral doses in man, in The Benzodiazepines. Edited by Garattini S, Musini E, Randall LO. New York, Raven, 1973, pp 165–173

Vestal RE, Wood AJJ: Influence of age and smoking on drug kinetics in man: studies using model compounds, in Handbook of Clinical Pharmacokinetics. Edited by Gibaldi M, Prescott L. Balgowlah, Australia, ADIS Health Science Press, 1983, pp 188–199

Vestergaard P, Amdisen A, Schou M: Clinically significant side effects of treatment: a survey of 237 patients in long-term treatment. Acta Psychiatr Scand 62:193–200, 1980

Villeneuve R, Langlier P, Bedard P: Estrogens, dopamine and dyskinesia. Can Psychiatr Assn J 28:391–394, 1983

Villeponteaux VA, Lydiard RB, Laraia MT, et al: The effects of pregnancy on preexisting panic disorder. J Clin Psychiatry 53:201–203, 1992

Vinarova E, Uhlir V, Stika L, et al: Side effects of lithium administration. Activas Nervosa Superior 14:105–107, 1972

Vinarova E, Vinar O, Kalvach Z: Smokers need higher levels of neuroleptic drugs. Biol Psychiatry 19:1265–1268, 1984

von Kuhn R: The treatment of depressive states with G22355 (imipramine hydrochloride). Am J Psychiatry 115:459–464, 1958

Wagner G, Levin RJ: Effect of atropine and methylatropine on human vaginal blood flow, sexual arousal and climax. Acta Pharmacologica et Toxicologica 46:321–332, 1980

Wagner HR, Crutcher KA, Davis JN: Chronic estrogen treatment decreases beta-adrenergic responses in rat cerebral cortex. Brain Res 71:147–151, 1979

Wald A, Van Thiel DH, Hoechstetter L, et al: Gastrointestinal transit: the effect of the menstrual cycle. Gastroenterol 80:1497–1500, 1981

Walker A, Bancroft J: Relationship between premenstrual symptoms and oral contraceptive use: a controlled study. Psychosom Med 52:86–96, 1990

Walker PW, Cole JO, Gardner EA, et al: Improvement in fluoxetine-associated sexual dysfunction in patients switched to bupropion. J Clin Psychiatry 54:459–465, 1993

Walle T, Byington RP, Furberg CD, et al: Biologic determinants of propranolol disposition: results from 1308 patients in the Beta-Blocker Heart Attack Trial. Clin Pharmacol Ther 38:509–518, 1985

Walle T, Walle UK, Conradi EC: Pathway-selective sex differences in the metabolic clearance of propranolol in human subjects. Clin Pharmacol Ther 46:257–263, 1989

Walle T, Walle UK, Mathur RS, et al: The metabolic clearance of propranalol is regulated by testosterone in women as well as in men (abstract). Clin Pharmacol Ther 51:180, 1992

Walle T, Walle UK, Fagan TC, et al: Influence of gender and sex steroid hormones on plasma binding of the propranalol enantiomers (abstract). Clin Pharmacol Ther 53:183, 1993

Wanberg KW, Horn JL: Alcoholism symptom pattern of men and women: a comparative study. Quarterly Journal of Studies on Alcohol 31:40–61, 1970

Wanwimolruk S, Patamasucon P, Lee EJD: Evidence for the polymorphic oxidation of debrisoquine in the Thai population. Br J Clin Pharmacol 29:244–247, 1990

Ward SA, Walle T, Walle UK, et al: Propranalol's metabolism is determined by both mephenytoin and debrisoquin hydroxylase activities. Clin Pharmacol Ther 45:72–79, 1989

Warrington SJ: Clinical implications of the pharmacology of sertraline. International Journal of Clinical Psychopharmacology 6 (suppl 2):11–21, 1991

Watt DC, Szulecka TK: The effect of sex, marriage and age at first admission on the hospitalization of schizophrenia during 2 years following discharge. Psychol Med 9:529–539, 1979

Weber WW: The acetylator genes and drug responses. New York, Oxford University Press, 1987

Weber WW, Hein DW: *N*-Acetylation pharmacogenetics. Pharmacologic Rev 37:26–79, 1985

Wedlund PJ, Aslanian WS, McAllister CB, et al: Mephenytoin hydroxylation deficiency in Caucasians: frequency of a new oxidative drug metabolism polymorphism. Clin Pharmacol Ther 36:773–780, 1984

Wedmann B, Schmidt G, Wegener M, et al: Effects of age and gender on fat-induced gallbladder contraction and gastric emptying of a caloric liquid meal: a sonographic study. Am J Gastroenterol 86:1765–1770, 1991

Wehr TA, Sack DA, Rosenthal NE, et al: Rapid cycling affective disorder: contributing factors and treatment processes in 51 patients. Am J Psychiatry 145:179–184, 1988

Weiland NG: Estradiol selectively regulates agonist binding sites on the NMDA receptor complex in the CA1 region of the hippocampus. Endocrinology 131:662–668, 1992

Weinstein MR: Lithium treatment of women during pregnancy and in the post-delivery period, in Handbook of Lithium Therapy. Edited by Jonson FN. Lancaster, UK, MTP Press, 1980, pp 421–429

Weis WF, Muller GO, Lyell H, et al: Materno-fetal cholinesterase inhibitor poisoning. Anesth Analg 62:233–235, 1983

Weisner C: The epidemiology of combined alcohol and drug use within treatment agencies: a comparison by gender. J Stud Alcohol 54:268–274, 1993

Weiss RD, Mirin SM, Michael JL, et al: Psychopathology in chronic cocaine abusers. Am J Drug Alcohol Abuse 12:17–26, 1986

Weiss RD, Mirin SM, Griffin ML, et al: Personality disorders in cocaine dependence. Compr Psychiatry 34:145–149, 1993

Weissman MM, Klerman GL: Sex differences and the epidemiology of depression. Arch Gen Psychiatry 34:98–111, 1977

Weissman MM, Leaf PJ, Livingston-Bruce M, et al: The epidemiology of dysthymia in five communities: rates, risks, comorbidity, and treatment. Am J Psychiatry 145:815–819, 1988

Weizman A, Morgenstern H, Kaplan B, et al: Up-regulatory effect of triphasic oral contraceptive on [^{3}H]imipramine binding sites. Psychiatry Res 23:23–29, 1988

Welner A, Reich T, Robin E: Obsessive-compulsive neurosis record, follow-up and family studies, I: inpatient record study. Compr Psychiatry 17:527–539, 1976

Westermeyer J, Harrow M: Predicting outcome in schizophrenics and non-schizophrenics of both sexes: the Zigler-Phillips Social Competence Scale. J Abnorm Psychol 95:406–409, 1986

Westland-Danielsson A, Gould E, McEwen BS: Thyroid hormone causes sexually distinct neurochemical and morphological alterations in rat septal-diagonal band neurons. J Neurochem 56:119–128, 1991

Wettstein RM: Psychiatry and the law, in The American Psychiatric Press Textbook of Psychiatry. Edited by Talbott JA, Hales RE, Yudofsky SC. Washington, DC, American Psychiatric Press, 1988, pp 1059–1084

Wettstein RM: Psychiatric malpractice, in American Psychiatric Press Review of Psychiatry, Vol 8. Edited by Tasman A, Hales RE, Frances AJ. Washington, DC, American Psychiatric Press, 1989, pp 392–408

Whalley LJ, Blain DG, Prime JK: Haloperidol secreted in breast milk. BMJ 282:1746–1747, 1981

White K, Goldenberg I, Yonkers KA, et al: The infrequency of pure culture diagnoses among anxiety disorders (abstract). Clin Neuropharmacol 15 (suppl 1B):56B, 1992

Whitehead W, Cheskin L, Heller B, et al: Evidence for exacerbation of irritable bowel syndrome during menses. Gastroenterol 98:1485–1489, 1990

Whitelaw AGL, Cummings AJ, McFadyen IF: Effect of maternal lorazepam on the neonate. BMJ 282:1106–1108, 1981

Wilcox AJ, Baird DD, Weinberg CR, et al: The use of biochemical assays in epidemiologic studies of reproduction. Environ Health Perspect 75:29–35, 1987

Wilkinson GR, Kurata D: The uptake of diphenylhydantoin by the human erythrocyte and its application to the estimation of plasma binding, in Drug Interactions. Edited by Mortselli PL, Garattini S, Cohen SN. New York, Raven, 1974, pp 289–297

Wilkinson GR, Guengerich FP, Branch RA: Genetic polymorphism of S-mephenytoin hydroxylation. Pharmacol Ther 43:53–76, 1989

Williams P, Murray J, Clare A: A longitudinal study of psychotropic drug prescription. Psychol Med 12:201–206, 1982

Wilson JD, Brauwald E, Isselbacher KJ (eds): Harrison's Principles of Internal Medicine, 12th Edition. New York, McGraw-Hill, 1991

Wilson JG: Current status of teratology, general principles and mechanisms derived from animal studies, in Handbook of Teratology, General Principles and Etiology, Vol 1. Edited by Wilson JG, Fraser FC. New York, Plenum, 1977, pp 47–74

Wilson JR, Erwin VG, DeFries JC, et al: Ethanol dependence in mice: direct and correlated responses to ten generations of selective breeding. Behav Genet 14:235–256, 1984

Wilson K: Sex-related differences in drug disposition in man. Clin Pharmacokinet 9:189–202, 1984

Wilson K, Oram M, Horth CE, et al: The influence of the menstrual cycle on the metabolism and clearance of methaqualone. Br J Clin Pharmacol 14:333–339, 1982

Wilson MA, Roy EJ: Pharmacokinetics of imipramine are affected by age and sex in rats. Life Sciences 38:711–718, 1986

Wilson MA, Dwyer K, Roy E: Direct effects of ovarian hormones on antidepressant binding sites. Brain Res Bull 22:181–185, 1989

Winfield I, George LK, Swartz M, et al: Sexual assault and psychiatric disorders among a community sample of women. Am J Psychiatry 147:335–341, 1990

Wirz-Justice A, Chappuis-Arndt E: Sex specific differences in clomipramine inhibition of serotonin uptake in human platelets. Eur J Pharmacol 40:21–25, 1976

Wirz-Justice A, Puhringer W, Hole G, et al: Monoamine oxidase and free tryptophan in human plasma: normal variations and their implications for biochemical research in affective disorders. Pharmakopsychiatrie Neuropsychopharmakologie 8:310–317, 1975

Wise MG, Ward SC, Townsend-Parchman W, et al: Case report of ECT during high-risk pregnancy. Am J Psychiatry 141:99–101, 1984

Wise PM, Weiland NG, Scarbrough K, et al: Changing hypothalamopituitary function: its role in aging of the female reproductive system. Horm Res 31:39–44, 1989

Wisner KL, Perel JM: Psychopharmacologic agents and electroconvulsive therapy during pregnancy and the puerperium, in Psychiatric Consultation in Childbirth Settings. Edited by Cohen PL. New York, Plenum, 1988, pp 165–206

Wisner KL, Perel JM: Serum nortriptyline levels in nursing mothers and their infants. Am J Psychiatry 148:1234–1236, 1991

Wisner KL, Wheeler SB: Prevention of recurrent postpartum major depression. Hosp Community Psychiatry 45:1191–1196, 1994

Wisner KL, Perel JM, Wheeler SM: Tricyclic dose requirements across pregnancy. Am J Psychiatry 150:1541–1542, 1993

Witten CL, Bradbury JT: Hemodilution as a result of estrogen therapy: estrogenic effects in the human female. Proc Soc Exp Biol Med 78:626–629, 1951

Wolf DP, Blasco L, Khan MA, et al: Human cervical mucus, II: changes in viscoelasticity during the ovulatory menstrual cycle. Fertil Steril 28:47–52, 1977

Wolf FM: Meta-Analysis: Quantitative Methods for Research Synthesis. Beverly Hills, CA, Sage, 1986

Wolff PH: Ethnic difference in alcohol sensitivity. Science 175:449–450, 1972

Wolff PH: Vasomotor sensitivity to alcohol in diverse mongoloid population. Am J Hum Genet 25:193–199, 1973

Wolkin A, Jeager J, Brodie JD, et al: Persistence of cerebral metabolic abnormalities in chronic schizophrenia as determined by positron emission tomography. Am J Psychiatry 142:564–571, 1985

Wolters-Everhardt E, Vemer H, Thomas C, et al: Ultrasound versus laparoscopy in the diagnosis of the LUF syndrome, in Ovulation and Its Disorders (Studies in Fertility and Sterility). Edited by Thompson W, Harrison RF, Bonnar J. Boston, MA, MTP Press, 1984, pp 13–19

Wong WH, Freedman RI, Levan NE, et al: Changes in the capillary filtration coefficient of cutaneous vessels in women with premenstrual tension. Am J Obstet Gynecol 114:950–953, 1972

Wood AJJ, Zhou HH: Ethnic differences in drug disposition and responsiveness. Clin Pharmacokinet 20:1–24, 1991

Wood C, Larsen L, Williams R, et al: Menstrual characteristics in 2,343 women attending the Shepard Foundation. Aust N Z J Obstet Gynaecol 19:107–110, 1979

Woods JR, Plessinger MA, Clark KE: Effect of cocaine on uterine blood flow and fetal oxygenation. JAMA 257:957–961, 1987

Woolhouse NM, Andoh B, Mahgoub A, et al: Debrisoquin hydroxylation polymorphism among Ghanaians and Caucasians. Clin Pharmacol Ther 26:584–591, 1979

Woolley CS, Gould E, Frankfurt M, et al: Naturally occurring fluctuations in dendritic spine density on adult hippocampal pyramidal neurons. J Neurosci 10:4035–4039, 1990

World Health Organization: Temporal relationships between ovulation and defined changes in the concentration of plasma estradiol-17b, luteinizing hormone, follicle stimulating hormone, and progesterone, I: probit analysis. Am J Obstet Gynecol 138:383–390, 1980

World Health Organization: Temporal relationships between ovulation and defined changes in the concentration of plasma estradiol-17b, luteinizing hormone, follicle stimulating hormone, and progesterone, II: histologic dating. Am J Obstet Gynecol 139:886–895, 1981

World Health Organization: Temporal relationships between indices of the fertile period. Fertil Steril 39:647–655, 1983

Wright RA, Krinsky S, Fleeman C, et al: Gastric emptying and obesity. Gastroenterol 84:747–751, 1983

Xu XM, Jiang WD: Debrisoquine hydroxylation and sulfamethazine acetylation in a Chinese population. Acta Pharmacologica Sinica 11:387–388, 1990

Yager J: Bethanechol chloride can reverse erectile and ejaculatory dysfunction induced by tricyclic antidepressant and mazinol: case report. J Clin Psychiatry 47:210–211, 1986

Yamagata S, Ishimori A, Sato H, et al: Secretory function of the stomach of Japanese with endoscopically normal gastric mucosa. Gastroenterol Jap 10:162–167, 1975

Yamaguchi K, Okuda K, Yonemitsu H, et al: Cyclic premenstrual unconjugated hyperbilirubinemia: report of two cases. Ann Intern Med 83:514–517, 1975

Yassa R: Sexual disorders in the course of clomipramine treatment: a report of three cases. Can J Psychiatry 27:148–149, 1982

Yassa R, Jeste DV: Gender difference in tardive dyskinesia: a critical review of the literature. Schizophr Bull 18:701–709, 1992

Yassa R, Ananth J, Cordozo S, et al: Tardive dyskinesia in an outpatient population: prevalence and predisposing factors. Can J Psychiatry 28:391–394, 1983

Yasunami M, Chen CS, Yoshida A: A human alcohol dehydrogenase gene (ADH6) encoding an additional class of isozyme. Proc Natl Acad Sci U S A 88:7610–7614, 1991

Yeh SVH: Urinary excretion of morphine and its metabolites in morphine dependent subjects. J Pharmacol Exp Ther 192:201–210, 1975

Yen SSC: Chronic anovulation due to CNS-hypothalamic-pituitary dysfunction, in Reproductive Endocrinology. Edited by Yen SSC, Jaffe R. Philadelphia, PA, WB Saunders, 1991, pp 631–688

Yeragani VK: Anorgasmia associated with desipramine (letter). Can J Psychiatry 33:76, 1987

Yin J, Kaplitt MG, Kwong AD: In vivo promoter analysis for detecting an estrogen effect on preproenkephalin (PPE) transcription in hypothalamic neurons. Endocrine Society Abstracts 76:560, 1994

Yoder MC, Belik J, Lannon RA, et al: Infants of mothers treated with lithium during pregnancy have an increased incidence of prematurity, macrosomia and perinatal mortality. Pediatr Res 18:163A, 1984

Yonkers KA: Panic disorder in women. Journal of Women's Health 3:481–486, 1994

Yonkers KA, Gurguis G: Gender differences in the prevalence and expression of anxiety disorders, in Gender and Psychopathology. Edited by Seeman MV. Washington, DC, American Psychiatric Press, 1995, pp 113–130

Yonkers KA, Kando JC, Cole JO, et al: Gender differences in pharmacokinetics and pharmacodynamics in psychotropic medication. Am J Psychiatry 149:587–595, 1992a

Yonkers KA, Ellison SM, Shera DM, et al: Pharmacotherapy observed in a large prospective longitudinal study in anxiety disorders. Psychopharmacol Bull 28:131–137, 1992b

Yoshida A, Huang IY, Ikawa M: Molecular abnormality of an inactive aldehyde dehydrogenase variant commonly found in Orientals. Proc Natl Acad Sci U S A 81:258–261, 1984

Yoshida A, Ward RJ, Peters TJ: Cytosolic aldehyde dehydrogenase (ALDH$_1$) variants found in alcohol flushers. Ann Hum Genet 53:1–7, 1989

Yoshida A, Hsu LC, Yasunami M: Genetics of human alcohol-metabolizing enzymes. Prog Nucleic Acid Res Mol Biol 40:255–287, 1991

Yoshikawa T, Sugiyama Y, Sawada Y, et al: Effect of late pregnancy on salicylate, diazepam, warfarin, and propranolol binding: use of florescent probes. Clin Pharmacol Ther 36:201–208, 1984

Young RC: Plasma nor₁-chlorpromazine concentrations. Effects of age, race, and sex. Ther Drug Monit 8:23–26, 1986

Yue QY, Svensson JO, Alm C, et al: Interindividual and interethnic differences in the demethylation and glucuronidation of codeine. Br J Clin Pharmacol 28:629–637, 1989

Yue QY, Svensson JO, Sjoqvist F, et al: A comparison of the pharmacokinetics of codeine and its metabolites in healthy Chinese and Caucasian extensive hydroxylators of debrisoquin. Br J Clin Pharmacol 31:643–647, 1991

Yussman MA, Taymor ML: Serum levels of follicle stimulating hormones and luteinizing hormone and of plasma progesterone related to ovulation by corpus luteum biopsy. J Clin Endocrinol Metab 30:396–399, 1970

Zajecka J, Fawcett J, Schaff M, et al: The role of serotonin in sexual dysfunction: fluoxetine-associated orgasm dysfunction. J Clin Psychiatry 52:66–68, 1991

Zalzstein E, Koran G, Einarson T, et al: A case-control study on the association between first trimester exposure to lithium and Ebstein's anomaly. Am J Cardiol 65:817–818, 1990

Zetin M, Garber D, Cramer M: A simple mathematical model for predicting lithium dose requirements. J Clin Psychiatry 44:144–145, 1983

Zhou H, Adedoyin A, Wilkinson GR: Differences in plasma binding of drugs between Caucasian and Chinese subjects. Clin Pharmacol Ther 48:10–17, 1990

Zhu YS, Freidin M, Pfaff DW: DNA binding of hypothalamic and pituitary nuclear proteins on BRE and proenkephalin (Penk) promoter. Society for Neuroscience Abstracts 20:53, 1994

Ziegler VE, Biggs JT: Tricyclic plasma levels: effects of age, race, sex and smoking. JAMA 238:2167–2169, 1977

Zigler E, Levine J: Premorbid competence in schizophrenia: what is being measured? J Consult Clin Psychol 49:96–105, 1981

Zigun JR, Daniel DG, Kleinman JR, et al: Ventricular enlargement in schizophrenia: is there really a gender effect? (letter). Arch Gen Psychiatry 49:995, 1992

Zilleruelo I, Espinoza E, Ruiz I: Influence of the assessment of the severity on the frequency of adverse drug reactions (ADRs). International Journal of Clinical Pharmacology, Therapy, and Toxicology 25:328–333, 1987

Zimmerman M, Coryell W, Corenthal C, et al: A self-report scale to diagnose major depressive disorder. Arch Gen Psychiatry 43:1076–1081, 1986

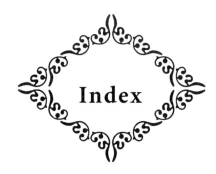

Index

*Page numbers printed in **boldface** type refer to tables or figures.*